Imaging and Cancer Screening

Editor

DUSHYANT V. SAHANI

RADIOLOGIC CLINICS OF NORTH AMERICA

www.radiologic.theclinics.com

Consulting Editor
FRANK H. MILLER

November 2017 • Volume 55 • Number 6

ELSEVIER

1600 John F. Kennedy Boulevard • Suite 1800 • Philadelphia, Pennsylvania, 19103-2899

http://www.theclinics.com

RADIOLOGIC CLINICS OF NORTH AMERICA Volume 55, Number 6
November 2017 ISSN 0033-8389, ISBN 13: 978-0-323-54899-1

Editor: John Vassallo (j.vassallo@elsevier.com)
Developmental Editor: Donald Mumford

Radiologic Clinics of North America (ISSN 0033-8389) is published bimonthly by Elsevier Inc., 360 Park Avenue South, New York, NY 10010-1710. Months of issue are January, March, May, July, September, and November. Periodicals postage paid at New York, NY and additional mailing offices. Subscription prices are USD 474 per year for US individuals, USD 831 per year for US institutions, USD 100 per year for US students and residents, USD 551 per year for Canadian individuals, USD 1062 per year for Canadian institutions, USD 680 per year for international individuals, USD 1062 per year for international institutions, and USD 315 per year for Canadian and international students/residents. To receive student and resident rate, orders must be accompanied by name of affiliated institution, date of term and the signature of program/residency coordinatior on institution letterhead. Orders will be billed at individual rate until proof of status is received. Foreign air speed delivery is included in all *Clinics* subscription prices. All prices are subject to change without notice. **POSTMASTER:** Send address changes to *Radiologic Clinics of North America*, Elsevier Health Sciences Division, Subscription Customer Service, 3251 Riverport Lane, Maryland Heights, MO63043. **Customer Service: Telephone: 1-800-654-2452** (U.S. and Canada); **1-314-447-8871** (outside U.S. and Canada). **Fax: 1-314-447-8029. E-mail: journalscustomerservice-usa@ elsevier.com (for print support); journalsonlinesupport-usa@elsevier.com (for online support)**.

Reprints. For copies of 100 or more of articles in this publication, please contact the Commercial Reprints Department, Elsevier Inc., 360 Park Avenue South, New York, New York 10010-1710. Tel.: +1-212-633-3874; Fax: +1-212-633-3820; E-mail: reprints@elsevier.com.

Radiologic Clinics of North America also published in Greek Paschalidis Medical Publications, Athens, Greece.

Radiologic Clinics of North America is covered in *MEDLINE/PubMed (Index Medicus)*, *EMBASE/Excerpta Medica*, *Current Contents/Life Sciences*, *Current Contents/Clinical Medicine*, *RSNA Index to Imaging Literature*, *BIOSIS*, *Science Citation Index*, and *ISI/BIOMED*.

Contributors

CONSULTING EDITOR

FRANK H. MILLER, MD
Chief, Body Imaging Section and Fellowship
Program, Medical Director of MRI, Professor,
Department of Radiology, Northwestern
University Feinberg School of Medicine,
Chicago, Illinois, USA

EDITOR

DUSHYANT V. SAHANI, MD, FACR
Director, Computed Tomography,
Massachusetts General Hospital, Associate
Professor, Radiology, Division of Abdomen
Imaging, Department of Radiology, Harvard
University, Boston, Massachusetts, USA

AUTHORS

ELIZABETH KAGAN ARLEO, MD
Associate Professor, Division of Breast
Imaging, Department of Radiology, Weill
Cornell Medical College, Weill Cornell
Medicine, New York, New York, USA

KRISTINE S. BURK, MD
Department of Radiology, Massachusetts
General Hospital, Boston, Massachusetts, USA

ALBERTO DIAZ DE LEON, MD
Assistant Professor, Department of Radiology,
The University of Texas Southwestern Medical
Center, Dallas, Texas, USA

JENNIFER S. DRUKTEINIS, MD
Associate Member, Division of Breast Imaging,
Department of Diagnostic Imaging, H. Lee
Moffitt Cancer Center & Research Institute,
Associate Professor, University of South
Florida, Tampa, Florida, USA

DAVID T. FETZER, MD
Assistant Professor, Department of Radiology,
The University of Texas Southwestern Medical
Center, Dallas, Texas, USA

FLORIAN J. FINTELMANN, MD, FRCPC
Thoracic Imaging and Intervention,
Department of Radiology, Massachusetts
General Hospital, Boston, Massachusetts,
USA

JOEL G. FLETCHER, MD
Department of Radiology, Mayo Clinic,
Rochester, Minnesota, USA

PHOEBE E. FREER, MD
Associate Professor, Division of Breast
Imaging, Department of Radiology, Huntsman
Cancer Institute, University of Utah, Salt Lake
City, Utah, USA

MICHAEL S. GEE, MD, PhD
Department of Radiology, Massachusetts
General Hospital, Boston, Massachusetts,
USA

MATTHEW D. GILMAN, MD
Thoracic Imaging and Intervention,
Department of Radiology, Massachusetts
General Hospital, Boston, Massachusetts,
USA

RAVI V. GOTTUMUKKALA, MD
Department of Radiology, Massachusetts
General Hospital, Boston, Massachusetts,
USA

STEPHANIE HANSEL, MD, MS
Department of Gastroenterology and
Hepatology, Mayo Clinic, Rochester,
Minnesota, USA

**ALISON C. HARRIS, BSc(Hons), MBChB,
FRCR, FRCPC**
Clinical Associate Professor, Department of
Radiology, Vancouver General Hospital,
Vancouver, British Columbia, Canada

AYA KAMAYA, MD
Associate Professor, Department of Radiology,
Stanford University, Stanford, California, USA

VENKATA S. KATABATHINA, MD
Department of Radiology, The University of
Texas Health Science Center at San Antonio,
San Antonio, Texas, USA

JIN SIL KIM, MD
Department of Radiology and Research
Institute of Radiology, University of Ulsan
College of Medicine, ASAN Medical Center,
Seoul, South Korea

YUKO KONO, MD, PhD
Clinical Associate Professor, Departments of
Medicine and Radiology, University of
California San Diego, San Diego, California,
USA

SUSANNA I. LEE, MD, PhD
Associate Professor, Radiology,
Massachusetts General Hospital, Harvard
Medical School, Boston, Massachusetts, USA

INGA T. LENNES, MD, MPH, MBA
Massachusetts General Hospital Cancer
Center, Boston, Massachusetts, USA

QIAN LI, MD
Department of Radiology, Massachusetts
General Hospital, Harvard Medical School,
Boston, Massachusetts, USA

XUEYING LIN, MD
Department of Ultrasound, Fujian Medical
University Union Hospital, Fuzhou, Fujian,
China

GRACE C. LO, MD
Department of Radiology, Massachusetts
General Hospital, Boston, Massachusetts, USA

KATHRYN P. LOWRY, MD
Assistant Professor, Radiology, University
of Washington School of Medicine, Seattle
Cancer Care Alliance, Seattle, Washington,
USA

SHAUNAGH McDERMOTT, MD
Thoracic Imaging and Intervention, Department
of Radiology, Massachusetts General Hospital,
Boston, Massachusetts, USA

CHRISTINE O. MENIAS, MD
Professor, Department of Radiology, Mayo
Clinic, Scottsdale, Arizona, USA

BETHANY L. NIELL, MD, PhD
Section Chief, Division of Breast Imaging,
Department of Diagnostic Imaging, H. Lee
Moffitt Cancer Center & Research Institute,
Associate Professor, University of South
Florida, Tampa, Florida, USA

SEONG HO PARK, MD, PhD
Department of Radiology and Research
Institute of Radiology, University of Ulsan
College of Medicine, ASAN Medical Center,
Seoul, South Korea

IVAN PEDROSA, MD, PhD
Associate Professor, Radiology and Advanced
Imaging Research Center, Department of
Radiology, The University of Texas
Southwestern Medical Center, Dallas, Texas,
USA

PERRY J. PICKHARDT, MD
Professor of Radiology, Chief, Gastrointestinal
Imaging, Department of Radiology, University
of Wisconsin School of Medicine and Public
Health, Madison, Wisconsin, USA

SRINIVASA R. PRASAD, MD
Department of Radiology, The University of
Texas MD Anderson Cancer Center, Houston,
Texas, USA

SHUCHI K. RODGERS, MD
Department of Radiology, Clinical Assistant
Professor, Sidney Kimmel Medical College,
Thomas Jefferson University, Einstein Medical
Center, Philadelphia, Pennsylvania, USA

DUSHYANT V. SAHANI, MD, FACR
Director, Computed Tomography,
Massachusetts General Hospital, Associate
Professor, Radiology, Division of Abdomen
Imaging, Department of Radiology, Harvard
University, Boston, Massachusetts, USA

ANTHONY E. SAMIR, MD, MPH
Department of Radiology, Massachusetts
General Hospital, Harvard Medical School,
Boston, Massachusetts, USA

KUMAR SANDRASEGARAN, MD
Professor, Department of Radiology, Indiana
University School of Medicine, Indianapolis,
Indiana, USA

YUHONG SHAO, MD
Department of Ultrasound, Peking University
First Hospital, Beijing, China

JO-ANNE O. SHEPARD, MD
Thoracic Imaging and Intervention, Department
of Radiology, Massachusetts General Hospital,
Boston, Massachusetts, USA

CLAUDE SIRLIN, MD
Professor, Liver Imaging Group, Department of
Radiology, University of California San Diego,
San Diego, California, USA

ASHISH P. WASNIK, MD
Associate Professor, Department of Radiology,
University of Michigan Health System, Ann
Arbor, Michigan, USA

ROBERT JARED WEINFURTNER, MD
Assistant Member, Division of Breast
Imaging, Department of Diagnostic
Imaging, H. Lee Moffitt Cancer Center &
Research Institute, Assistant Professor,
University of South Florida, Tampa, Florida,
USA

FEIXIANG XIANG, MD
Department of Ultrasound, Union Hospital,
Tongji Medical College, Huazhong
University of Science and Technology,
Wuhan, China

Contents

The goal of screening is to detect breast cancers when still curable to decrease breast cancer–specific mortality. Breast cancer screening in the United States is routinely performed with mammography, supplemental digital breast tomosynthesis, ultrasound, and/or MR imaging. This article aims to review the most commonly used breast imaging modalities for screening, discuss how often and when to begin screening with specific imaging modalities, and examine the pros and cons of screening. By the article's end, the reader will be better equipped to have informed discussions with patients and medical professionals regarding the benefits and disadvantages of breast cancer screening.

This article explains the rationale of lung cancer screening with low-dose computed tomography and provides a practical approach to all relevant aspects of a lung cancer screening program. Imaging protocols, patient eligibility criteria, facility readiness, and reimbursement criteria are addressed step by step. Diagnostic criteria and Lung-RADS (Lung Computed Tomography Screening Reporting and Data System) nodule management pathways are illustrated with examples. Pearls and pitfalls for interpretation of lung cancer screening of low-dose chest computed tomography are discussed.

Despite being readily preventable, colorectal cancer ranks second behind only lung cancer in overall mortality. However, this situation could be reversed if screening tests that effectively detect advanced adenomas and early cancers were broadly applied. Computed tomographic colonography (CTC) reflects an ideal balance of minimal invasiveness with high-level performance, assuming all facets of the examination are appropriately addressed. Unfortunately, this promising screening test remains grossly underused. This article details the technical and interpretive approaches used by one successful CTC screening program.

Given the high prevalence, increasing incidence, and significant morbidity and mortality related to hepatocellular carcinoma (HCC), a robust and cost-effective screening and surveillance program is needed. Most societies recommend ultrasound for HCC screening, despite lack of standardization in imaging acquisition, reporting content and language, and follow-up recommendations. The American College of Radiology Ultrasound Liver Imaging Reporting and Data System (US LI-RADS) fills this unmet need by providing standardization in the use of ultrasound in at-risk patients. It is anticipated that ultrasound LI-RADS will improve the performance of ultrasound for HCC screening and surveillance and unify management recommendations.

Biliary cancers include gallbladder cancer (GBC) and cholangiocarcinoma (CCA). GBC may appear as a mass replacing the gallbladder, thickened gallbladder wall, or polypoid lesion in the gallbladder. Gallbladder polyps with low risk of GBC (eg, 6-mm to 10-mm polyps without other risk factors) are screened with sonography. In general, polyps smaller than 5 mm are ignored and those larger than 10 mm require surgical consideration. Screening for CCA is less well-established. On imaging, CCA may be divided into mass-forming, periductal infiltrating, and intraductal types. This article discusses the current state of screening and diagnosis of GBC and CCA.

Given the low disease prevalence of both exocrine and endocrine cancers in the general population, screening is not recommended. However, in as many as 25% of cases there is a precursor lesion or an identifiable genetic predisposition. For these patients at increased risk, screening with imaging is recommended. Multidetector computed tomography, MR imaging, or MR cholangiopancreatography, and endoscopic ultrasound examination can be used as screening modalities. Recent advances in dual-energy computed tomography and total body MR imaging have increased the suitability of these noninvasive modalities as first-line imaging screening options.

Renal cell carcinoma (RCC) exhibits a diverse and heterogeneous disease spectrum, but insight into its molecular biology has provided an improved understanding of potential risk factors, oncologic behavior, and imaging features. Computed tomography (CT) and MR imaging may allow the identification and preoperative subtyping of RCC and assessment of a response to various therapies. Active surveillance is a viable management option in some patients and has provided further insight into the natural history of RCC, including the favorable prognosis of cystic neoplasms. This article reviews CT and MR imaging in RCC and the role of screening in selected high-risk populations.

Ovarian cancer has a high mortality, attributed to its typically advanced stage at detection. Despite much effort to identify an effective approach for ovarian cancer screening, to date no screening test has proven to reduce ovarian cancer mortality.

The natural history of ovarian cancer is reviewed as well as data from the largest trials of ovarian cancer screening. Currently, no North American society recommends routine ovarian cancer screening; some societies recommend consideration of screening with pelvic ultrasound and CA-125 in women at high risk, although its use in this setting is not supported by data demonstrating a mortality benefit.

Ultrasound is the first-line diagnostic tool for diagnosis of thyroid diseases. The low aggressiveness of many thyroid cancers coupled with high sensitivity of sonography can lead to cancer diagnosis and treatment with no effect on outcomes. Ultrasound is recognized as the most important driver of thyroid cancer overdiagnosis. Ultrasound should not be used as a general screening tool and should be reserved for patients at high risk of thyroid cancer and in the diagnostic management of incidentally discovered thyroid nodules. With prescreening risk stratification and application of consensus criteria for nodule biopsy, the value of the diagnostic ultrasound can be maximized.

Delayed diagnosis of small bowel cancers frequently occurs and may arise because of many factors, including low incidence of disease, difficult endoscopic access, lack of mucosal mass or abnormality, subtle radiologic features, and low index of clinical suspicion. As small bowel cancers are rare and their causes are largely unknown, routine population-based screening of asymptomatic patients to find precursor lesions or early cancers is ineffective. However, targeted screening/surveillance strategies are used in specific at-risk and symptomatic patient populations. This article reviews issues regarding early diagnosis of small bowel cancers, with focus on state-of-the-art cross-sectional imaging techniques.

There is a wide spectrum of mendelian disorders that predispose patients to an increased risk of benign as well as malignant tumors. Hereditary cancer syndromes are characterized by the early onset of diverse, frequently advanced malignancies in specific organ systems in multiple family members, posing significant challenges to diagnosis and management. A better understanding of the genetic abnormalities and pathophysiology that underlie these disorders has led to contemporary paradigms to screen, allowing early diagnosis, and has improved targeted therapies to aid in management. This article reviews select hereditary cancer syndromes with an emphasis on imaging-based screening and surveillance strategies.

PROGRAM OBJECTIVE

The objective of the *Radiologic Clinics of North America* is to keep practicing radiologists and radiology residents up to date with current clinical practice in radiology by providing timely articles reviewing the state of the art in patient care.

TARGET AUDIENCE

Practicing radiologists, radiology residents, and other health care professionals who provide patient care utilizing radiologic findings.

LEARNING OBJECTIVES

Upon completion of this activity, participants will be able to:
1. Review the imaging and screening for cancer of the gall bladder, bile ducts, and kidney.
2. Discuss imaging techniques for colorectal cancer and cancer of the small bowel.
3. Recognize screening tools for breast and ovarian cancer.

ACCREDITATION

The Elsevier Office of Continuing Medical Education (EOCME) is accredited by the Accreditation Council for Continuing Medical Education (ACCME) to provide continuing medical education for physicians.

The EOCME designates this enduring material for a maximum of 15 *AMA PRA Category 1 Credit*(s)™. Physicians should claim only the credit commensurate with the extent of their participation in the activity.

All other health care professionals requesting continuing education credit for this enduring material will be issued a certificate of participation.

DISCLOSURE OF CONFLICTS OF INTEREST

The EOCME assesses conflict of interest with its instructors, faculty, planners, and other individuals who are in a position to control the content of CME activities. All relevant conflicts of interest that are identified are thoroughly vetted by EOCME for fair balance, scientific objectivity, and patient care recommendations. EOCME is committed to providing its learners with CME activities that promote improvements or quality in healthcare and not a specific proprietary business or a commercial interest.

The planning committee, staff, authors and editors listed below have identified no financial relationships or relationships to products or devices they or their spouse/life partner have with commercial interest related to the content of this CME activity:

Elizabeth Kagan Arleo, MD; Kristine S. Burk, MD; Alberto Diaz de Leon, MD; Jennifer S. Drukteinis, MD; David T. Fetzer, MD; Florian J. Fintelmann, MD, FRCPC; Joel G. Fletcher, MD; Anjali Fortna; Phoebe E. Freer, MD; Michael S. Gee, MD, PhD; Matthew D. Gilman, MD; Ravi V. Gottumukkala, MD; Stephanie Hansel, MD, MS; Alison C. Harris, BSc(Hons), MBChB, FRCR, FRCPC; Aya Kamaya, MD; Venkata S. Katabathina, MD; Jim Sil Kim, MD; Yuko Kono, MD, PhD; Inga T. Lennes, MD, MPH, MBA; Qian Li, MD; Xueying Lin, MD; Grace C. Lo, MD; Leah Logan; Kathryn P. Lowry, MD; Shaunagh McDermott, MD; Christine O. Menias, MD; Bethany L. Niell, MD, PhD; Seong Ho Park, MD, PhD; Ivan Pedrosa, MD, PhD; Srinivasa R. Prasad, MD; Shuchi K. Rodgers, MD; Dushyant V. Sahani, MD; Anthony E. Samir, MD, MPH; Yuhong Shao, MD; Jo-Anne O. Shepard, MD; Claude Sirlin, MD; Karthik Subramaniam; John Vassallo; Ashish P. Wasnik, MD; Robert Jared Weinfurtner, MD; Feixiang Xiang, MD.

The planning committee, staff, authors and editors listed below have identified financial relationships or relationships to products or devices they or their spouse/life partner have with commercial interest related to the content of this CME activity:

Susanna I. Lee, MD, PhD has an employment affiliation with Wolters Kluwer.

Perry J. Pickhardt, MD is a consultant/advisor for Bracco and Check-Cap, and has stock ownership in VirtuoCTC; SHINE Medical Technologies; Elucent Medical; and Cellectar Biosciences.

Kumar Sandrasegaran, MD is a consultant/advisor for Geurbet LLC.

UNAPPROVED/OFF-LABEL USE DISCLOSURE

The EOCME requires CME faculty to disclose to the participants:
1. When products or procedures being discussed are off-label, unlabelled, experimental, and/or investigational (not US Food and Drug Administration [FDA] approved); and
2. Any limitations on the information presented, such as data that are preliminary or that represent ongoing research, interim analyses, and/or unsupported opinions. Faculty may discuss information about pharmaceutical agents that is outside of FDA-approved labelling. This information is intended solely for CME and is not intended to promote off-label use of these medications. If you have any questions, contact the medical affairs department of the manufacturer for the most recent prescribing information.

TO ENROLL

To enroll in the PET Clinics Continuing Medical Education program, call customer service at 1-800-654-2452 or sign up online at http://www.theclinics.com/home/cme. The CME program is available to subscribers for an additional annual fee of USD $315.

METHOD OF PARTICIPATION

In order to claim credit, participants must complete the following:

1. Complete enrolment as indicated above.
2. Read the activity.
3. Complete the CME Test and Evaluation. Participants must achieve a score of 70% on the test. All CME Tests and Evaluations must be completed online.

CME INQUIRIES/SPECIAL NEEDS

For all CME inquiries or special needs, please contact elsevierCME@elsevier.com.

RADIOLOGIC CLINICS OF NORTH AMERICA

THE CLINICS ARE AVAILABLE ONLINE!
Access your subscription at:
www.theclinics.com

Preface
Imaging and Cancer Screening

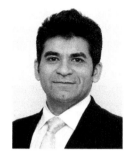

Dushyant V. Sahani, MD, FACR
Editor

Cancer remains a major public health issue, representing a leading cause of morbidity and mortality worldwide. The estimated 14 million new cases of cancer diagnosed in 2012 worldwide are expected to increase to 24 million by 2030. Breast, prostate, and lung cancers will remain the leading cancer diagnoses, but thyroid cancer is projected to unseat colorectal cancer as the fourth leading cancer diagnosis by 2030, and melanoma and uterine cancer will become the fifth and sixth most common cancers, respectively. Lung cancer is projected to remain the top cancer killer throughout this time period. However, pancreas and liver cancers are projected to surpass breast, prostate, and colorectal cancers to become the second and third leading causes of cancer-related death by 2030, respectively.

Despite advancements in chemotherapeutic agents and development of novel treatment strategies, the cure for most cancers remains elusive, and at present, we have only witnessed survival benefit for a few cancers. The need for action is especially critical in countries undergoing economic transition, which are currently ill equipped to provide the necessary patient care and will bear the disproportionate impact of the projected increase in the future cancer burden.

The American Cancer Society (ACS) estimates that more than half of all cancer deaths could be prevented if people adopted cancer-prevention measures, including receiving routine checkups, living a healthy lifestyle, and having an awareness of the early signs of cancer. Cancer screening tests are recommended to the public at certain baseline ages to detect and remove cancer in its earliest and most curable stage. Screening tests are recommended to large numbers of healthy people; therefore, any potential harm from the tests has to be outweighed by the potential benefits. Discovery of association between genetic mutations, a risk factor, and cancers such as BRCA with breast and ovarian cancers and VHL in renal cell carcinoma and neuroendocrine tumors highlights the importance of screening high-risk individuals to detect precursor lesions or early-stage cancer.

The role of imaging as a screening tool has been established by the ACS for three out of the four most common cancers, for example, breast, lung, and colorectal region. Breast cancer is the posterchild for the importance and success of screening, and dedicated mammography programs have reported a decrease in mortality by more than 40%. Clinical trials have recently confirmed the benefits of low-dose computed tomography (CT) for lung cancer screening. Recently, the US Preventive Services Task Force has approved CT colonography as an effective and safe screening modality for colorectal cancer. The American Association for the Study of Liver Diseases also adopted different imaging modalities from ultrasound to MR imaging for surveillance of hepatocellular carcinoma. Imaging is also being explored to screen high-risk populations for thyroid, pancreatic, ovarian, and renal cancers. Owing to the limitations of prostate-specific antigen in prostate cancer detection, MR is being evaluated for screening for prostate cancer in high-risk patients and for guiding tissue sampling and treatment delivery.

Imaging thus forms one of the main pillars in comprehensive cancer care from screening to

Radiol Clin N Am 55 (2017) xiii–xiv
http://dx.doi.org/10.1016/j.rcl.2017.09.001
0033-8389/17/© 2017 Published by Elsevier Inc.

radiologic.theclinics.com

management to follow-up. Advancement in imaging technology, development of safer CT scanners, faster MR protocols, and an approved lexicon for standardized reporting have significantly improved the universal appeal and ubiquity of imaging in the past decade. With promising results from research in functional imaging, new contrast agents, imaging biomarkers, and radiomics, the role of imaging in cancer care is only likely to increase. Cognizance of value of imaging, eligible patient population, cost-effectiveness, and local expertise influences the choice and use of imaging as a screening tool. The limited availability of monetary resources for health care is poised to shift the emphasis of expenditure from treatment to screening, especially in developed nations. However, successful imaging-based cancer screening will require a dedicated collaborative effort and a service-line model with involvement of various stakeholders, including referring physicians, to reap the full benefits of a program.

This issue of the *Radiologic Clinics of North America* has assembled leading experts with years of clinical and research experience in using imaging techniques as screening tests. Moreover, several authors are part of the taskforce responsible for developing such screening guidelines.

Dushyant V. Sahani, MD, FACR
Division of Abdomen Imaging
Department of Radiology
Massachusetts General Hospital
Harvard University
55 Fruit Street, White 270
Boston, MA 02114, USA

E-mail address:
dsahani@mgh.harvard.edu

Screening for Breast Cancer

Bethany L. Niell, MD, PhD[a],*, Phoebe E. Freer, MD[b], Robert Jared Weinfurtner, MD[a], Elizabeth Kagan Arleo, MD[c], Jennifer S. Drukteinis, MD[a]

KEYWORDS

- Screening • Mammography • Ultrasound • MR imaging • Cancer detection rate

KEY POINTS

- Early detection with screening mammography significantly reduces breast cancer deaths by 20% to 40%.
- Annual screening mammography of women aged 40 to 84 prevents more deaths from breast cancer than biennial screening of women 50 to 74 years old.
- Currently, it is recommended that supplemental screening with ultrasound or MR imaging be performed in addition to mammography.
- The American Cancer Society recommends annual screening mammography and supplemental screening MR imaging for women with an estimated lifetime risk of breast cancer ≥20%, *BRCA* mutation carriers, first-degree relatives of *BRCA* mutation carriers who remain untested, women with a history of mediastinal irradiation between the ages of 10 and 30, and women with certain genetic syndromes.

INTRODUCTION

In the United States in 2017, an estimated 255,180 new breast cancer cases will be diagnosed.[1] In 2013, breast cancer deaths totaled 773,100 person-years of life lost, with each death averaging 19 years of life lost.[2] The goal of screening is to find cancers when still curable (ie, smaller and node-negative) to decrease breast cancer–specific mortality. Since screening mammography became widespread in the United States during the 1980s, age-adjusted breast cancer mortality in women has steadily decreased (Fig. 1). This article aims to review the most commonly used breast imaging modalities for screening, discuss how often and when to begin screening with specific imaging modalities, and examine the pros and cons of screening. By the end of this article, the reader will be better equipped to have informed discussions with patients and medical professionals regarding the benefits and disadvantages of breast cancer screening.

SCREENING MAMMOGRAPHY

Early detection of breast cancer with screening mammography significantly reduces the risk of death from the disease.[3,4] The strongest evidence is provided by randomized controlled trials (RCTs), and pooled estimates show that screening mammography can reduce breast cancer mortality by at least 20%.[5] Eight RCTs have been performed and published. The first was initiated in 1963, the Health Insurance Plan (HIP) trial.[6] It recruited 62,000 women ages 40 to 64 from the HIP of greater New York and half were invited to

Disclosure Statement: The authors have nothing to disclose.
[a] Division of Breast Imaging, Department of Diagnostic Imaging, H. Lee Moffitt Cancer Center and Research Institute, 12902 USF Magnolia Drive, Tampa, FL 33612-9416, USA; [b] Division of Breast Imaging, Department of Radiology, University of Utah Hospitals, Huntsman Cancer Institute, 2000 Circle of Hope Drive, Salt Lake City, UT 84112, USA; [c] Division of Breast Imaging, Department of Radiology, Weill Cornell Medical College, Weill Cornell Medicine, 425 East 61st Street, New York, NY 10065, USA
* Corresponding author.
E-mail address: bethany.niell@moffitt.org

radiologic.theclinics.com

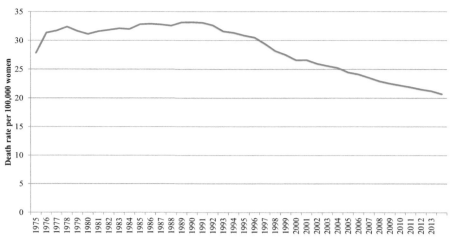

Fig. 1. Age-adjusted breast cancer death rate in American women decreased after the widespread introduction of screening mammography in the 1980s. (*Data from* the Surveillance, epidemiology, and end results [SEER] program from 1975–2013 and US Mortality Files, National Center for Health Statistics, Centers for Disease Control and Prevention. Rates are per 100,000 and are age-adjusted to the 2000 US population (19 age groups - Census P25-1130).)

undergo annual clinical breast examination and screening mammography. Breast cancer mortality was reduced by 22% among those invited to screen (**Table 1**).[3,7,8]

> Pooled estimates from RCTs demonstrate that screening mammography can reduce breast cancer mortality by at least 20%.

In the late 1970s, 2 trials in Sweden, the Swedish Two-County trial and Malmö investigated the effect of screening mammography without physical examination. The Swedish Two-County trial consisted of 133,065 women ages 40 to 74, who were randomized into a group invited to single-view screening mammography and a control group. Screening intervals were 24 months for ages 40 to 49, and 33 months for those 50 to 74.[9] After 3 decades of follow-up, invitation to screening resulted in a 27% to 31% reduction in breast cancer mortality, with only 45% of prevented breast cancer deaths occurring in the first 10 years. At 10 years of follow-up, 1303 women were needed to screen for 7 years to save 1 life. At 20 years, 577 women were needed to screen, and at 29 years, 519 women were needed to screen to save 1 life.[10] The observed number of prevented breast cancer deaths increases with follow-up duration, providing evidence that estimates of absolute benefit and number needed to screen requires trial follow-up intervals exceeding 20 years. Malmö recruited approximately 31,000 to each group, women ages 45 to 70 (MMST1) and ages 43 to 49 (MMST2). Invitation to screening

at 18-month to 24-month intervals resulted in a 22% reduction in breast cancer mortality.[11]

The Edinburgh trial evaluated the efficacy of mammography and CBE in 3 cohorts of women recruited between 1978 and 1985. Patients were randomized by clinical practice to biennial single-view mammography (initial screening round was 2-view) plus annual CBE versus CBE alone.[12] With 14 years of follow-up from 28,628 women offered screening and 26,026 controls, invitation to screening decreased breast cancer mortality by 21% to 29%.[13] The Stockholm trial included 40,000 women invited to biennial screening and 20,000 women as controls.[14] The Swedish Two-County trial was already showing significant benefit; the Stockholm trial was terminated after only 2 rounds of screening with single-view mammography and showed no statistically significant mortality reduction (see **Table 1**).

The Canadian National Breast Screening Trials in women ages 40 to 49 (CNBSS-1) and 50 to 59 (CNBSS-2) investigated the efficacy of CBE and screening mammography on breast cancer mortality reduction.[15,16] Women were asked to volunteer to participate, and following CBE, approximately 50,000 volunteers were included in CNBSS-1 and 40,000 in CNBSS-2.[15,16] At 7 years of follow-up in CNBSS-1, women invited to screening had 36% *greater* mortality from breast cancer than control women. At 25 years of follow-up, breast cancer mortality was identical in the mammography and control arms.[17] Flawed study design and suboptimal image quality and interpretation may explain why the Canadian National Breast Screening Trials are outliers compared with other RCTs (see **Table 1**). In the

Table 1
Evidence for mortality reduction from screening mammography

Trial or Data	%	Mortality Reduction 95% Confidence Interval
HIP RCT[3,8]	22	0–39
Malmo RCT[11]	22	5–35
Swedish Two-County RCT[10]	27	11–41
Edinburgh RCT[13]	21	−2–40
Stockholm RCT[3,11]	10	−28–37
NBSS1 and NBSS2 RCTs[17]	1	−12–12
Gothenburg RCT[21]	23	0–40
Overall RCTs[3]	20	14–27
European service screening Invited vs not invited[22]	25	24–31
European service screening Screened vs not screened[22]	38	31–44
Canadian service screening[23]	40	33–48
European case control studies Screened vs not screened[22]	48	35–58

Abbreviations: HIP, Health Insurance Plan; NBSS, National Breast Screening Trial; RCT, randomized controlled trial.

first round of screening, significantly more women with palpable and advanced (lymph node–positive) breast cancer were randomized to the screening arm. For women with 4 or more positive nodes, the ratio between those assigned to the screening group compared with the control group was 19:5, and 17 of the 19 had palpable cancers despite the trials' intention to evaluate *screening* mammography. These data suggest flawed randomization.[18] Among women in the CNBSS-1 control group diagnosed with breast cancer, the greater than 90% 5-year survival is higher than the less than 80% survival reported in the United States and Canada during a similar time period, which may be in part due to the flawed randomization process and the recruitment of volunteers.[18] Due in part to the high survival in the control arm, the CNBSS trials lacked statistical power to demonstrate a 40% breast cancer mortality reduction, let alone a more reasonable 20% to 30% reduction as expected from other RCT trial data.[18] An external review judged more than 50% of the mammograms as poor or unacceptable, and the CNBSS's own radiologist revealed that 42% of missed cancers were visible on a previous mammogram.[18,19]

The most recent RCT in mammography started in 1982 in Gothenburg, Sweden. Approximately 52,000 women aged 39 to 59 years were randomized, and the screening arm offered 2-view mammography every 18 months.[20] After 14 years of follow-up, women ages 39 to 59 invited to screening had a 23% mortality reduction.[21]

RCTs provide the strongest evidence for mortality reduction; however, RCTs underestimate the expected benefit because some women invited to screening do not actually undergo screening (noncompliance) and some women in the control group go outside the study to obtain a screening mammogram (contamination). Service screening studies use large, population-based screening programs and measure outcomes from women who actually undergo screening. European service screening data demonstrate a 38% reduction in breast cancer mortality among women who underwent screening, compared with a 25% reduction among women invited to screen.[22] Canadian service screening data demonstrate a 40% reduction in mortality and a 44% mortality reduction in women ages 40 to 49 who underwent screening.[23] Case control studies compare how often and when screening was done in 2 groups of women, those who died from breast cancer (cases), and those who are alive (matched controls). A meta-analysis of European case control studies demonstrated a 48% decrease in breast cancer mortality in women screened, and a case control study in Western Australia showed a 52% reduction.[22,24]

> RCTs underestimate the potential benefit of screening mammography because some women invited to screening do not actually undergo screening (noncompliance) and some women in the control group go outside the study to obtain a screening mammogram (contamination).

> Service screening studies measure outcomes from women who *actually* undergo screening in large, population-based screening programs. Among women who underwent screening in Europe and Canada, breast cancer mortality was decreased by 38% and 40%, respectively.

PERFORMANCE BENCHMARKS FOR SCREENING MAMMOGRAPHY

Screening mammography detects 2 to 8 cancers per 1000 mammograms.[25–27] The sensitivity of mammography decreases in women with dense breasts, measuring 30% to 64% for extremely dense breasts compared with 76% to 98% for fatty breasts.[28–33] Decreased sensitivity in denser breasts is attributable to the concept of masking. Cancers have similar x-ray attenuation as dense fibroglandular tissue, resulting in obscuration of the tumor.[31] With this limitation, supplemental screening modalities have been investigated.

DIGITAL BREAST TOMOSYNTHESIS

Digital breast tomosynthesis (DBT) is a digital mammogram technique in which tomosynthesis images are constructed from a series of low-dose images acquired as the x-ray source moves over the breast, which reduces the impact of overlapping breast tissue. Eliminating tissue overlap increases conspicuity of lesions while reducing false positives due to tissue summation. DBT detects malignancies occult on digital mammography (Fig. 2).[34] Two major prospective clinical trials have been performed comparing full-field digital mammography (FFDM) to FFDM with DBT. In 12,621 screening examinations in the Oslo Tomosynthesis Screening Trial, tomosynthesis with FFDM increased the invasive cancer detection rate by 40% and decreased false positives by 15%, compared with FFDM alone.[35] In 7292 Italian women enrolled in the Screening with Tomosynthesis or Mammography (STORM) trial, DBT increased the cancer detection rate from 5.3 to 8.1 per 1000 examinations with a simultaneous 17% reduction in recall rate.[36] Retrospective analysis of 173,663 FFDM-DBT and 281,187 FFDM examinations from 13 sites in the United States demonstrated a 29% increase in cancer detection rate with a concomitant 15% decrease in recall rate compared with FFDM alone.[37]

> DBT increases cancer detection and decreases recall rate, compared with digital mammography.

A synthesized mammogram can be created by summing and filtering a stack of reconstructed DBT images, resulting in an FFDM equivalent image and an examination with roughly half the dose of a standard combined FFDM and DBT examination.[38]

CONTRAST-ENHANCED MAMMOGRAPHY AND DIGITAL BREAST TOMOSYNTHESIS

Neovascularity causes tumors to enhance, usually more so than the surrounding normal parenchyma, following administration of intravenous contrast agents. Contrast-enhanced spectral mammography (CESM) or DBT acquires FFDM or DBT images following intravenous iodine-based contrast media injection. A recent meta-analysis of CESM demonstrated very high sensitivity (98%) but limited specificity (58%).[39] At this time, CESM and CE-DBT remain active areas of research and are not currently recommended for screening.

SCREENING ULTRASOUND

Ultrasound has shown utility in detecting breast cancer as a supplemental screening modality since the 1980s.[40,41] Compared with screening mammography alone, screening ultrasound in combination with mammography can increase cancer detection (additional cancer detection rate [ACDR]) but at the cost of increased callbacks ("recall rate") and a large number of biopsies needed to identify 1 breast cancer (positive predictive value 3 [PPV_3] = number of cancers detected/number of biopsies performed).[42–45] In patients at increased risk of developing breast cancer, supplemental screening ultrasound can detect an additional 4.2 cancers per 1000 women with 11 cancers per 100 biopsies performed (PPV_3 = 11%), compared with a PPV_3 of 29% for mammography alone in the first year of screening ultrasound.[42,43] PPV_3 may increase in subsequent screening rounds (as high as 16%) while maintaining an ACDR of 2.3 to 3.7 per 1000 in subsequent years.[43,46] As expected, screening ultrasound in women with breast density as their only risk factor detects fewer cancers and requires more biopsies per cancer detected, with ACDR of 3.2 per 1000 in the first year and PPV_3 of 6.5% to 6.7%.[44,45] In a recent meta-analysis, supplemental screening ultrasound demonstrated a PPV_3 of 2% to 8% and ACDR of 4.4 per 1000 with a recall rate of 14%.[47] Because ultrasound detects masked breast cancers obscured by breast parenchyma on mammography, screening ultrasound halves the rate of interval cancers (cancers that present within 1 year of a negative screening mammogram).[48] In women with dense breasts and a negative screening mammogram, supplemental screening with ultrasound had an ACDR of 7.1 per 1000 compared with 4 per 1000 for DBT with similar recall rates.[49]

> Screening ultrasound detects 2 to 4 additional cancers per 1000 examinations but requires many recalls and a large number of biopsies needed to identify each breast cancer.

In addition to the drawbacks of increased recalls and lower PPV, another disadvantage to whole breast ultrasound is acquisition time and interpretation time. Screening ultrasound trials report a 10-minute to 20-minute acquisition time and 7-minute to 10-minute interpretation time.[42,50,51] Screening ultrasound with automated whole breast units yields similar results to screening with hand-held whole breast ultrasound performed by a radiologist or a breast technologist.[47]

SCREENING BREAST MR IMAGING

Breast MR imaging with gadolinium is highly sensitive (≥90%) for the detection of breast cancer.[52–54] Although initial reports suggested lower sensitivity for the detection of ductal carcinoma in situ (DCIS), advances in image quality and

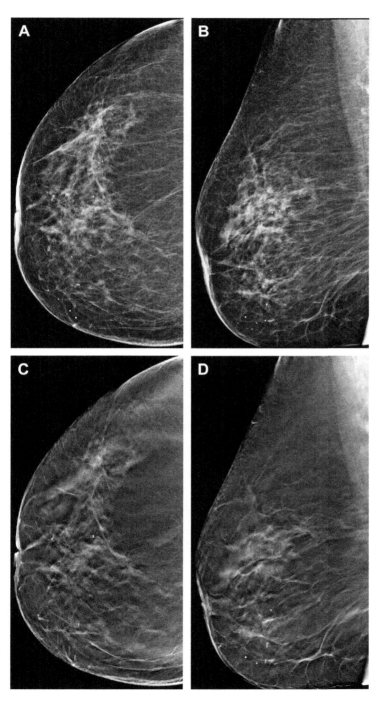

Fig. 2. Increased lesion conspicuity on DBT images increases cancer detection rate on DBT compared with FFDM. (A) CC and (B) MLO FFDM images show scattered fibroglandular densities in the right breast without definite abnormality. Selected CC (C) and MLO (D) tomosynthesis slices demonstrate architectural distortion in the right upper central breast. Targeted ultrasound demonstrated no sonographic correlate. Pathology from tomosynthesis-guided percutaneous biopsy yielded invasive ductal carcinoma. CC, craniocaudal; MLO, mediolateral oblique.

image interpretation have resulted in 98% and 85% sensitivities for high-grade and non–high-grade DCIS, respectively.[55] In prospective trials of asymptomatic high-risk women, screening MR imaging was more sensitive (90%–93%) than clinical breast examination (18%), mammography (33%–50%), ultrasonography (37%–52%), or mammography combined with ultrasonography (48%–63%).[52,54,56] Up to 31% to 52% of MR imaging–detected breast cancers were detected only on MR imaging (**Fig. 3**).[52,54,56]

The cancer yield of MR imaging is approximately 14 to 30 per 1000 high-risk women screened.[43,52,53]

In addition to its utility in asymptomatic women, breast MR imaging detects *contralateral* cancers in 3.1% of women with newly diagnosed breast cancer and a negative contralateral mammogram.[57]

High-risk women undergoing annual screening mammography and supplemental screening MR imaging do not benefit from the addition of screening ultrasound.[52,54,56] However, women undergoing annual screening mammography and supplemental screening ultrasound do benefit from the addition of MR imaging. In women with dense breasts and elevated breast cancer risk

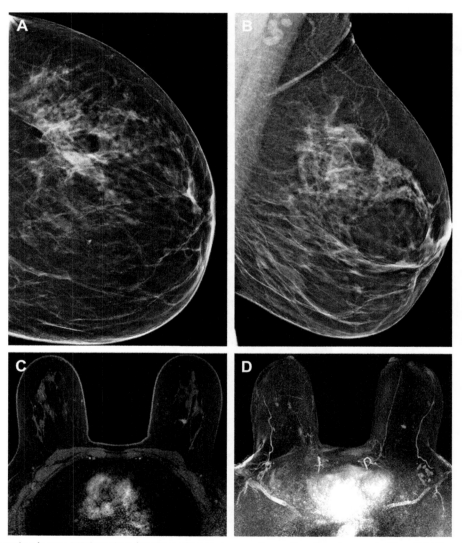

Fig. 3. Screening breast MR imaging detects malignancies occult on other imaging modalities. (*A*) CC and (*B*) MLO FFDM images of the left breast demonstrate no suspicious findings. (*C*) Early postcontrast T1-weighted fat subtracted axial and (*D*) maximum intensity projection images from screening breast MR imaging demonstrate a 7-mm enhancing mass with spiculated margins in the left breast at 12 o'clock 10 cm from the nipple. Pathology from an MR imaging–guided percutaneous breast biopsy yielded invasive ductal carcinoma (grade 1).

who underwent 3 rounds of annual screening ultrasound and mammography, cancer detection rate increased from 11.4 per 1000 for mammography plus ultrasound to 26.1 per 1000 with the addition of a single MR imaging screen (ACDR of 14.7/1000 for MR imaging).[43] MR imaging–detected breast cancers often exhibit underlying pathologic markers of biologic aggressiveness; for example, MR imaging better detects intermediate and high-grade DCIS in addition to small and node-negative invasive tumors, suggesting that MR imaging–detected cancers are less likely to contribute to overdiagnosis.[52,53] Screening MR imaging also results in a near zero rate of interval cancers.[52] Despite the benefits of screening MR imaging, fewer than half of documented *BRCA* mutation carriers and fewer than one-third of women with a ≥20% lifetime risk have received screening breast MR imaging.[58]

> Screening breast MR imaging demonstrates high sensitivity for the detection of breast cancer. Up to one-half of MR imaging–detected breast cancers are seen only on MR imaging.

Disadvantages of breast MR imaging include the need for intravenous gadolinium contrast administration, the lack of data regarding decreased breast cancer–specific mortality, expense and lack of availability, as well as decreased specificity. In published studies to date, the specificity of MR imaging with mammography was lower than mammography alone (range 73%–97% vs 91%–100%).[59] However, recent data suggest that the specificity of MR imaging when added to mammography approaches 96.0% to 97.6%, compared with 99.0% for mammography alone, for experienced readers.[52,54] With regard to expense, supplemental screening MR imaging in patients with elevated breast cancer risk was 2.5 times more expensive per life-year gained with an estimated mortality reduction of 25% compared with 17% with mammography alone.[60] To address the expense and resource limitations, an abbreviated screening breast MR imaging protocol can be acquired in 3 minutes, requires an average of 28 seconds to read, and demonstrates equivalent diagnostic accuracy to the 17-minute acquisition complete protocol.[61] A prospective, multicenter trial of abbreviated screening breast MR imaging is currently planned. Ongoing and future research efforts will investigate noncontrast screening breast MR imaging using diffusion-weighted imaging.

ADDITIONAL BREAST IMAGING MODALITIES

Positron emission mammography (PEM) remains investigational but uses mild compression with acquisitions in 2 views, similar to mammography. Data from experienced readers suggest sensitivity of 90% to 96%, although PEM may not reliably detect lower-grade malignancies and has a higher radiation dose than mammography, limiting its screening utility.[62–67] Breast-specific gamma imaging (BSGI) uses a radiotracer, most commonly ^{99m}Tc-sestamibi, which accumulates in tumor more than normal breast tissue. To date, no large prospective studies have been performed, and BSGI is not currently recommended for screening. BSGI demonstrates sensitivity greater than 90% and specificity of 60% to 80%,[68–72] but the examination is limited by long examination time and high radiation dose.[68,73]

Breast thermography cannot and should not be used to diagnose breast cancer due to unacceptably low sensitivity (61%) and specificity (74%).[74,75]

BREAST CANCER SCREENING GUIDELINES

The US Preventive Services Task Force (USPSTF), the American Cancer Society (ACS), and the American College of Radiology (ACR) are the 3 main organizations that have issued evidence-based guidelines for breast cancer screening in the average-risk woman based on estimates of risk versus benefits (**Table 2**).[5,76,77] All 3 organizations agree that screening mammography saves lives, and, at a minimum, should be performed in women 50 to 74. All 3 guidelines recognize that annual mammography should remain an option for each woman starting at the age of 40 because all 3 organizations acknowledge that annual screening mammography beginning at age 40 saves the most lives from breast cancer.

> The USPSTF, ACS, and ACR are the 3 main organizations that have issued evidence-based guidelines for breast cancer screening in average-risk women. All 3 guidelines state that annual mammography should remain an option for women starting at age 40 because annual screening mammography beginning at age 40 saves the most lives from breast cancer.

The ACR and Society of Breast Imaging recommend that women at average risk of breast cancer begin annual screening mammography at age 40 and stop screening when life expectancy is less than 5 to 7 years on the basis of age or comorbid

Table 2
Screening mammography guidelines for average-risk women

	Age to Start	How Often	Age to Stop	Comment
American College of Radiology	40+	Annual	Continue as long as in good health	
American Cancer Society	45–54 \n 55+	Annual \n Biennial	Until approximately 10 y of life left	Option to start screening 40–44; if start at 40, recommend annual screening 40–54
US Preventive Services Task Force	50–74 (Category B recommendation)	Biennial	≥75	Individual decision to start screening at ages 40–49 (Category C)

conditions and/or when abnormal results of screening would not be acted on due to similar reasons.[78]

The USPSTF recommendation (2009 and 2016) is biennial screening mammography for women aged 50 to 74 years (B recommendation). The decision to start screening mammography in women before age 50 years should be an individual one. Women who place a higher value on the potential benefit than the potential harms may choose to begin biennial screening between the ages of 40 and 49 years (C recommendation). The USPSTF concludes that the current evidence is insufficient to assess the balance of benefits and harms of screening mammography in women aged 75 years or older (I statement).[77] The Task Force defines a B recommendation as one in which "there is high certainty that the net benefit is moderate or there is moderate certainty that the net benefit is moderate to substantial."[77] Under the Patient Protection and Affordable Care Act, "insurers now must cover evidence-based services for adults that have a rating of 'A' or 'B' in the current USPSTF."[79] Based on the USPSTF recommendations, private insurers will cover biennial screening mammography beginning at age 40; however, women ages 40 to 49 or older than 75 who choose routine screening, as well as women of any age who want to be screened annually may not be guaranteed coverage. As a result, Congress recently enacted the Consolidated Appropriations Act, which included language from the Protecting Access to Lifesaving Screenings Act (PALS) (H.R.3339) to delay implementation of the USPSTF recommendations for 2 years and thus allow women continued access to screening mammography in the interim.[80]

The ACS recommends that women with an average risk of breast cancer should undergo regular screening mammography starting at age 45 years (strong recommendation). Women aged 45 to 54 years should be screened annually (qualified recommendation). Women 55 years and older should transition to biennial screening or have the opportunity to continue screening annually (qualified recommendation). Women should have the opportunity to begin annual screening between the ages of 40 and 44 years (qualified recommendation). Women should continue screening mammography as long as their overall health is good and they have a life expectancy of 10 years or longer (qualified recommendation).[5] The ACS defines a strong recommendation as one for which "most individuals in this situation would want the recommended course of action, and only a small proportion would not" and a qualified recommendation as one for which "the majority of individuals in this situation would want the suggested course of action, but many would not."[5]

The National Comprehensive Cancer Network (NCCN) and the American Congress of Obstetricians and Gynecologists (ACOG) agree with the ACR, recommending mammography screening starting at age 40 and continuing annually, regardless of risk.[81,82] The American College of Surgeons Oncology Group recommends following the ACS guidelines. The American Academy of Family Physicians and American College of Physicians both recommend following the USPSTF guidelines.[83,84]

WOMEN WITH DENSE BREASTS

Approximately 40% to 50% of women undergoing screening mammography have dense breasts (higher ratio of fibroglandular and stromal elements relative to fatty tissue).[85] The definition of "dense" is subjective by the radiologist and demonstrates moderate variability between radiologists with 17% of patients being recategorized into dense versus nondense on subsequent mammograms.[86] Women with dense breasts have a 1.2-fold to 2.1-fold higher risk of breast cancer compared with the average woman.[87] Because dense tissue causes a "masking" phenomenon and obscures underlying cancers, women with dense breasts have more interval cancers (a cancer diagnosed within 12 months of a negative screening mammogram). The interval cancer rate is as much as 17-fold higher in women with extremely dense breasts compared with women with the fattiest breasts.[88]

As of December 5, 2016, 28 states have enacted legislation that requires radiologists to notify patients of their breast density. Although the wording of the individual laws varies, most encourage a patient to discuss with her referring provider whether she would benefit from supplemental screening tests. Individual clinical practices may choose to offer supplemental screening ultrasound, or other tests, to women with dense breasts, given the increased cancer detection (Fig. 4). However, supplemental screening for dense breasts remains controversial due to the high frequencies of false-positive recall and false-positive biopsy compared with mammography.[89] Compared with mammography alone, supplemental ultrasound is predicted to prevent 0.36 additional cancer deaths and lead to an additional 354 biopsies per 1000 women screened biennially for 25 years.[90] As such, screening ultrasound is unlikely to be considered cost-effective.[90] The ACR recommends supplemental screening ultrasound in women with dense breasts and an elevated risk of breast cancer who cannot undergo MR imaging.[91]

> Clinicians may choose to offer supplemental screening ultrasound, or other tests, to women with dense breasts, given the increased cancer detection. However, this remains controversial due to the high frequencies of false-positive recall and false-positive biopsy compared with mammography.

DBT may have its largest incremental cancer detection benefit over digital mammography in women with heterogeneously dense breasts and, when accessible, may thus be preferred over

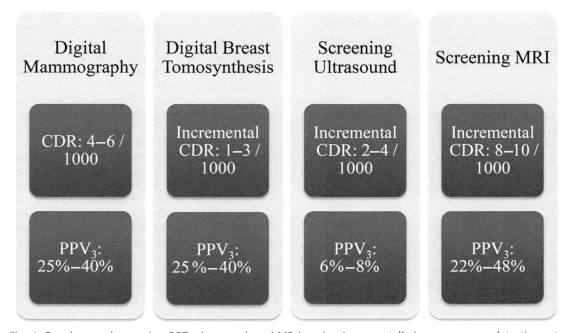

Digital Mammography	Digital Breast Tomosynthesis	Screening Ultrasound	Screening MRI
CDR: 4–6 / 1000	Incremental CDR: 1–3 / 1000	Incremental CDR: 2–4 / 1000	Incremental CDR: 8–10 / 1000
PPV_3: 25%–40%	PPV_3: 25%–40%	PPV_3: 6%–8%	PPV_3: 22%–48%

Fig. 4. Supplemental screening DBT, ultrasound, and MR imaging incrementally increase cancer detection rate (CDR) when added to digital mammography in women with dense breasts. PPV_3 is the positive predictive value of biopsy and equals the number of cancers detected divided by the number of breast biopsies performed. (*Data from* Tice JA, Ollendorf DA, Lee JM, et al. The comparative clinical effectiveness and value of supplemental screening tests following negative mammography in women with dense breast tissue. Institute for Clinical and Economic Review; 2013. Available at: https://icer-review.org/wp-content/uploads/2016/01/ctaf-final-report-dense-breast-imaging-11.04.2013-b.pdf.)

standard digital mammography.[92] It should be noted, however, that the benefit of DBT in improving cancer detection does not persist in the fewer than 10% women who have extremely dense breasts.[92]

"RISK-BASED" OR "PERSONALIZED" OR "TAILORED" SCREENING

In the emerging era of precision medicine, it is unlikely that there will be a "one-size-fits-all" approach to breast cancer screening. Women at increased risk of breast cancer may benefit from supplemental screening with imaging examinations, such as DBT, MR imaging, or ultrasound. Supplemental screening should be in addition to, and not as a replacement for, annual mammography.

The 20% to 40% reduction in breast cancer mortality was observed in screening mammography RCTs and service screening studies in women irrespective of risk. Existing data do not support the assertion that average-risk women do not benefit from screening. The idea that only high-risk women should begin screening mammography at age 40 ignores the fact that 75% of women diagnosed with breast cancer at ages 40 to 49 do not have a strong family history or extremely dense breast tissue.[93] Ongoing research studies, including the WISDOM trial, will evaluate the effects of increased screening including supplemental screening modalities in high-risk women, while other studies are evaluating decreasing mammography screening in low-risk or average-risk women.[94]

> Average-risk women benefit from screening mammography.

SCREENING AVERAGE-RISK OR LOW-RISK WOMEN

Women who have less than 15% lifetime risk of breast cancer should continue to be offered screening mammography annually starting at the age of 40 per ACR guidelines. The ACS and the USPSTF, who advise routinely starting screening at a later date (45–50), acknowledge that the most lives are saved from breast cancer when screening starts at 40 and is performed annually.[5,77] Women of average or low risk require no additional supplemental screening in addition to mammography, although the NCCN recommends that tomosynthesis be considered (Category 1 recommendation) in all women starting at 40.[81] The ACS and NCCN recommend against MR imaging or supplemental screening in women with a <15% lifetime risk of breast cancer. NCCN guidelines state there is "insufficient evidence" to routinely recommend supplemental screening tests such as ultrasound or MR imaging in women who have dense breasts who are otherwise of low or average risk.[81] The USPSTF states there is a dearth of evidence to recommend supplemental screening tests in women of average risk and dense breasts.[47,77]

SCREENING INTERMEDIATE-RISK WOMEN

Women with an intermediate risk of breast cancer (15% to <20% lifetime risk) include women with a prior personal history of breast cancer, lobular neoplasia, and other atypias. Some consider women with dense breasts in the intermediate-risk category. For women with 15% to less than 20% lifetime risk, the 2007 ACS guidelines state that there was insufficient evidence to recommend for or against supplemental breast MR imaging.[95] Subsequently published studies in women with a personal history of breast cancer or a personal history of atypia on prior breast biopsy suggest that these 2 groups of women demonstrate similar ACDR (~14–15 cancers per 1000 MR imaging examinations) on supplemental screening breast MR imaging as high-risk women.[96–104] The ACR appropriateness criteria ranks supplemental screening MR imaging in intermediate-risk women as 7 and supplemental ultrasound as 5 on a scale of 1 (not recommended) to 9 (highly recommended).[76]

SCREENING HIGH-RISK WOMEN

Since 2007, the ACS has recommended annual screening mammography and supplemental screening MR imaging for women with an estimated lifetime risk of breast cancer ≥20%, BRCA mutation carriers, first-degree relatives of BRCA mutation carriers who remain untested, women with a history of mediastinal irradiation between the ages of 10 and 30, and women with certain genetic syndromes (Li-Fraumeni, Cowden, Bannayan-Riley-Ruvalcaba).[95] Many statistical models have been developed to assess breast cancer risk, such as the Gail and modified Gail models, Claus, BOADICEA (Breast and Ovarian Analysis of Disease Incidence and Carrier Estimation Algorithm), Tyrer-Cuzick (TC), and BRCAPRO. Existing models have been calibrated to estimate population risk but demonstrate only moderate accuracy in discriminating each woman's individual risk.[105] To determine eligibility for screening breast MR imaging, the ACS specifically recommends using BRCAPRO or TC or other models that incorporate first-degree and second-degree relatives to estimate breast cancer risk.[95,106] The ACS recommends against using models with limited family history input (eg, Gail or modified Gail).

The ACS recommends annual screening mammography and supplemental screening MR imaging for the following women:

- Estimated lifetime risk of breast cancer ≥20%
- BRCA mutation carriers
- First-degree relatives of BRCA mutation carriers who remain untested
- Mediastinal irradiation between the ages of 10 and 30
- Certain genetic syndromes

The NCCN guidelines mirror the ACS and include the recommendation to start MR imaging at age 25 and mammography at age 30, or 10 years before the first-degree relative was diagnosed, whichever comes later.[95] If a woman is unable to undergo breast MR imaging (eg, secondary to pacemaker or other implantable non–MR imaging compatible device, prior contrast anaphylaxis, or severe claustrophobia not responsive to treatment), she may be offered whole breast screening ultrasound as an adjunct to mammography.[76] Screening ultrasound does not add value or incremental cancer detection in women who are already receiving both annual mammography and MR imaging.[52,54,107]

Screening ultrasound does not add value or incremental cancer detection in women who are already receiving both annual mammography and MR imaging.

No data or specific recommendations exist regarding the best way to schedule annual mammography and MR imaging. As a result, some high-risk women choose to obtain mammography and MR imaging around the same time, whereas others choose to alternate mammography and MR imaging every 6 months.

CONTROVERSIES REGARDING SCREENING MAMMOGRAPHY IN AVERAGE-RISK WOMEN
Benefits and "Harms" of Screening

Individuals and different professional organizations disagree about the relative benefits and harms of screening mammography, resulting in hotly debated controversies. Breast cancer–specific mortality reduction is the primary benefit of screening mammography, but not the only one. Earlier detection and treatment of breast cancers results not only in decreased breast cancer deaths but also decreased treatment-related morbidity; that is, fewer mastectomies and less frequent and less toxic chemotherapy.[108,109] Women diagnosed with localized breast cancer commonly have the option of breast-conserving therapy, which is associated with few surgical side effects and postoperative upper body impairments, less chronic pain, better body image, and less psychological distress.[110–112] Women with localized disease are more likely to be eligible for sentinel lymph node biopsy, which compared with axillary dissection, is associated with less upper body morbidity and a lower risk of lymphedema.[113] Smaller and less advanced cancers can be effectively treated without chemotherapy, which has a broad range of side effects, including cardiac toxicity, premature menopause, and an increased risk of blood disorders.[114–116]

"Harms" of screening mammography include false-positive results and associated anxiety, overdiagnosis and overtreatment, and radiation risk. Before considering each individually, it is important to note that both false positives and overdiagnosis are a risk of any and all screening tests. Neither is unique to screening mammography.

When to Begin and End Screening Mammograms and at What Frequency

Patients and clinicians grapple with 3 possible ages (40, 45, and 50) at which to begin screening mammography and 2 possible frequencies (annual or biennial) with several different permutations based on the ACR, ACS, and USPSTF guidelines (see **Table 2**). All 3 guidelines recognize that annual mammography should remain an option for each woman starting at the age of 40 because all 3 organizations acknowledge that annual screening mammography beginning at age 40 saves the most lives from breast cancer. Annual screening mammography of women ages 40 to 84 prevents more deaths from breast cancer (39.6% mortality reduction) than biennial screening of women 50 to 74 years old (which has only a 23.2% mortality reduction).[117] Rapidly growing cancers may become lethal in the interval between screening rounds, so an increased screening frequency has the potential to detect more aggressive tumors before lethality. Premenopausal women diagnosed with breast cancer on biennial screening mammography (23–26 months) are 21% to 28% more likely to have larger tumors or higher-stage tumors compared with premenopausal women with breast cancer detected at annual (11–14 months) screening.[118]

> Premenopausal women diagnosed with breast cancer on biennial screening mammography are significantly more likely to have larger tumors or higher-stage tumors compared with premenopausal women with breast cancer detected at annual screening.

The debate to begin screening at age 40 or 50 exists because age 50 was chosen as a surrogate for menopause, and age-stratified analyses (40–49 vs >50) within individual studies were underpowered to detect significant mortality reduction in younger women. After combining data from multiple RCTs, a meta-analysis showed that screening mammography decreases breast cancer deaths by 18% to 29% in women ages 40 to 49, similar to breast cancer mortality reduction in women older than 50.[119] Approximately 1 in 6 women will be diagnosed with breast cancer before the age of 50, and 40% of the person-years of life lost from breast cancer deaths are in women diagnosed in their 40s or younger.[2] In part because the absolute risk of developing breast cancer within the next 5 years is similar in women ages 45 to 49 (0.9%) and 50 to 54 (1.1%) but lower in women ages 40 to 44 (0.6%), the ACS suggested 45 as an alternative age criterion to begin screening mammography in 2015 despite the lack of difference in mortality reduction.[5]

False-Positive Mammograms

A "false positive" is a test result that suggests the presence of a disease when the disease is not present. For women who begin annual screening mammography at age 40, the cumulative probability of a false-positive recall over a 10-year period is 61%.[120] On average, an individual woman ages 40 to 49 who undergoes annual screening mammography will experience 1 false-positive mammogram every 10 years and 1 false-positive biopsy every 149 years.[117] Biennial screening reduces false-positive mammograms by one-third compared with annual screening because of the smaller number of mammograms performed.[85,120]

> On average, an individual woman aged 40 to 49 who undergoes annual screening mammography will experience 1 false-positive mammogram every 10 years.

Although false-positive mammograms are a downside to screening, most women recalled from screening mammography require only additional imaging. Women are willing to tolerate far higher false-positive rates than actually occur in clinical practice, suggesting that the "harm" of false positives may be overemphasized.[121]

Overdiagnosis

Overdiagnosis is defined as a diagnosis by screening of a cancer that never would have become symptomatic in the woman's lifetime or never would have been detected if screening had not taken place. The conversation regarding overdiagnosis largely pertains to DCIS, as nonprogressive invasive disease has not to our knowledge been documented in the peer-reviewed literature. Overdiagnosis and overtreatment of DCIS remain controversial; however, detection and treatment of DCIS has been shown to decrease subsequent invasive malignancies. A recent study of more than 5 million women who underwent screening mammography demonstrated that for every 3 screen-detected cases of DCIS, there was 1 fewer invasive interval breast cancer in the subsequent 3 years.[122]

The USPSTF acknowledged that "methods for estimating overdiagnosis at a population level are not well established" and because of the "lack of consensus concerning the optimal method for calculating the magnitude of overdiagnosis," the USPSTF acknowledged a very wide range of estimates in the available literature (0% to 54%) but emphasized an estimate of approximately 20%.[77,123] In studies with adequate adjustment for confounders and baseline incremental increase in breast cancer incidence, the frequency of overdiagnosis is estimated at 1% to 10%.[124] Regardless of the frequency of overdiagnosis, an "overdiagnosed" cancer will persist on imaging regardless of screening interval or age at initial screening. Decreasing the screening frequency and delaying onset of screening (from 40 to 45 or 50) will delay the timing of overdiagnosis but will not decrease the degree of overdiagnosis. Therefore, overdiagnosis should not be used to determine when to start screening or how often to screen.

> Decreasing screening frequency or delaying onset of screening (from age 40 to later) will not decrease the degree of overdiagnosis.

Radiation Risk

The 2016 USPSTF recommendations state that "...radiation-induced breast cancer and resulting death can also occur, although the number of both of these events is predicted to be low."[77] At most, 2 to 11 deaths due to radiation-induced cancer may occur per 100,000 women screened[125] and additional publications estimate the risk of a fatal radiation-induced breast cancer due to screening mammography for a woman in her forties is 1 in 76,000 to 97,000 and too large to estimate for a women in her eighties.[117]

False-Negative Mammograms and "False Reassurance"

Mammograms do not detect all breast cancers and should not be used to tell a woman that she does not have breast cancer. The probability of a missed breast cancer increases with age, averaging once every 667 years for a woman older than 70 and once every 1000 years for a woman aged 40 to 49.[117]

Decreased Breast Cancer Mortality: Is It Secondary to Screening or Improved Treatment?

The incidence of breast cancer has been steadily increasing in the United States, with an annual percent change of 0.8% to 2.3% per year with similar increases observed in other countries.[126] However, between 1990 and 2000, breast cancer mortality in women decreased 24% in the United States (see **Fig. 1**). The decrease in breast cancer mortality despite increasing incidence is attributable to a combination of screening mammography and improved treatment options.[127] American men, who presumably have access to similar treatment regimens as women but do not have access to screening mammography, had a breast cancer mortality in 2013 which is identical to 1990.[2] In Sweden, women aged 40 to 69 who underwent screening experienced a 44% reduction in breast cancer mortality, compared with only a 16% mortality reduction in women ages 40 to 69 not exposed to screening and a 27% mortality reduction in women ages 20 to 39 who were not offered screening.[128] Improved treatment alone does not account for the dramatic decrease in breast cancer mortality.

Does Screening Decrease the Incidence of Late-Stage Breast Cancer?

Recall that breast cancer incidence had been increasing in the United States, with an annual percentage change (APC) of 0.8% to 2.3%.[126] An APC *estimate* of 1.3% for women older than 40 coincides with the 40-year APC of 1.2% *actually observed* in the Connecticut Tumor Registry. Assuming an APC of 1.3%, the incidence of late-stage breast cancer decreased 37% in 2007 to 2009 compared with 1977 to 1979 with a concomitant increase in early-stage breast cancers.[126] Publications that claim that screening mammography has not resulted in decreased late-stage cancers have consistently failed to account for the underlying interval increase in breast cancer incidence.[129,130]

SUMMARY

The ACS, ACR, and the USPSTF, as well as every medical professional organization, to our knowledge, agree that screening mammography significantly decreases breast cancer mortality. Although screening mammography is covered as a preventive care benefit without cost sharing under the Patient Protection and Affordable Care Act, nearly one-third of US women older than 40 are not receiving regular screening mammograms. In 2013, fewer than 66% of women older than 40 in the United States had a screening mammogram in the preceding 2 years, compared with fewer than 69% of women older than 50.[131] The lack of a national consensus on screening frequency and age to begin screening may contribute to the low compliance. After reviewing this article, clinicians should feel empowered to engage women in informed discussions regarding the pros and cons of regular screening mammography, as well as supplemental screening in high-risk women. By educating our patients on the importance of breast cancer screening and early detection, we can continue to decrease the number of lives unnecessarily lost to breast cancer each year.

> Screening mammography is underused, resulting in unnecessary breast cancer deaths.

REFERENCES

1. American Cancer Society. Cancer facts and figures 2017. Atlanta (GA): American Cancer Society; 2017.
2. Howlader N, Noone AM, Krapcho M, et al, editors. SEER cancer statistics review, 1975-2013. Bethesda (MD): National Cancer Institute; 2016. Available at: http://seer.cancer.gov/csr/1975_2013/. based on November 2015 SEER data submission, posted to the SEER web site.
3. Smith RA, Duffy SW, Gabe R, et al. The randomized trials of breast cancer screening: what have we learned? Radiol Clin North Am 2004;42(5):793–806, v.
4. Tabar L, Yen AM, Wu WY, et al. Insights from the breast cancer screening trials: how screening affects the natural history of breast cancer and

implications for evaluating service screening programs. Breast J 2015;21(1):13–20.

5. Oeffinger KC, Fontham ET, Etzioni R, et al. Breast cancer screening for women at average risk: 2015 guideline update from the American Cancer Society. JAMA 2015;314(15):1599–614.

6. Shapiro S, Strax P, Venet L. Periodic breast cancer screening in reducing mortality from breast cancer. JAMA 1971;215(11):1777–85.

7. Shapiro S, Venet W, Strax P, et al. Periodic screening for breast cancer: the Health Insurance Plan project and its sequelae, 1963–1986. Baltimore (MD): Johns Hopkins University Press; 1988.

8. Shapiro S. Periodic screening for breast cancer: the HIP randomized controlled trial. Health insurance plan. J Natl Cancer Inst Monogr 1997;(22): 27–30.

9. Tabar L, Fagerberg CJ, Gad A, et al. Reduction in mortality from breast cancer after mass screening with mammography. Randomised trial from the Breast Cancer Screening Working Group of the Swedish National Board of Health and Welfare. Lancet 1985;1(8433):829–32.

10. Tabar L, Vitak B, Chen TH, et al. Swedish two-county trial: impact of mammographic screening on breast cancer mortality during 3 decades. Radiology 2011;260(3):658–63.

11. Nystrom L, Andersson I, Bjurstam N, et al. Long-term effects of mammography screening: updated overview of the Swedish randomised trials. Lancet 2002;359(9310):909–19.

12. Roberts MM, Alexander FE, Anderson TJ, et al. Edinburgh trial of screening for breast cancer: mortality at seven years. Lancet 1990;335(8684):241–6.

13. Alexander FE, Anderson TJ, Brown HK, et al. 14 years of follow-up from the Edinburgh randomised trial of breast-cancer screening. Lancet 1999; 353(9168):1903–8.

14. Frisell J, Lidbrink E, Hellstrom L, et al. Followup after 11 years–update of mortality results in the Stockholm mammographic screening trial. Breast Cancer Res Treat 1997;45(3):263–70.

15. Miller AB, Baines CJ, To T, et al. Canadian National Breast Screening Study: 2. Breast cancer detection and death rates among women aged 50 to 59 years. CMAJ 1992;147(10):1477–88.

16. Miller AB, Baines CJ, To T, et al. Canadian National Breast Screening Study: 1. Breast cancer detection and death rates among women aged 40 to 49 years. CMAJ 1992;147(10):1459–76.

17. Miller AB, Wall C, Baines CJ, et al. Twenty five year follow-up for breast cancer incidence and mortality of the Canadian National Breast Screening Study: randomised screening trial. BMJ 2014;348:g366.

18. Kopans DB, Feig SA. The Canadian National Breast Screening Study: a critical review. AJR Am J Roentgenol 1993;161(4):755–60.

19. Baines CJ, McFarlane DV, Miller AB. The role of the reference radiologist. Estimates of inter-observer agreement and potential delay in cancer detection in the national breast screening study. Invest Radiol 1990;25(9):971–6.

20. Bjurstam N, Bjorneld L, Duffy SW, et al. The Gothenburg Breast Cancer Screening Trial: preliminary results on breast cancer mortality for women aged 39-49. J Natl Cancer Inst Monogr 1997;(22):53–5.

21. Bjurstam N, Bjorneld L, Warwick J, et al. The Gothenburg Breast Screening Trial. Cancer 2003; 97(10):2387–96.

22. Broeders M, Moss S, Nystrom L, et al. The impact of mammographic screening on breast cancer mortality in Europe: a review of observational studies. J Med Screen 2012;19(Suppl 1):14–25.

23. Coldman A, Phillips N, Wilson C, et al. Pan-Canadian study of mammography screening and mortality from breast cancer. J Natl Cancer Inst 2014; 106(11) [pii:dju261].

24. Nickson C, Mason KE, English DR, et al. Mammographic screening and breast cancer mortality: a case-control study and meta-analysis. Cancer Epidemiol Biomarkers Prev 2012;21(9):1479–88.

25. Lee CS, Bhargavan-Chatfield M, Burnside ES, et al. The national mammography database: preliminary data. AJR Am J Roentgenol 2016;206(4):883–90.

26. Miglioretti DL, Ichikawa L, Smith RA, et al. Criteria for identifying radiologists with acceptable screening mammography interpretive performance on basis of multiple performance measures. AJR Am J Roentgenol 2015;204(4):W486–91.

27. D'Orsi CJ, Sickles EA, Mendelson EB, et al. ACR BI-RADS® Atlas, breast imaging reporting and data system. 5th edition. Reston (VA): American College of Radiology; 2013.

28. Carney PA, Miglioretti DL, Yankaskas BC, et al. Individual and combined effects of age, breast density, and hormone replacement therapy use on the accuracy of screening mammography. Ann Intern Med 2003;138(3):168–75.

29. van der Waal D, Ripping TM, Verbeek AL, et al. Breast cancer screening effect across breast density strata: a case-control study. Int J Cancer 2017; 140(1):41–9.

30. Mandelson MT, Oestreicher N, Porter PL, et al. Breast density as a predictor of mammographic detection: comparison of interval- and screen-detected cancers. J Natl Cancer Inst 2000;92(13):1081–7.

31. Wang AT, Vachon CM, Brandt KR, et al. Breast density and breast cancer risk: a practical review. Mayo Clin Proc 2014;89(4):548–57.

32. Kolb TM, Lichy J, Newhouse JH. Comparison of the performance of screening mammography, physical examination, and breast US and evaluation of factors that influence them: an analysis of 27,825 patient evaluations. Radiology 2002;225(1):165–75.

33. Brem RF, Lenihan MJ, Lieberman J, et al. Screening breast ultrasound: past, present, and future. AJR Am J Roentgenol 2015;204(2):234–40.

34. Niklason LT, Christian BT, Niklason LE, et al. Digital tomosynthesis in breast imaging. Radiology 1997; 205(2):399–406.

35. Skaane P, Bandos AI, Gullien R, et al. Comparison of digital mammography alone and digital mammography plus tomosynthesis in a population-based screening program. Radiology 2013;267(1):47–56.

36. Ciatto S, Houssami N, Bernardi D, et al. Integration of 3D digital mammography with tomosynthesis for population breast-cancer screening (STORM): a prospective comparison study. Lancet Oncol 2013;14(7):583–9.

37. Friedewald SM, Rafferty EA, Conant EF. Breast cancer screening with tomosynthesis and digital mammography-reply. JAMA 2014;312(16):1695–6.

38. Zuley ML, Guo B, Catullo VJ, et al. Comparison of two-dimensional synthesized mammograms versus original digital mammograms alone and in combination with tomosynthesis images. Radiology 2014;271(3):664–71.

39. Tagliafico AS, Bignotti B, Rossi F, et al. Diagnostic performance of contrast-enhanced spectral mammography: systematic review and meta-analysis. Breast 2016;28:13–9.

40. Lapayowker MS, Revesz G. Thermography and ultrasound in detection and diagnosis of breast cancer. Cancer 1980;46(4 Suppl):933–8.

41. Sickles EA, Filly RA, Callen PW. Breast cancer detection with sonography and mammography: comparison using state-of-the-art equipment. AJR Am J Roentgenol 1983;140(5):843–5.

42. Berg WA, Blume JD, Cormack JB, et al. Combined screening with ultrasound and mammography vs mammography alone in women at elevated risk of breast cancer. JAMA 2008; 299(18):2151–63.

43. Berg WA, Zhang Z, Lehrer D, et al. Detection of breast cancer with addition of annual screening ultrasound or a single screening MRI to mammography in women with elevated breast cancer risk. JAMA 2012;307(13):1394–404.

44. Hooley RJ, Greenberg KL, Stackhouse RM, et al. Screening US in patients with mammographically dense breasts: initial experience with Connecticut Public Act 09-41. Radiology 2012;265(1):59–69.

45. Weigert J, Steenbergen S. The Connecticut experiment: the role of ultrasound in the screening of women with dense breasts. Breast J 2012;18(6): 517–22.

46. Weigert J, Steenbergen S. The Connecticut experiments second year: ultrasound in the screening of women with dense breasts. Breast J 2015;21(2): 175–80.

47. Melnikow J, Fenton JJ, Whitlock EP, et al. Supplemental screening for breast cancer in women with dense breasts: a systematic review for the U.S. Preventive Services Task Force. Ann Intern Med 2016;164(4):268–78.

48. Ohuchi N, Suzuki A, Sobue T, et al. Sensitivity and specificity of mammography and adjunctive ultrasonography to screen for breast cancer in the Japan Strategic Anti-cancer Randomized Trial (J-START): a randomised controlled trial. Lancet 2016;387(10016):341–8.

49. Tagliafico AS, Calabrese M, Mariscotti G, et al. Adjunct screening with tomosynthesis or ultrasound in women with mammography-negative dense breasts: interim report of a prospective comparative trial. J Clin Oncol 2016;34:1882–8.

50. Kelly KM, Dean J, Comulada WS, et al. Breast cancer detection using automated whole breast ultrasound and mammography in radiographically dense breasts. Eur Radiol 2010;20(3):734–42.

51. Skaane P, Gullien R, Eben EB, et al. Interpretation of automated breast ultrasound (ABUS) with and without knowledge of mammography: a reader performance study. Acta Radiol 2015;56(4):404–12.

52. Kuhl C, Weigel S, Schrading S, et al. Prospective multicenter cohort study to refine management recommendations for women at elevated familial risk of breast cancer: the EVA trial. J Clin Oncol 2010; 28(9):1450–7.

53. Lehman CD. Role of MRI in screening women at high risk for breast cancer. J Magn Reson Imaging 2006;24(5):964–70.

54. Sardanelli F, Podo F, Santoro F, et al. Multicenter surveillance of women at high genetic breast cancer risk using mammography, ultrasonography, and contrast-enhanced magnetic resonance imaging (the high breast cancer risk Italian 1 study): final results. Invest Radiol 2011;46(2):94–105.

55. Kuhl CK, Schrading S, Bieling HB, et al. MRI for diagnosis of pure ductal carcinoma in situ: a prospective observational study. Lancet 2007; 370(9586):485–92.

56. Riedl CC, Luft N, Bernhart C, et al. Triple-modality screening trial for familial breast cancer underlines the importance of magnetic resonance imaging and questions the role of mammography and ultrasound regardless of patient mutation status, age, and breast density. J Clin Oncol 2015;33(10): 1128–35.

57. Lehman CD, Gatsonis C, Kuhl CK, et al. MRI evaluation of the contralateral breast in women with recently diagnosed breast cancer. N Engl J Med 2007;356(13):1295–303.

58. Stout NK, Nekhlyudov L, Li L, et al. Rapid increase in breast magnetic resonance imaging use: trends from 2000 to 2011. JAMA Intern Med 2014;174(1): 114–21.

59. Warner E, Messersmith H, Causer P, et al. Systematic review: using magnetic resonance imaging to screen women at high risk for breast cancer. Ann Intern Med 2008;148(9):671–9.

60. Saadatmand S, Tilanus-Linthorst MM, Rutgers EJ, et al. Cost-effectiveness of screening women with familial risk for breast cancer with magnetic resonance imaging. J Natl Cancer Inst 2013;105(17): 1314–21.

61. Kuhl CK, Schrading S, Strobel K, et al. Abbreviated breast magnetic resonance imaging (MRI): first postcontrast subtracted images and maximum-intensity projection—a novel approach to breast cancer screening with MRI. J Clin Oncol 2014; 32(22):2304–10.

62. Avril N, Adler LP. F-18 fluorodeoxyglucose-positron emission tomography imaging for primary breast cancer and loco-regional staging. Radiol Clin North Am 2007;45(4):645–57, vi.

63. Berg WA, Madsen KS, Schilling K, et al. Comparative effectiveness of positron emission mammography and MRI in the contralateral breast of women with newly diagnosed breast cancer. AJR Am J Roentgenol 2012;198(1):219–32.

64. Berg WA, Weinberg IN, Narayanan D, et al. High-resolution fluorodeoxyglucose positron emission tomography with compression ("positron emission mammography") is highly accurate in depicting primary breast cancer. Breast J 2006;12(4): 309–23.

65. Hendrick RE. Radiation doses and cancer risks from breast imaging studies. Radiology 2010; 257(1):246–53.

66. Narayanan D, Madsen KS, Kalinyak JE, et al. Interpretation of positron emission mammography and MRI by experienced breast imaging radiologists: performance and observer reproducibility. AJR Am J Roentgenol 2011;196(4):971–81.

67. Yamamoto Y, Tasaki Y, Kuwada Y, et al. A preliminary report of breast cancer screening by positron emission mammography. Ann Nucl Med 2016;30(2):130–7.

68. Holbrook A, Newel MS. Alternative screening for women with dense breasts: breast-specific gamma imaging (molecular breast imaging). AJR Am J Roentgenol 2015;204(2):252–6.

69. Brem RF, Floerke AC, Rapelyea JA, et al. Breast-specific gamma imaging as an adjunct imaging modality for the diagnosis of breast cancer. Radiology 2008;247(3):651–7.

70. Weigert JM, Bertrand ML, Lanzkowsky L, et al. Results of a multicenter patient registry to determine the clinical impact of breast-specific gamma imaging, a molecular breast imaging technique. AJR Am J Roentgenol 2012;198(1):W69–75.

71. Rechtman LR, Lenihan MJ, Lieberman JH, et al. Breast-specific gamma imaging for the detection of breast cancer in dense versus nondense breasts. AJR Am J Roentgenol 2014;202(2):293–8.

72. Tadwalkar RV, Rapelyea JA, Torrente J, et al. Breast-specific gamma imaging as an adjunct modality for the diagnosis of invasive breast cancer with correlation to tumour size and grade. Br J Radiol 2012;85(1014):e212–6.

73. Hendrick RE, Tredennick T. Benefit to radiation risk of breast-specific gamma imaging compared with mammography in screening asymptomatic women with dense breasts. Radiology 2016; 281(2):583–8.

74. Isard HJ, Becker W, Shilo R, et al. Breast thermography after four years and 10000 studies. Am J Roentgenol Radium Ther Nucl Med 1972;115(4):811–21.

75. Williams KL, Phillips BH, Jones PA, et al. Thermography in screening for breast cancer. J Epidemiol Community Health 1990;44(2):112–3.

76. Mainiero MB, Lourenco A, Mahoney MC, et al. ACR appropriateness criteria breast cancer screening. J Am Coll Radiol 2013;10(1):11–4.

77. Siu AL, U.S. Preventive Services Task Force. Screening for breast cancer: U.S. Preventive Services Task Force Recommendation Statement. Ann Intern Med 2016;164(4):279–96.

78. Lee CH, Dershaw DD, Kopans D, et al. Breast cancer screening with imaging: recommendations from the Society of Breast Imaging and the ACR on the use of mammography, breast MRI, breast ultrasound, and other technologies for the detection of clinically occult breast cancer. J Am Coll Radiol 2010;7(1):18–27.

79. The Henry J. Kaiser Family Foundation. Preventive services covered by private health plans under the Affordable Care Act. 2015. Available at: http://kff.org. Accessed September 28, 2016.

80. Congress t. H.R.3339-protecting access to lifesaving screenings act (PALS Act). Available at: https://www.congress.gov/bill/114th-congress/house-bill/3339. Accessed September 28, 2016.

81. National Comprehensive Cancer Network Breast Cancer Screening and Diagnosis. NCCN Clinical Practice Guidelines in Oncology (NCCN Guidelines). Version 1.2016, 2016. Available at: https://www.nccn.org/professionals/physician_gls/pdf/breast-screening.pdf. Accessed December 13, 2016.

82. ACOG Statement on Breast Cancer Screening Guidelines. 2016. Available at: http://www.acog.org/About-ACOG/News-Room/Statements/2016/ACOG-Statement-on-Breast-Cancer-Screening-Guidelines. Accessed December 16, 2016.

83. American Academy of Family Physicians. Clinical preventive service recommendation. 2016. http://www.aafp.org/patient-care/clinical-recommendations/all/breast-cancer.html. Accessed December 19, 2016.

84. Wilt TJ, Harris RP, Qaseem A, High Value Care Task Force of the American College of Physicians. Screening for cancer: advice for high-value care from the American College of Physicians. Ann Intern Med 2015;162(10):718–25.

85. Kerlikowske K, Zhu W, Hubbard RA, et al. Outcomes of screening mammography by frequency, breast density, and postmenopausal hormone therapy. JAMA Intern Med 2013;173(9):807–16.

86. Sprague BL, Conant EF, Onega T, et al. Variation in mammographic breast density assessments among radiologists in clinical practice: a multicenter observational study. Ann Intern Med 2016; 165(7):457–64.

87. Sickles EA. The use of breast imaging to screen women at high risk for cancer. Radiol Clin North Am 2010;48(5):859–78.

88. Boyd NF, Guo H, Martin LJ, et al. Mammographic density and the risk and detection of breast cancer. N Engl J Med 2007;356(3):227–36.

89. Tice JA, Ollendorf DA, Lee JM, et al. The comparative clinical effectiveness and value of supplemental screening tests following negative mammography in women with dense breast tissue. Comparative Effectiveness Public Advisory Council web site. 2013. Available at: https://icer-review.org/wp-content/uploads/2016/02/CEPAC-Supplemental-Screening-for-Breast-Cancer-11-08-13.pdf. Accessed December 16, 2016.

90. Sprague BL, Stout NK, Schechter C, et al. Benefits, harms, and cost-effectiveness of supplemental ultrasonography screening for women with dense breasts. Ann Intern Med 2015;162(3):157–66.

91. Imaging ACoRCoPPB. ACR Practice Parameter for the performance of a breast ultrasound examination. 2016. Available at: https://www.acr.org/~/media/52D58307E93E45898B09D4C4D407DD76.pdf. Accessed January 19, 2017.

92. Rafferty EA, Durand MA, Conant EF, et al. Breast cancer screening using tomosynthesis and digital mammography in dense and nondense breasts. JAMA 2016;315(16):1784–6.

93. Price ER, Keedy AW, Gidwaney R, et al. The potential impact of risk-based screening mammography in women 40-49 years old. AJR Am J Roentgenol 2015;205(6):1360–4.

94. Wisdom study website. Available at: https://wisdom.secure.force.com/portal/. Accessed December 16, 2016.

95. Saslow D, Boetes C, Burke W, et al. American Cancer Society Guidelines for breast screening with MRI as an adjunct to mammography. CA Cancer J Clin 2007;57(2):75–89.

96. Brennan S, Liberman L, Dershaw DD, et al. Breast MRI screening of women with a personal history of breast cancer. AJR Am J Roentgenol 2010;195(2):510–6.

97. Friedlander LC, Roth SO, Gavenonis SC. Results of MR imaging screening for breast cancer in high-risk patients with lobular carcinoma in situ. Radiology 2011;261(2):421–7.

98. Giess CS, Poole PS, Chikarmane SA, et al. Screening breast MRI in patients previously treated for breast cancer: diagnostic yield for cancer and abnormal interpretation rate. Acad Radiol 2015; 22(11):1331–7.

99. King TA, Muhsen S, Patil S, et al. Is there a role for routine screening MRI in women with LCIS? Breast Cancer Res Treat 2013;142(2):445–53.

100. Lehman CD, Lee JM, DeMartini WB, et al. Screening MRI in women with a personal history of breast cancer. J Natl Cancer Inst 2016;108(3) [pii:djv349].

101. Port ER, Park A, Borgen PI, et al. Results of MRI screening for breast cancer in high-risk patients with LCIS and atypical hyperplasia. Ann Surg Oncol 2007;14(3):1051–7.

102. Schacht DV, Yamaguchi K, Lai J, et al. Importance of a personal history of breast cancer as a risk factor for the development of subsequent breast cancer: results from screening breast MRI. AJR Am J Roentgenol 2014;202(2):289–92.

103. Schwartz T, Cyr A, Margenthaler J. Screening breast magnetic resonance imaging in women with atypia or lobular carcinoma in situ. J Surg Res 2015;193(2):519–22.

104. Sung JS, Malak SF, Bajaj P, et al. Screening breast MR imaging in women with a history of lobular carcinoma in situ. Radiology 2011;261(2):414–20.

105. Amir E, Freedman OC, Seruga B, et al. Assessing women at high risk of breast cancer: a review of risk assessment models. J Natl Cancer Inst 2010; 102(10):680–91.

106. Smith RA, Cokkinides V, Brawley OW. Cancer screening in the United States, 2012: a review of current American Cancer Society guidelines and current issues in cancer screening. CA Cancer J Clin 2012;62(2):129–42.

107. Berg WA, Bandos AI, Mendelson EB, et al. Ultrasound as the primary screening test for breast cancer: analysis from ACRIN 6666. J Natl Cancer Inst 2015;108(4) [pii:djv367].

108. Maibenco D, Daoud Y, Phillips E, et al. Relationship between method of detection of breast cancer and stage of disease, method of treatment, and survival in women aged 40 to 49 years. Am Surg 1999; 65(11):1061–6.

109. Barth RJ Jr, Gibson GR, Carney PA, et al. Detection of breast cancer on screening mammography allows patients to be treated with less-toxic therapy. AJR Am J Roentgenol 2005;184(1):324–9.

110. Aerts L, Christiaens MR, Enzlin P, et al. Sexual functioning in women after mastectomy versus breast

conserving therapy for early-stage breast cancer: a prospective controlled study. Breast 2014;23(5):629–36.

111. Collins KK, Liu Y, Schootman M, et al. Effects of breast cancer surgery and surgical side effects on body image over time. Breast Cancer Res Treat 2011;126(1):167–76.

112. Crosbie J, Kilbreath SL, Dylke E, et al. Effects of mastectomy on shoulder and spinal kinematics during bilateral upper-limb movement. Phys Ther 2010;90(5):679–92.

113. Hayes SC, Johansson K, Stout NL, et al. Upper-body morbidity after breast cancer: incidence and evidence for evaluation, prevention, and management within a prospective surveillance model of care. Cancer 2012;118(8 Suppl):2237–49.

114. Ewertz M, Jensen AB. Late effects of breast cancer treatment and potentials for rehabilitation. Acta Oncol 2011;50(2):187–93.

115. Kaplan HG, Malmgren JA, Atwood MK. Increased incidence of myelodysplastic syndrome and acute myeloid leukemia following breast cancer treatment with radiation alone or combined with chemotherapy: a registry cohort analysis 1990-2005. BMC Cancer 2011;11:260.

116. Hughes KS, Schnaper LA, Bellon JR, et al. Lumpectomy plus tamoxifen with or without irradiation in women age 70 years or older with early breast cancer: long-term follow-up of CALGB 9343. J Clin Oncol 2013;31(19):2382–7.

117. Hendrick RE, Helvie MA. United States Preventive Services Task Force screening mammography recommendations: science ignored. AJR Am J Roentgenol 2011;196(2):W112–6.

118. Miglioretti DL, Zhu W, Kerlikowske K, et al. Breast tumor prognostic characteristics and biennial vs annual mammography, age, and menopausal status. JAMA Oncol 2015;1(8):1069–77.

119. Hendrick RE, Smith RA, Rutledge JH 3rd, et al. Benefit of screening mammography in women aged 40-49: a new meta-analysis of randomized controlled trials. J Natl Cancer Inst Monogr 1997;(22):87–92.

120. Hubbard RA, Kerlikowske K, Flowers CI, et al. Cumulative probability of false-positive recall or biopsy recommendation after 10 years of screening mammography: a cohort study. Ann Intern Med 2011;155(8):481–92.

121. Schwartz LM, Woloshin S, Sox HC, et al. US women's attitudes to false positive mammography results and detection of ductal carcinoma in situ: cross sectional survey. BMJ 2000;320(7250):1635–40.

122. Duffy SW, Dibden A, Michalopoulos D, et al. Screen detection of ductal carcinoma in situ and subsequent incidence of invasive interval breast cancers: a retrospective population-based study. Lancet Oncol 2016;17(1):109–14.

123. Nelson HD, Fu R, Cantor A, et al. Effectiveness of breast cancer screening: systematic review and meta-analysis to update the 2009 U.S. Preventive Services Task Force Recommendation. Ann Intern Med 2016;164(4):244–55.

124. Puliti D, Duffy SW, Miccinesi G, et al. Overdiagnosis in mammographic screening for breast cancer in Europe: a literature review. J Med Screen 2012;19(Suppl 1):42–56.

125. Nelson HD, Pappas M, Cantor A, et al. Harms of breast cancer screening: systematic review to update the 2009 U.S. Preventive Services Task Force recommendation. Ann Intern Med 2016;164(4):256–67.

126. Helvie MA, Chang JT, Hendrick RE, et al. Reduction in late-stage breast cancer incidence in the mammography era: implications for overdiagnosis of invasive cancer. Cancer 2014;120(17):2649–56.

127. Berry DA, Cronin KA, Plevritis SK, et al. Effect of screening and adjuvant therapy on mortality from breast cancer. N Engl J Med 2005;353(17):1784–92.

128. Tabar L, Yen MF, Vitak B, et al. Mammography service screening and mortality in breast cancer patients: 20-year follow-up before and after introduction of screening. Lancet 2003;361(9367):1405–10.

129. Bleyer A, Welch HG. Effect of three decades of screening mammography on breast-cancer incidence. N Engl J Med 2012;367(21):1998–2005.

130. Welch HG, Prorok PC, O'Malley AJ, et al. Breast-cancer tumor size, overdiagnosis, and mammography screening effectiveness. N Engl J Med 2016;375(15):1438–47.

131. National Center for Health Statistics. Health, United States, 2015: with special feature on racial and ethnic health disparities. Hyattsville (MD); 2016.

Lung Cancer Screening
Why, When, and How?

Florian J. Fintelmann, MD, FRCPC[a],*, Ravi V. Gottumukkala, MD[a],
Shaunagh McDermott, MD[a], Matthew D. Gilman, MD[a], Inga T. Lennes, MD, MPH, MBA[b],
Jo-Anne O. Shepard, MD[a]

KEYWORDS

• Screening • Lung cancer screening • Low-dose computed tomography • Lung-RADS

KEY POINTS

• Lung cancer screening with low-dose chest computed tomography (CT) is a public health recommendation.
• Eligibility criteria differ slightly between the Centers for Medicare and Medicaid Services (CMS) and private insurance companies.
• Lung cancer screening with low-dose chest CT is not simply a test but is a process that requires a structured approach and a multidisciplinary team.
• Findings on low-dose chest CT obtained for lung cancer screening are managed according to Lung-RADS (Lung Computed Tomography Screening Reporting and Data System), not Fleischner Society guidelines, because patients eligible for screening are at increased risk for lung cancer and have agreed to annual low-dose CT of the chest.
• Reimbursement for lung cancer screening services is contingent on meeting specifications in the 2015 CMS decision memo (for Medicare patients) and the 2013 United States Preventive Services Task Force recommendation statement (for private insurance companies).

INTRODUCTION

Lung cancer is the second most common malignancy in both men and women and about 222,500 new cases are expected in the United States in 2017.[1] Lung cancer accounts for more deaths than any other cancer in men and women, resulting in about 1 in 4 cancer deaths, with an estimated total of 155,870 deaths in the United States in 2017.[1] If diagnosed after symptoms occur, lung cancer has often spread to regional or distant sites, resulting in 5-year survival rates of only 28% and 4%, respectively.[2] Because lung cancer is curable if detected at an early stage and high-risk individuals can be identified, screening provides a reasonable approach to reduce deaths from lung cancer.

IMAGING TECHNIQUE

In 2011, the publication of the National Lung Screening Trial (NLST) established low-dose computed tomography (LDCT) of the chest as an effective lung cancer screening (LCS) tool. To date, the NLST is the largest randomized, prospective, multicenter LCS trial.[3] A total of 53,454 high-risk patients underwent 3 rounds of annual screening for lung cancer with either LDCT of the chest or conventional chest radiography (CXR) at 33 medical centers in the United States.[4] LDCT was defined as having an average whole-body effective dose of 1.5 mSv, about one-fifth that of a routine chest computed tomography (CT) scan.[3] The primary outcome was lung cancer

Disclosures: None of the authors have relevant conflicts of interests or funding sources to disclose.
[a] Thoracic Imaging and Intervention, Department of Radiology, Massachusetts General Hospital, 55 Fruit Street, Boston, MA 02114, USA; [b] Massachusetts General Hospital Cancer Center, 55 Fruit Street, Boston, MA 02114, USA
* Corresponding author.
E-mail address: fintelmann@mgh.harvard.edu

Radiol Clin N Am 55 (2017) 1163–1181
http://dx.doi.org/10.1016/j.rcl.2017.06.003

mortality, which was compared between the 2 arms of the trial. Secondary outcomes included incidence of lung cancer and causes of death other than lung cancer. A total of 1060 lung cancers were diagnosed in the CT group compared with 941 in the CXR group. There were nearly twice as many early-stage lung cancers (stage IA) detected in the LDCT group (40%) compared with the CXR group (21%). Among participants who underwent at least 1 screening test, there were 356 lung cancer deaths in the LDCT group compared with 442 deaths in the CXR group. This finding corresponds with rates of death from lung cancer of 247 and 309 deaths per 100,000 person-years in the LDCT and CXR groups, respectively, and translates into a 20% (95% confidence interval, 6.8–26.7; $P = .004$) relative reduction of lung cancer–specific mortality because of screening with LDCT. The number needed to screen with LDCT to prevent 1 death from lung cancer was 320. There were 1877 deaths in the LDCT group, compared with 2000 deaths in the CXR group, a 6.7% reduction in the rate of death from any cause caused by LDCT. The rate of lung cancer detection did not diminish between the screening years. However, fewer stage IV lung cancers were observed in the LDCT group than in the CXR group during the second and third screening rounds, which suggests that the diagnosis of earlier-stage cancers reduced the occurrence of later-stage cancers.

The NLST was the first trial to show a reduction of lung cancer–specific mortality caused by LDCT. Several observational studies, such as the Early Lung Cancer Project (ELCAP) and the Mayo Clinic CT study, had previously shown that screening with LDCT could identify early-stage asymptomatic lung cancers.[5,6] However, several randomized prospective trials conducted in Europe had not shown a mortality benefit, likely because the studies were underpowered.

The NLST investigators also reported a major disadvantage of screening with LDCT: a high false-positivity rate. Of participants in the LDCT arm, 39% had at least 1 positive screening result over the course of 3 years but 96% were false-positives.[3] Additional drawbacks included complications of diagnostic procedures, radiation exposure, overdiagnosis, financial costs, and anxiety.[7] With regard to complications from diagnostic procedures such as percutaneous needle biopsy, bronchoscopy, and surgical procedures, there were few major complications related to the work-up of nodules suspicious for lung cancer and a very low rate of complications in lesions that eventually were proved to be benign. The risk of radiation exposure is likely not a disadvantage for high-risk individuals. Data from the NLST models predict approximately 1 cancer death caused by cumulative radiation exposure per 2500 patients screened. Therefore, the benefit in preventing lung cancer deaths considerably outweighs the radiation risk, which, also, only manifests 10 to 20 years later.[8]

PATIENT ELIGIBILITY CRITERIA

Several American medical societies have since recommended LCS with LDCT.[9–12] Although the eligibility criteria vary, it is universally agreed that screening should be discontinued once a person develops a health problem that substantially limits life expectancy or the ability or willingness to undergo treatment (Table 1). The United States Preventive Services Task Force (USPSTF) formally recommended LCS of high-risk patients with LDCT in 2013.[7] As a result, commercial insurers are required to cover LCS for patients meeting the USPSTF eligibility criteria without cost sharing (deductible, copay, or coinsurance) based on a provision in the Patient Protection and Affordable Care Act (PPACA).[13] Individuals insured by the government plan administered by the Centers for Medicare and Medicaid Services (CMS) are eligible for LCS with LDCT as of 2015.[14]

Depending on the payer, reimbursement may depend on the characteristics of patients undergoing screening, a shared decision-making visit, facility infrastructure, the way LCS LDCT is ordered, the image acquisition technique, the qualifications of the interpreting radiologist, structured reporting, and the ability to share outcomes with a national registry. Table 2 summarizes the elements required for reimbursement by private payers (according to USPSTF criteria) and Medicare (CMS criteria). These elements are also emphasized throughout this article.

IMAGING PROTOCOLS

The American College of Radiology (ACR) and the Society of Thoracic Radiology (STR) released a joint practice parameter for the performance and reporting of LCS LDCT.[15] This document recommends equipment specifications and image acquisition parameters (Table 3). LCS LDCT of the chest is to be performed without any contrast material during a single breath hold in full inspiration. The scan should cover an area from the lung apices to the costophrenic angles. Scanners should be helical with at least 16 detector rows and a gantry rotation time of 500 milliseconds or faster. Radiation should not exceed a CT volumetric dose index (CTDIvol) of 3 mGy for a

Table 1
Eligibility criteria for lung cancer screening with low-dose computed tomography

Organization	Age (y)	Smoking History (Pack-years)	Years Since Quitting Smoking	Other
CMS	55–77	≥30	<15	—
USPSTF	55–80	≥30	<15	—
American Association for Thoracic Surgery				
Tier 1	55–79	≥30	—	Additional risk factor[a]
Tier 2	≥50	≥20	—	Lung cancer survivor >5 y
ACCP and ASCO	55–74	≥30	<15	—
American Cancer Society	55–74	≥30	<15	—
National Comprehensive Cancer Network				
Group 1	55–74	≥30	<15	—
Group 2	≥50	≥20	—	At least 1 additional risk factor[b]

Definition: 1 pack-year = having smoked an average of 1 pack of cigarettes per day for 1 year.
Abbreviations: ACCP, American College of Chest Physicians; ASCO, American Society of Clinical Oncology; CMS, Centers for Medicare & Medicaid Services; USPSTF, US Preventive Services Task Force.
[a] Additional risk factors for lung cancer defined by the American Association for Thoracic Surgery include chronic obstructive pulmonary disease, environmental and occupational exposures, any prior cancer or thoracic radiation, and genetic or family history.
[b] Additional risk factors for lung cancer defined by National Comprehensive Cancer Network include cancer history, lung disease history, family history of lung cancer, radon exposure, and occupational exposure.

standard-sized patient (170 cm and 70.3 kg [5′ 7″ and 155 lb]) with appropriate adjustments for smaller and larger patients. Slice thickness should be no more than 2.5 mm. Slice thickness and reconstruction interval up to 1 mm allows for better characterization of small nodules. Maximum intensity projection (MIP) reformats are recommended to increase the sensitivity of pulmonary nodule detection.

Of note, the only element required for CMS reimbursement is a CTDIvol less than or equal to 3 mGy for average-sized patients. Table 4 lists sample protocols that meet the specified requirements. Additional LCS LDCT protocols for 36 different scanners from 6 different manufacturers are available free of charge on the Web site of the American Association of Physicists in Medicine.[16]

FACILITY READINESS

It is important to understand that LCS with LDCT is not simply a test but is a process that requires a structured approach and a multidisciplinary team. It is therefore advantageous to form a lung screening program. In addition to the ACR-STR practice parameter referenced earlier, the American College of Chest Physicians and the American Thoracic Society have also issued statements regarding what they consider best practice for the

implementation of LCS programs in clinical practice.[17,18] Briefly, a team with members from pulmonology, radiology, thoracic surgery, interventional radiology, medical oncology, and radiation oncology is required to run an effective program that ensures that screening is properly performed; results are properly interpreted; and that disease, if detected, is managed appropriately (Table 5). There should be a clearly defined steering committee, departmental champions, and a patient navigator (Fig. 1).[19]

CMS requires that patients complete a shared decision-making visit before initiating the LCS process. Referring providers need to use at least 1 decision support tool and discuss the benefits and harms of screening with their patients, including overdiagnosis, false-positive test results, radiation exposure, importance of adherence to annual screening, impact of comorbidities, and ability and willingness to undergo diagnosis and/or treatment if a lung cancer is detected.[14] Patients should be encouraged during this visit to provide copies of any preexisting outside hospital imaging examinations so that they may be loaded onto the local picture archiving and communication system (PACS) for comparison.

CMS also requires that screening programs provide smoking cessation interventions for current smokers.[14] Smoking cessation has been shown

Table 2
Reimbursement criteria for Medicare and private insurance companies

	Medicare (CMS Coverage Decision Memo)	Private Insurers (USPSTF Guidelines)
Patient Eligibility Criteria		
Age (y)	55–77	55–80
Smoking History	≥30 pack-years of cigarette smoking Either currently smoking or quit within the last 15 y	
Symptoms	Asymptomatic; no symptoms suggestive of lung cancer	
Shared Decision-making Visit	Required: • Office visit with a physician or qualified nonphysician practitioner (physician assistant, nurse practitioner, or clinical nurse specialist) • Use of at least 1 decision aid • Discussion of benefits, harms, follow-up testing and importance of adherence, overdiagnosis, false-positive rate, cumulative radiation exposure, willingness and ability to undergo evaluation and treatment	Recommended
Ordering Information	Required: • Written order • Beneficiary date of birth • Smoking history (in pack-years) • Current smoking status and, if current nonsmoker, number of years since quitting • Statement that the patient does not have signs or symptoms of lung cancer • NPI number of the ordering provider	Not specified
Imaging Facility Criteria	Required: • Volumetric CT dose index ≤3.0 mGy for standard-sized patient, with appropriate reduction for small patients and increase for large patients • Provides smoking cessation interventions • Uses a standardized lung nodule classification and reporting system • Submit data to CMS-approved registry for each LDCT, according to guidelines specified by CMS	• Suggests that LDCT may be more effective in "clinical settings that have high rates of diagnostic accuracy using LDCT, appropriate follow-up protocols for positive results, and clear criteria for doing invasive procedures"[7] • Smoking cessation counseling is recommended
Interpreting Radiologist Criteria	Required: • Training in radiology and radiation safety • Board certified or eligible for board certification by the ABR (or equivalent) • Supervision and interpretation of at least 300 chest CTs in the past 3 y • Compliant with CME according to ACR standards	—

Abbreviations: ABR, American Board of Radiology; ACR, American College of Radiology; CME, continuing medical education; CMS, Centers for Medicare & Medicaid Services; LDCT, low-dose computed tomography; NPI, national provider identifier; USPSTF, United States Preventive Services Task Force.

Adapted from Wiener RS, Gould MK, Arenberg DA, et al. An official American Thoracic Society/American College of Chest Physicians policy statement: implementation of low-dose computed tomography lung cancer screening programs in clinical practice. Am J Respir Crit Care Med 2015;192(7):881–91.

Table 3
Lung cancer screening low-dose chest computed tomography acquisition parameters as per American College of Radiology–Society of Thoracic Radiology 2014 practice parameters

Parameter	Specification	Comments
Scanner type	Multidetector helical (spiral) with ≥16 detector rows	Nonhelical and single-detector scanners are not appropriate for LCS
Contrast	None	No intravenous or oral contrast
Patient instructions	Single breath hold in full inspiration	—
CTDIvol	<3 mGy for a standard-sized patient	CTDIvol should be reduced for smaller-sized patients and increased for larger-sized patients
kV	—	Should be set in combination with mAs to meet CTDIvol specifications
mAs	—	Should be set in combination with kV to meet CTDIvol specifications
Gantry rotation time	≤0.5 s	—
Pitch	—	Should be set with other technical parameters to achieve single-breath-hold scan and CTDIvol specifications
Reconstructed image width (nominal width of reconstructed image along z-axis)	≤2.5 mm	≤1-mm slice thickness and reconstruction interval preferred to allow better characterization of small lung nodules
Reconstructed image spacing (distance between 2 reconstructed images)	≤slice width	Reconstruction intervals equal to or less than the slice thickness
Additional reconstructions	Maximum intensity projection	CT scanner and/or the viewing platform should be capable of generating maximum intensity projection

Abbreviations: CTDIvol, CT volumetric dose index; LCS, lung cancer screening.

to be more beneficial to patients than screening with LDCT because tobacco use remains the major modifiable risk factor for lung cancer and results in a 20-fold relative increase in risk of lung cancer.[20]

Another element required for a successful LCS program is information technology (IT) support. CMS reimbursement depends on documentation of specific data elements each time LCS LDCT is ordered (see **Table 2**). Specifically, orders for CMS beneficiaries must contain beneficiary date of birth; pack-year smoking history (number); current smoking status and, for former smokers, the number of years since smoking cessation; a statement that the beneficiary is asymptomatic (no signs or symptoms of lung cancer); and National Provider Identifier (NPI) of the ordering practitioner. Attestation that a shared decision-making visit has taken place is also required for the initial LCS service. **Fig. 2** shows how IT can facilitate compliance by integrating these elements into a physician order entry system.

CMS reimbursement is also tied to the screening program's ability to share data with a national registry. Specifically, smoking history, radiation dose, and downstream care, including interventions and resulting complications, are some of the elements that are collected. So far the ACR Lung Cancer Screening Registry is the only CMS-approved registry and several vendors have reported being able

Table 4
Sample scanner protocols for low-dose chest computed tomography

	Siemens 128 with SAFIRE	GE 64 with ASIR
Anatomic Coverage	Lung apices through costophrenic sulci	
Patient Instructions	Full inspiration, breath hold	
Mode	Helical	
Rotation Time (s)	0.4	0.4
Collimation (mm)	128 × 0.6	64 × 0.625
Slice Thickness (mm)	3	2.5
Reconstruction Interval (mm)	2	2.5
Pitch	1.1	1.375
Table Speed (mm/s)	38	55
kV	120	120
Algorithm/Kernel	I31f	Detail
Noise and Radiation Dose Reduction Techniques	SAFIRE 3 Care kV off CARE Dose 4D off	ASIR 50%
Fixed mAs (Weight Based)	<90 kg (200 lb): 25 >90 kg (200 lb): 30	≤61 kg (135 lb): 40 62–90 kg (136–200 lb): 60 >90 kg (200 lb): 80
Reformats (Skin to Skin)	Slice Thickness/Interval (mm)	
Axial	1/0.8	1.25/1
Sagittal and Coronal	2/2	2.5/2.5
Axial MIP	5/2.5	5/2.5

Abbreviations: ASIR, adaptive statistical iterative reconstruction; MIP, maximum intensity projection; SAFIRE, sinogram affirmed iterative reconstruction.

to successfully upload data to the registry.[21] In addition to data sharing at the national level, a local database needs to be maintained for real-time tracking of the number of enrolled patients, patient satisfaction, and other outcomes of interest. IT support is required to guarantee that patients are reliably followed over many years. An interface with the radiology information system enables patient navigators to efficiently identify and contact non-compliant patients and providers, and some commercial solutions allow the generation of notification letters. Although patient notification of CT results is not a CMS requirement, it is considered best practice by the ACR.[22]

IMAGING FINDINGS

Images should be reviewed on a PACS workstation with the goal to detect signs of early lung cancer, such as pulmonary nodules, and to identify

Table 5
Lung cancer screening program team members

Hospital Leadership	Referring Providers	Nodule Management Experts	Support Staff
• Management • Finance • Public relations • Human resources	• Primary care providers • Specialists	• Interventional pulmonology • Interventional radiology • Medical oncology • Pulmonology • Radiation oncology • Radiology • Thoracic surgery	• Patient navigator • Smoking cessation • Information technology

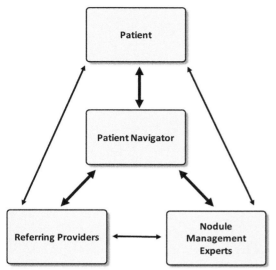

Fig. 1. The central role of the patient navigator in a lung cancer screening program. Arrows indicate flow of information.

potentially significant incidental findings. Nodules should be examined on contiguous thin-cut images (≤1 mm thickness) to determine the nodule morphology because this has implications for the nodule management algorithm. MIP images should be reviewed to increase the sensitivity for nodule detection.[23,24] All nodules need to be compared with the baseline screening examination and any preexisting imaging studies to determine whether they are growing or stable.

List: Pearls for interpretation of lung cancer screening low-dose chest computed tomography

- Examine nodules on contiguous thin-cut images (≤1 mm thickness) to determine the nodule type and ensure that the correct nodule management algorithm is applied
- Review MIP images to increase sensitivity for nodule detection
- Compare all nodules with the baseline screening examination and any preexisting imaging studies

---

The most common differential diagnoses for a solitary noncalcified pulmonary nodule include both benign and malignant causes (**Box 1**).

If available, use of computer-assisted detection (CAD) of nodules and volumetric assessment of nodule volume is encouraged (**Fig. 3**).[15] A recent study found that CAD systems detected up to 70% of lung cancers missed by radiologists. However, CAD systems missed about 20% of cancers

identified by radiologists. Therefore, the most appropriate role, at least for now, is for CAD to be used as a second reader.[25] It is hoped that volumetric nodule measurements and risk calculators will ultimately reduce the need for follow-up imaging and invasive procedures.[26]

A variety of findings other than pulmonary nodules can also be expected on LCS LDCT. Common diagnoses include emphysema, bronchitis, infection, bronchiectasis, and sometimes pulmonary fibrosis (**Box 2**).

DIAGNOSTIC CRITERIA

The diagnostic criteria for LCS LDCT are provided by the Lung CT Screening Reporting and Data System (Lung-RADS) Version 1.0 (**Fig. 4**). The ACR developed this clinical decision-orientated reporting system in order to standardize LCS LDCT reporting and management recommendations, reduce confusion in LCS CT interpretation, and facilitate outcome monitoring.[27] Lung-RADS differs from Fleischner Society guidelines because screened patients are at increased risk for lung cancer and have agreed to return for annual chest CT. Contrary to the NLST investigators, Lung-RADS triages nodules on LCS LDCT based on morphology (solid, nonsolid, or subsolid) in addition to size.

Morphology is classified as solid, part solid, and nonsolid. A solid nodule has homogeneous soft tissue attenuation. A nonsolid (ground-glass) nodule manifests as hazy increased attenuation in the lung that does not obliterate the bronchial and vascular margins. A part-solid nodule consists of both ground-glass and solid soft tissue attenuation components. Size corresponds to the average diameter rounded to the nearest whole number as measured on lung windows. Increase in size by at least 1.5 mm on serial examinations is proof of growth as per Lung-RADS criteria. The management recommendations for a particular nodule (nodule care pathway) are determined by the morphology and size (see **Fig. 4**). Other than in a table, Lung-RADS care pathways can also be visualized as flowcharts.[28]

Category 0 corresponds to incomplete information caused by suboptimal technique or missing prior examinations. Category 1 corresponds to definitely benign nodules, such as calcified granulomas (**Fig. 5**) and hamartomas (**Fig. 6**), or no nodules. The management recommendation is to continue annual screening with LDCT in 12 months. Category 2 nodules have a very low likelihood of becoming a clinically active cancer because of size or lack of growth and should undergo annual screening with LDCT in 12 months (**Fig. 7**). Category 3 nodules are probably benign and include nodules with a low (1-2%) likelihood

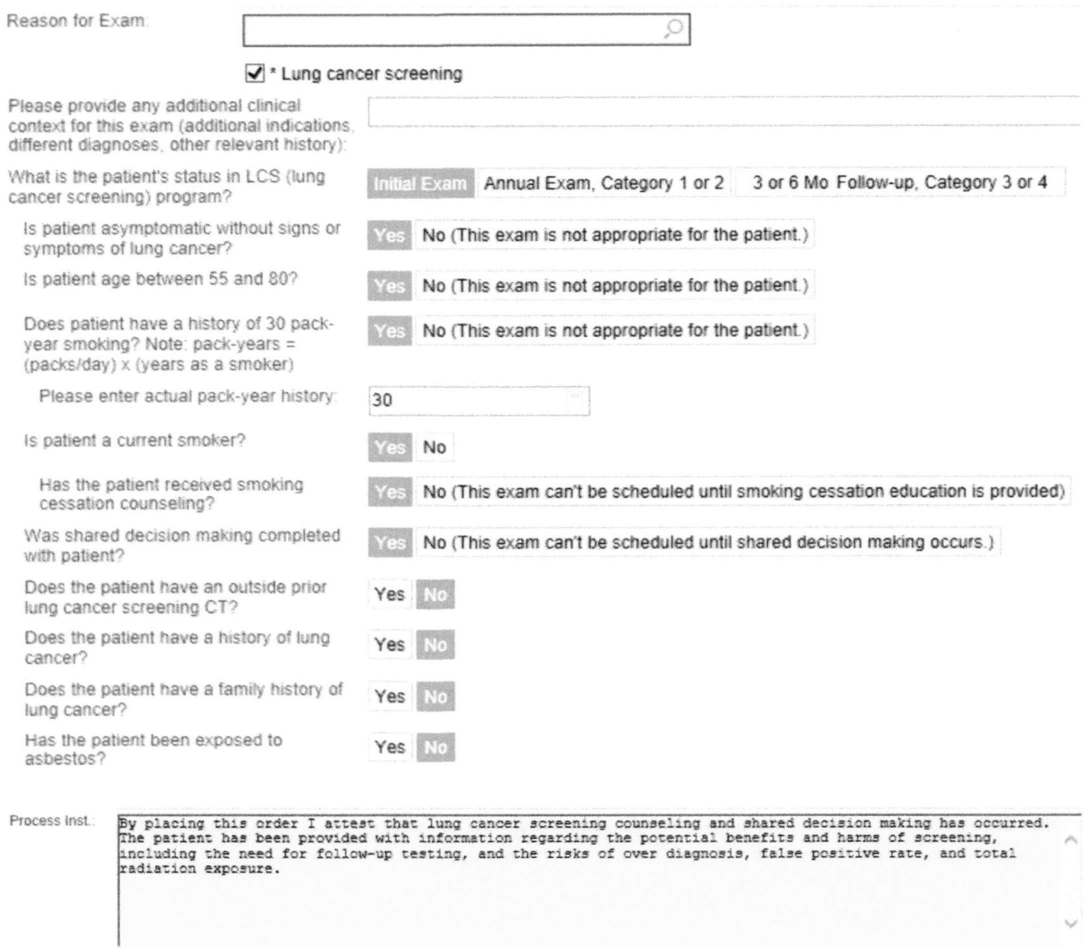

Reason for Exam: [🔍]

☑ * Lung cancer screening

Please provide any additional clinical context for this exam (additional indications, different diagnoses, other relevant history): [   ]

What is the patient's status in LCS (lung cancer screening) program?
[Initial Exam] [Annual Exam, Category 1 or 2] [3 or 6 Mo Follow-up, Category 3 or 4]

Is patient asymptomatic without signs or symptoms of lung cancer?
[Yes] No (This exam is not appropriate for the patient.)

Is patient age between 55 and 80?
[Yes] No (This exam is not appropriate for the patient.)

Does patient have a history of 30 pack-year smoking? Note: pack-years = (packs/day) x (years as a smoker)
[Yes] No (This exam is not appropriate for the patient.)

Please enter actual pack-year history: [30   ]

Is patient a current smoker?
[Yes] No

Has the patient received smoking cessation counseling?
[Yes] No (This exam can't be scheduled until smoking cessation education is provided)

Was shared decision making completed with patient?
[Yes] No (This exam can't be scheduled until shared decision making occurs.)

Does the patient have an outside prior lung cancer screening CT?
Yes [No]

Does the patient have a history of lung cancer?
Yes [No]

Does the patient have a family history of lung cancer?
Yes [No]

Has the patient been exposed to asbestos?
Yes [No]

Process Inst.: By placing this order I attest that lung cancer screening counseling and shared decision making has occurred. The patient has been provided with information regarding the potential benefits and harms of screening, including the need for follow-up testing, and the risks of over diagnosis, false positive rate, and total radiation exposure.

Fig. 2. Screenshot of computer physician order entry system shows how questions require referring providers to document the necessary elements to assess patient eligibility. Information can be electronically shared with the national registry.

> **Box 1**
> **Common differential diagnosis for solid noncalcified pulmonary nodule**
>
> *Benign*
> Granuloma (noncalcified)
> Hamartoma
> Intrapulmonary lymph node
> Focal pneumonia
> Focal scarring
>
> *Malignant*
> Lung cancer
> Solitary metastasis from extrathoracic malignancy

of becoming a clinically active cancer. Management recommendation is to obtain LDCT in 6 months. Category 3 nodules that remain unchanged at follow-up should be reclassified as category 2 nodules (**Fig. 8**). Category 4 nodules are suspicious, with a probability of malignancy of at least 5%. Management recommendations include LDCT in 3 months for category 4A, and CT with or without contrast, PET/CT, or tissue sampling for category 4B (**Figs. 9** and **10**).

The presence of suspicious features triggers the addition of the Lung-RADS X modifier to a category 3 or 4 nodule. Suspicious features include spiculation of a solid nodule, rapid enlargement of ground-glass nodule with a doubling time of less than 1 year, or additional findings such as lymphadenopathy (**Fig. 11**). If a radiologist sees suspicious features, addition of the Lung-RADS X

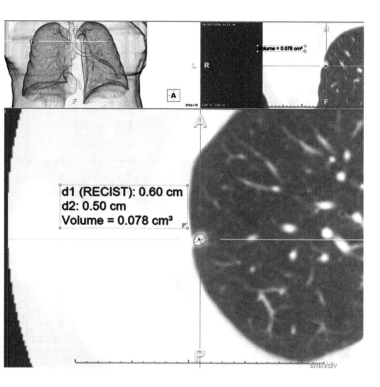

d1 (RECIST): 0.60 cm
d2: 0.50 cm
Volume = 0.078 cm³

Fig. 3. Screenshot of CAD system shows the ability to generate a volumetric measurement.

Box 2
Spectrum of possible incidental findings on lung cancer screening low-dose chest computed tomography

Pulmonary

- Emphysema
- Bronchitis
- Bronchiectasis
- Interstitial lung disease

Nonpulmonary

- Coronary artery disease or other cardiac findings
- Aortic aneurysm, abdominal > thoracic
- Thyroid nodules
- Renal calculi
- Liver disease (steatosis, cirrhosis)
- Chronic pancreatitis

Extrathoracic neoplasms

- Renal
- Liver
- Adrenal
- Pancreas
- Breast
- Lymphoma

---

modifier changes the designation of a nodule to 4X, which indicates a probability of malignancy higher than 15%. Management is the same as for category 4B lesions: additional diagnostic testing with contrast-enhanced CT, PET/CT, and/or tissue sampling (**Fig. 12**). Of note, the Lung-RADS category of the most concerning nodule determines the specific management recommendation (**Fig. 13**).

List: Lung-RADS for lung cancer screening low-dose chest computed tomography

- Lung-RADS is the structured reporting system for the interpretation of LCS CT examinations
- Lung-RADS differs from Fleischner Society guidelines because screened patients are at increased risk for lung cancer and have agreed to return for annual chest CT
- Lung-RADS triages nodules based on morphology (solid, nonsolid, or subsolid), size, and suspicious features
- Lung-RADS provides numeric categories that associate findings with management recommendations (nodule care pathways)
- The Lung-RADS category of the most concerning nodule determines the specific management recommendation

Category	Category Descriptor	Category	Findings	Management	Probability of Malignancy	Estimated Population Prevalence
Incomplete	-	0	prior chest CT examination(s) being located for comparison part or all of lungs cannot be evaluated	Additional lung cancer screening CT images and/or comparison to prior chest CT examinations is needed	n/a	1%
Negative	No nodules and definitely benign nodules	1	no lung nodules nodule(s) with specific calcifications: complete, central, popcorn, concentric rings and fat containing nodules			

Benign Appearance or Behavior	Nodules with a very low likelihood of becoming a clinically active cancer due to size or lack of growth	2	solid nodule(s):
			    <6 mm
			    new <4 mm
			part solid nodule(s):
			    <6 mm total diameter on baseline screening
			non solid nodule(s) (pure groundglass):
			    <20 mm OR
			    ≥20 mm and unchanged or slowly growing
			category 3 or 4 nodules unchanged for ≥3 mo
				Continue annual screening with LDCT in 12 mo	<1%	90%

Probably Benign	Probably benign finding(s) - short term follow up suggested; includes nodules with a low likelihood of becoming a clinically active cancer	3	solid nodule(s):
			    ≥6 to <8 mm at baseline OR
			    new 4 mm to <6 mm
			part solid nodule(s)
			    ≥6 mm total diameter with solid component <6 mm OR
			    new <6 mm total diameter
			non solid nodule(s) (pure groundglass) ≥20 mm on baseline CT or new
				6 mo LDCT	1%–2%	5%

Suspicious	Findings for which additional diagnostic testing and/or tissue sampling is recommended	4A	solid nodule(s):
			    ≥8 to <15 mm at baseline OR
			    growing <8 mm OR
			    new 6 to <8 mm
			part solid nodule(s):
			    ≥6 mm with solid component ≥6 mm to <8 mm OR
			    with a new or growing <4 mm solid component
			endobronchial nodule
				3 mo LDCT; PET/CT may be used when there is a ≥8 mm solid component	5%–15%	2%

		4B	solid nodule(s)
			    ≥15 mm OR
			    new or growing, and ≥8 mm
			part solid nodule(s) with:
			    a solid component ≥8 mm OR
			    a new or growing ≥4 mm solid component
				chest CT with or without contrast, PET/CT and/or tissue sampling depending on the *probability of malignancy and comorbidities. PET/CT may be used when there is a ≥8 mm solid component.	>15%	2%

		4X	Category 3 or 4 nodules with additional features or imaging findings that increases the suspicion of malignancy			

Other	Clinically Significant or Potentially Clinically Significant Findings (non lung cancer)	S	modifier - may add on to category 0–4 coding	As appropriate to the specific finding	n/a	10%
Prior Lung Cancer	Modifier for patients with a prior diagnosis of lung cancer who return to screening	C	modifier - may add on to category 0–4 coding	-	-	-

IMPORTANT NOTES FOR USE:

1) Negative screen: does not mean that an individual does not have lung cancer

2) Size: nodules should be measured on lung windows and reported as the average diameter rounded to the nearest whole number; for round nodules only a single diameter measurement is necessary

3) Size Thresholds: apply to nodules at first detection, and that grow and reach a higher size category

4) Growth: an increase in size of >1.5 mm

5) Exam Category: each exam should be coded 0–4 based on the nodule(s) with the highest degree of suspicion

6) Exam Modifiers: S and C modifiers may be added to the 0–4 category

7) Lung Cancer Diagnosis: Once a patient is diagnosed with lung cancer, further management (including additional imaging such as PET/CT) may be performed for purposes of lung cancer staging; this is no longer screening

8) Practice audit definitions: a negative screen is defined as categories 1 and 2; a positive screen is defined as categories 3 and 4

9) Category 4B Management: this is predicated on the probability of malignancy based on patient evaluation, patient preference and risk of malignancy; radiologists are encouraged to use the McWilliams and colleagues[26] assessment tool when

10) Category 4X: nodules with additional imaging findings that increase the suspicion of lung cancer, such as spiculation, GGN that doubles in size in 1 y, enlarged lymph nodes etc

11) Nodules with features of an intrapulmonary lymph node should be managed by mean diameter and the 0–4 numerical category classification

12) Category 3 and 4A nodules that are unchanged on interval CT should be coded as category 2, and individuals returned to screening in 12 mo

13) LDCT: low dose chest CT

Link to McWilliams Lung Cancer Risk Calculator

Upon request from the authors at: http://www.brocku.ca/lung-cancer-risk-calculator

At UptoDate http://www.uptodate.com/contents/calculator-solitary-pulmonary-nodule-malignancy-risk-brock-university-cancer-prediction-equation

Fig. 4. Lung-RADS Version 1.0 assessment categories. (*From* American College of Radiology. Lung CT Screening Reporting and Data System (Lung-RADS). Available at: http://www.acr.org/Quality-Safety/Resources/LungRADS. Accessed February 22, 2017; with permission.)

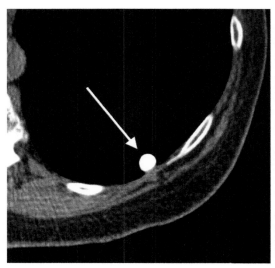

Fig. 5. Axial LCS LDCT image (mediastinal window) of a 68-year-old man shows a 12-mm left lower lobe nodule (*white arrow*) with homogeneous dense calcification, compatible with a benign granuloma. Appropriate designation would be Lung-RADS category 1 and management would be to return to annual LDCT screening in 12 months.

If a finding other than lung cancer requires some form of clinical or imaging evaluation before the next lung screening examination, it can be considered a potentially clinically significant finding and should trigger the Lung-RADS S modifier. S can be added to Lung-RADS categories 0 to 4. Although visual assessment of the degree of coronary artery calcifications on LCS LDCT has been shown to correlate with patient outcomes, there is no universally accepted comprehensive list of clinically significant findings.[29,30] Aneurysms and other cancers (including esophageal, breast, thyroid, and lymphoma) should definitely be included (Fig. 14). The ACR has released white papers on managing incidentally detected thyroid nodules and on incidental findings on abdominal CT which could be applied to incidental findings on LCS LDCT.[31,32] The Lung-RADS C modifier indicates that a patient has had lung cancer in the past; it can be added to any category.

Of note, Lung-RADS is expected to evolve as data of LCS programs are analyzed. New and updated versions will be published by the ACR and radiologists need to ensure that they are using the most up-to-date version of Lung-RADS.[22]

REPORTING LUNG CANCER SCREENING LOW-DOSE COMPUTED TOMOGRAPHY EXAMINATIONS

CMS specifies that physicians who want to claim reimbursement for the interpretation of LCS CT examinations need to be trained in diagnostic radiology

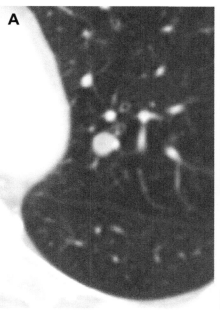
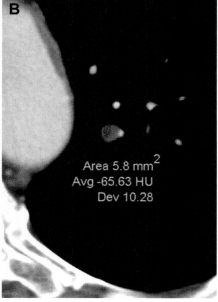

Area 5.8 mm^2
Avg -65.63 HU
Dev 10.28

Fig. 6. Axial contrast-enhanced chest CT image of a 63-year-old man shows an 8-mm left upper lobe nodule in lung window (*A*) and mediastinal window (*B*). The nodule contains fat (−66 Hounsfield units), compatible with a benign hamartoma. In the setting of LCS, the appropriate designation for this lesion would be Lung-RADS category 1. Management would be to return to annual screening with LDCT in 12 months.

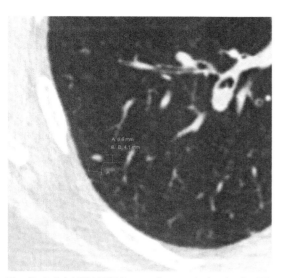

Fig. 7. Axial LCS LDCT image (lung window) of a 72-year-old man at baseline screening examination shows a right lower lobe solid noncalcified nodule. The average of the longest and shortest total axial diameters (A and B) rounded to the nearest whole number is 5 mm, making the appropriate designation Lung-RADS category 2. Management would be to return to annual screening with LDCT in 12 months.

and radiation safety. Such physicians must be board certified or eligible for board certification by the American Board of Radiology (ABR) or an equivalent organization. Supervision or interpretation of at least

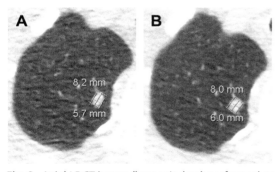

Fig. 8. Axial LDCT image (lung window) performed as the baseline LCS examination in a 55-year-old woman shows a right upper lobe solid nodule (A). The average of the longest and shortest axial diameters rounded to the nearest whole number is 7 mm, making this a Lung-RADS category 3 lesion, and management would be to follow up with LDCT in 6 months. Axial chest CT image (lung window) performed at 6 months (B) shows that the nodule is unchanged. It would now be downgraded to Lung-RADS category 2. Appropriate management would be to return to annual screening with LDCT in 12 months.

300 chest CT cases in the preceding 3 years as well as participation in continuing medical education is also required (see **Table 2**).[14]

CMS requires that LCS LDCT be reported using a structured format. The goal is to clearly communicate the pertinent findings to the ordering provider, define what constitutes a positive finding on the LDCT, and recommend nodule management based on the nodule care pathways accepted by the program. An LCS CT report should contain the following items: technique, comparison date, findings, impression, and a specific management recommendation (**Box 3**). The ACR-STR practice parameters suggest the following descriptors for each nodule: location (lobe and segment with series/image number), size, attenuation (soft tissue, type of calcification, fat), morphology (solid, nonsolid [ground glass], and part solid [containing both solid and nonsolid components]), and margins (ie, smooth, lobulated, spiculated). Any interval change should be compared with prior examinations, with particular attention to the most remote study.

MANAGEMENT OF IMAGING FINDINGS

A screening program needs to have predefined nodule care pathways in order to manage screen-detected lung nodules. In addition, there needs to be knowledge regarding nodule characterization with PET/CT and minimally invasive surgical approaches.

In our program, all category 4 nodules are seen in a dedicated pulmonary nodule clinic (**Fig. 15**). Before scheduling a patient into the nodule clinic, the patient's existing team is reviewed to ensure that they do not already have a pulmonologist or thoracic surgeon because the goal of any multidisciplinary program should be to add value rather than duplicate efforts. A comprehensive review of a patient's history, imaging studies, and other results is performed and then discussed with all relevant specialists in the same session. The key is the simultaneous review of imaging studies as a group and collaboration in creating a treatment plan for each patient. Although there is an upfront commitment of time from the team members, the payoff is that patients only see the most appropriate provider. For example, pulmonologists should not see patients who need surgical intervention and surgeons should not see patients who would never be surgical candidates. In addition to providing input on the management of pulmonary nodules, the nodule clinic provides a platform to reinforce smoking cessation. After the initial consultation, follow-up visits and imaging are scheduled by the nodule clinic and the

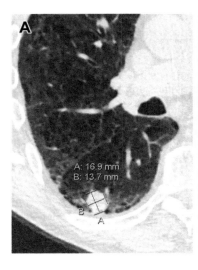
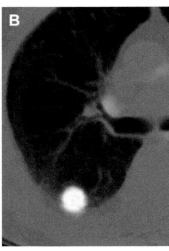

Fig. 9. Axial LCS LDCT image (*A*; lung window) of a 75-year-old man at baseline screening examination shows a right lower lobe solid nodule. The average of the longest and shortest total axial diameters (A and B) rounded to the nearest whole number is 16 mm, making the appropriate designation Lung-RADS category 4B. Subsequent PET/CT (*B*) showed intense fluorodeoxyglucose (FDG) uptake, highly suspicious for malignancy. Because of extensive comorbidities, the patient was referred to radiation oncology for treatment.

navigator ensures that recommendations are followed and updates the team if there is a change in a patient's health status.[33]

The decision to perform PET/CT depends on the probability of malignancy, and the size and morphology of the nodule. Lung-RADS suggests PET/CT for solid nodules greater than 8 mm, or part-solid nodules with a solid component greater than 8 mm (categories 4A, 4B, and 4X). Solid nodules less than 8 mm are unlikely to be malignant,

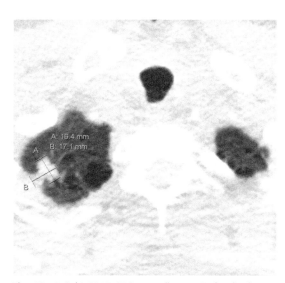

Fig. 10. Axial LCS LDCT image (lung window) of a 61-year-old man shows a lobulated right apical nodule contiguous with apical pleural thickening. The average of the longest and shortest axial diameters (A and B) rounded to the nearest whole number is 17 mm, making this a Lung-RADS category 4B lesion. Subsequent PET/CT (not shown) showed intense FDG uptake and right upper lobe lobectomy confirmed squamous cell carcinoma.

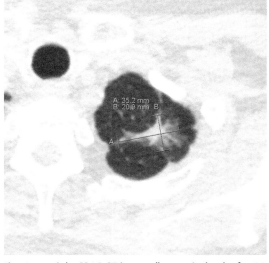

Fig. 11. Axial LCS LDCT image (lung window) of a 74-year-old man shows a spiculated, subsolid left apical nodule. The average of the longest and shortest total axial diameters (A and B) rounded to the nearest whole number is 28 mm, and the average diameter of the solid component is 11 mm, making this a Lung-RADS category 4B lesion. Spiculation increases suspicion for malignancy and the designation is Lung-RADS category 4X. Subsequent PET/CT (not shown) showed intense FDG uptake within the nodule, and percutaneous needle biopsy confirmed adenocarcinoma.

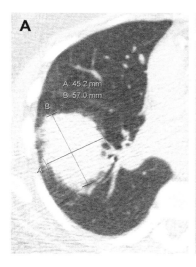

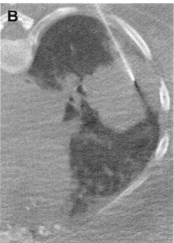

Fig. 12. Axial LCS LDCT image with patient supine (*A*; lung window) of a 72-year-old woman at baseline screening examination shows a right lower lobe mass. The appropriate designation is Lung-RADS category 4X. Axial CT image with the patient in the prone position (*B*) shows the introducer during percutaneous needle biopsy of the lesion. Pathology confirmed adenocarcinoma.

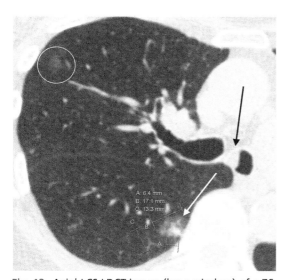

Fig. 13. Axial LCS LDCT image (lung window) of a 76-year-old woman at baseline screening examination shows a subsolid nodule in the right lower lobe (*white arrow*). The average of the longest and shortest total axial diameters (B and C) rounded to the nearest whole number is 15 mm. The solid component measures 6 mm (A); a single measurement is sufficient in this case given that the solid component is round. Appropriate designation would be Lung-RADS category 4A. A 9-mm right upper lobe pure ground-glass nodule (*circle*) is also present; however, the most concerning nodule determines the Lung-RADS category. The endobronchial filling defect in the proximal left mainstem bronchus (*black arrow*) would be a Lung-RADS category 4A lesion. The patient underwent PET/CT (not shown) and FDG uptake in the part-solid nodule triggered a needle biopsy, which confirmed adenocarcinoma. The endobronchial filling defect had resolved at the time of follow-up, compatible with secretions.

are difficult to biopsy, and are not reliably characterized with PET/CT, and therefore follow-up by CT is recommended. Subsolid nodules may be falsely negative on PET because a critical mass of metabolically active malignant cells is required for detection by PET. Solid nodules greater than 8 mm or part-solid nodules with a solid component greater than 8 mm can be more reliably

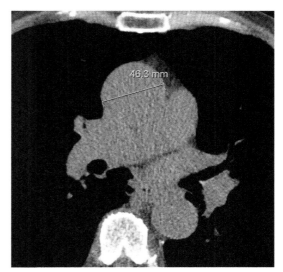

Fig. 14. Axial LCS LDCT image (mediastinal window) of a 68-year-old man reveals an incidental ascending thoracic aortic aneurysm measuring 4.6 cm in the axial plane at the level of the right pulmonary artery. No pulmonary nodules were identified. The aneurysm represents a clinically significant finding and the appropriate designation would be Lung-RADS category 1S.

Box 3
Example of a structured report for a lung cancer screening low-dose chest computed tomography examination using Lung-RADS

Technique

CT scan of the chest without intravenous contrast, using low-dose lung cancer screening protocol.

Comparison

None

Findings

Lines/tubes: None.

Lungs and airways: The central airways are patent. There is mild diffuse bronchial wall thickening, suggestive of bronchitis. There is centrilobular and paraseptal emphysema. No pulmonary nodules are identified.

Pleura: The pleural spaces are clear.

Base of neck, heart, and mediastinum: The thyroid gland is unremarkable. No supraclavicular, mediastinal, hilar, or axillary lymphadenopathy is seen. The heart and pericardium are within normal limits.

Soft tissues: Normal.

Abdomen: This study was performed without contrast and with lower than standard dose. These factors reduce the sensitivity for detection of small lesions in the upper abdomen. Given these technical limitations, no focal lesion is seen within the visualized liver, spleen, pancreas, kidneys, and adrenal glands.

Bones: The visualized bony thorax is within normal limits.

Impression

No pulmonary nodules identified. Emphysema and bronchitis.

Lung-RADS category: 1 (negative).

   Explanation of the Lung-RADS categories can be found at: http://www.acr.org/~/media/ACR/Documents/PDF/QualitySafety/Res0urces/LungRADS/AssessmentCategories

Recommendation

Continue annual screening with low-dose chest CT in 12 months.

This report has been forwarded to an automated communication system that will electronically notify appropriate providers of potentially important findings.

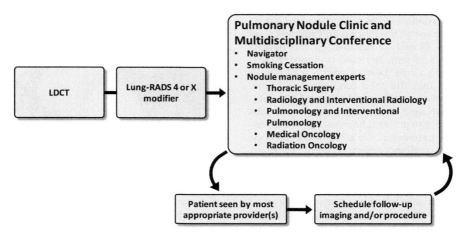

Fig. 15. The role of the pulmonary nodule clinic in the management of Lung-RADS category 4 lesions.

characterized by PET/CT and are also more likely to be successfully diagnosed by percutaneous needle biopsy. False-negative PET/CT of large nodules is a potential pitfall. Slow tumor metabolism in minimally invasive adenocarcinoma, mucinous adenocarcinoma, and carcinoid tumors may result in absent fluorodeoxyglucose (FDG) uptake. False-positive PET/CT is another pitfall and can occur with infectious and inflammatory conditions, including pneumonia, mycobacterial disease, rheumatoid nodules, and sarcoidosis. If less than 6 weeks pass between LDCT and PET/CT, infectious and inflammatory nodules likely do not have enough time to resolve or decrease in size.

Tissue sampling is recommended for solid nodules greater than 15 mm, new or growing nodules that are greater than 8 mm, part-solid nodules with a solid component greater than 8 mm, or a new or growing solid component greater than 4 mm (category 4B or 4X nodules). Tissue sampling can be performed using imaging or bronchoscopic guidance, or with a surgical biopsy.

Potential pitfalls in the management of findings on LCS LDCT also include lung cancers associated with cystic airspaces.[34] This uncommon manifestation of lung cancer is not specifically mentioned in Lung-RADS but accounted for 23% (5 out of 22) of missed cancers in a European LCS trial.[35] Lung cancer should be considered in cases of cystic lesions with wall thickening, increasing septations, and/or mural nodularity (**Fig. 16**).[36] In addition, lung cancer can sometimes present without a pulmonary nodule or mass (**Fig. 17**).

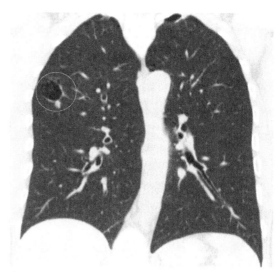

Fig. 16. Coronal LCS LDCT (lung window) of a 62-year-old man at baseline screening examination shows a cystic airspace with a mural nodule in the right upper lobe (*circle*). The overall lesion has a mean diameter of 31 mm and the nodular solid component along its inferior aspect measures 11 mm. Although the solid nodule would qualify for Lung-RADS category 4A, the presence of a cystic component further raises suspicion for lung cancer. Appropriate designation would be Lung-RADS category 4X. Right upper lobectomy confirmed adenocarcinoma.

List: Pitfalls in the management of findings on lung cancer screening low-dose chest computed tomography

- Carcinoid and low-grade adenocarcinomas including subcentimeter ground-glass nodules may show none or only minimal FDG uptake. CT features (size, growth, density, spiculation, location) are thus more important in guiding management

- PET/CT performed within 6 weeks after detection of a suspicious pulmonary nodule may be false-positive because of an infectious or inflammatory process

- Lung-RADS does not specifically mention lung cancers associated with cystic airspaces; lung cancer should be considered in cases of cystic lesions with wall thickening and/or mural nodularity

- On rare occasions, lung cancer can present with lymphadenopathy and/or pleural effusion but without a pulmonary nodule or mass

---

The need to maximize the sensitivity of Lung-RADS while curbing the number of false-positive results has triggered many efforts to identify biomarkers that can help with risk stratification of screen-detected nodules. Potential targets include airway epithelium (including buccal mucosa), sputum, exhaled breath, and blood. The underlying rationale of a diagnostic biomarker based on biological fluids is that molecular alterations within cancer cells lead to the synthesis of distinct molecular compounds, which, if detected, may signify the presence of cancerous transformation. Ideally, the presence of biomarkers in an LCS participant should help in making the decision whether to intervene on a nodule that is nonspecific on imaging.

WHAT REFERRING PROVIDERS NEED TO KNOW

The referring provider needs to know whether or not pulmonary nodule(s) are present, the degree of suspicion for any screen-detected nodules, and whether or not significant incidental findings are present. Most importantly, a clear management recommendation needs to be provided for every LCS LDCT so that the referring provider can identify

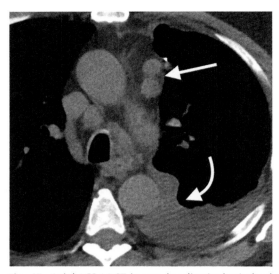

Fig. 17. Axial LCS LDCT image (mediastinal window) of a 72-year-old man at baseline screening examination shows mediastinal lymphadenopathy (*straight arrow*) and a moderate left pleural effusion (*curved arrow*). In any patient, lymphadenopathy and pleural effusion are suspicious for malignancy. No pulmonary nodule or mass was identified, so the significant finding leads to the designation of Lung-RADS 1S. Transbronchial lymph node biopsy confirmed metastatic lung adenocarcinoma.

the appropriate nodule care pathway. The Lung-RADS category provides all of this information.

Furthermore, it is helpful for referring providers to understand the logistics of the local lung screening program in order to facilitate management of imaging findings. A Web site with the contact information of the patient navigator and a list of frequently asked questions should be made available.[28]

SUMMARY

Although LCS with LDCT represents a valuable opportunity to reduce lung cancer mortality in high-risk patients, it is not simply a test but is a process that requires a structured approach and a multidisciplinary team. Standardized imaging protocols, structured reporting with Lung-RADS, and well-defined care pathways are required to realize the potential of LDCT. Management decisions should be made by a team of lung nodule management experts. Adherence to the requirements set forth by CMS and the USPSTF ensures reimbursement for LDCT examinations. Because the clinical practice of LCS is expected to evolve, radiologists are encouraged to periodically check for updates on the ACR's Lung Cancer Screening Resources Web site.[22]

REFERENCES

1. Cancer Facts & Figures 2017. Am Cancer Soc. 2017. Available at: https://www.cancer.org/research/cancer-facts-statistics/all-cancer-facts-figures/cancer-facts-figures-2017.html. Accessed February 18, 2017.
2. SEER stat fact sheets: lung and bronchus cancer. Surveillance, Epidemiology, and End Results Program. 2017. Available at: https://seer.cancer.gov/statfacts/html/lungb.html. Accessed February 18, 2017.
3. Aberle D, Adams A, Berg C. Reduced lung-cancer mortality with low-dose computed tomographic screening. N Engl J Med 2011;365:395–409.
4. National Lung Screening Trial Research Team, Aberle DR, Berg CD, Black WC, et al. The National Lung Screening Trial: overview and study design. Radiology 2011;258(1):243–53.
5. Swensen SJ, Jett JR, Hartman TE, et al. Lung cancer screening with CT: Mayo Clinic experience. Radiology 2003;226(3):756–61.
6. Henschke CI, McCauley DI, Yankelevitz DF, et al. Early lung cancer action project: overall design and findings from baseline screening. Lancet 1999;354(9173):99–105.
7. Moyer VA. Screening for lung cancer: U.S. Preventive Services Task Force recommendation statement. Ann Intern Med 2014;160(5):330–8.
8. Bach PB, Mirkin JN, Oliver TK, et al. Benefits and harms of CT screening for lung cancer: a systematic review. JAMA 2012;307(22):2418–29.
9. Jaklitsch MT, Jacobson FL, Austin JHM, et al. The American Association for Thoracic Surgery guidelines for lung cancer screening using low-dose computed tomography scans for lung cancer survivors and other high-risk groups. J Thorac Cardiovasc Surg 2012;144(1):33–8.
10. Detterbeck FC, Mazzone PJ, Naidich DP, et al. Screening for lung cancer: diagnosis and management of lung cancer, 3rd ed: American College of Chest Physicians evidence-based clinical practice guidelines. Chest 2013;143(5 Suppl):e78S–92S.
11. Wender R, Fontham ETH, Barrera E, et al. American Cancer Society lung cancer screening guidelines. CA Cancer J Clin 2013;63(2):106–17.
12. Wood DE, Kazerooni E, Baum SL, et al. Lung cancer screening, version 1.2015: featured updates to the NCCN guidelines. J Natl Compr Canc Netw 2015;13(1):23–34 [quiz: 34]. Available at: http://www.ncbi.nlm.nih.gov/pubmed/25583767. Accessed August 11, 2015.
13. FAQs about Affordable Care Act Implementation Part XII. United States Department of Labor. 2013. Available at: http://www.dol.gov/ebsa/faqs/faq-aca12.html. Accessed February 18, 2017.

14. Decision Memo for Screening for Lung Cancer with Low Dose Computed Tomography (LDCT) (CAG-00439N). Centers Medicare Medicaid Serv. 2015. Available at: http://www.cms.gov/medicare-coverage-database/details/nca-decision-memo.aspx?NCAId= 274. Accessed February 18, 2017.

15. Kazerooni EA, Austin JHM, Black WC, et al. ACR-STR practice parameter for the performance and reporting of lung cancer screening thoracic computed tomography (CT): 2014 (Resolution 4). J Thorac Imaging 2014;29(5):310–6.

16. Lung Cancer Screening Protocols Version 4.0. Am Assoc Phys Med. 2016. Available at: http://www.aapm.org/pubs/CTProtocols/documents/LungCancerScreeningCT.pdf. Accessed February 18, 2017.

17. Wiener RS, Gould MK, Arenberg DA, et al. An official American Thoracic Society/American College of Chest Physicians policy statement: implementation of low-dose computed tomography lung cancer screening programs in clinical practice. Am J Respir Crit Care Med 2015;192(7):881–91.

18. Mazzone P, Powell CA, Arenberg D, et al. Components necessary for high quality lung cancer screening: American College of Chest Physicians and American Thoracic Society policy statement. Chest 2014;147(2):295–303.

19. McKee BJ, McKee AB, Kitts AB, et al. Low-dose computed tomography screening for lung cancer in a clinical setting: essential elements of a screening program. J Thorac Imaging 2015;30(2): 115–29.

20. Villanti AC, Jiang Y, Abrams DB, et al. A cost-utility analysis of lung cancer screening and the additional benefits of incorporating smoking cessation interventions. PLoS One 2013;8(8):e71379.

21. Lung Cancer Screening Registry. Am Coll Radiol. Available at: https://www.acr.org/Quality-Safety/National-Radiology-Data-Registry/Lung-Cancer-Screening-Registry. Accessed February 18, 2017.

22. Lung Cancer Screening Resources. Am Coll Radiol. Available at: http://www.acr.org/Quality-Safety/Resources/Lung-Imaging-Resources. Accessed December 18, 2016.

23. Donnelly EF. Technical parameters and interpretive issues in screening computed tomography scans for lung cancer. J Thorac Imaging 2012;27(4):224–9.

24. Ebner L, Roos JE, Christensen JD, et al. Maximum-intensity-projection and computer-aided-detection algorithms as stand-alone reader devices in lung cancer screening using different dose levels and reconstruction kernels. AJR Am J Roentgenol 2016;207(2):282–8.

25. Liang M, Tang W, Xu DM, et al. Low-dose CT screening for lung cancer: computer-aided detection of missed lung cancers. Radiology 2016; 281(1):279–88.

26. McWilliams A, Tammemagi MC, Mayo JR, et al. Probability of cancer in pulmonary nodules detected on first screening CT. N Engl J Med 2013;369(10): 910–9.

27. Lung Imaging Reporting and Data System (Lung-RADS) Version 1.0. Am Coll Radiol. 2014. Available at: http://www.acr.org/Quality-Safety/Resources/LungRADS. Accessed February 18, 2017.

28. Fintelmann FJ, Bernheim A, Digumarthy SR, et al. The 10 pillars of lung cancer screening: rationale and logistics of a lung cancer screening program. Radiographics 2015;35:1893–908.

29. Chiles C, Duan F, Gladish GW, et al. Association of coronary artery calcification and mortality in the national lung screening trial: a comparison of three scoring methods. Radiology 2015;276(1):82–90.

30. Bernheim A, Auffermann WF, Stillman AE. The dubious value of coronary calcium scoring on lung cancer screening CT. J Am Coll Radiol 2016;14(3): 343–4.

31. Hoang JK, Langer JE, Middleton WD, et al. Managing incidental thyroid nodules detected on imaging: white paper of the ACR incidental thyroid findings committee. J Am Coll Radiol 2015;12(2):143–50.

32. Berland LL, Silverman SG, Gore RM, et al. Managing incidental findings on abdominal CT: white paper of the ACR incidental findings committee. J Am Coll Radiol 2010;7(10):754–73.

33. Campo MJ, Lennes IT. Managing patients with screen-detected nodules: the nodule clinic. Semin Roentgenol 2017;52(3):161–5.

34. Farooqi AO, Cham M, Zhang L, et al. Lung cancer associated with cystic airspaces. AJR Am J Roentgenol 2012;199(4):781–6.

35. Scholten ET, Horeweg N, de Koning HJ, et al. Computed tomographic characteristics of interval and post screen carcinomas in lung cancer screening. Eur Radiol 2014;25(1):81–8.

36. Fintelmann FJ, Brinkmann JK, Jeck WR, et al. Lung cancers associated with cystic airspaces: natural history, pathologic correlation, and mutational analysis. J Thorac Imaging 2017;32:176–88.

Imaging and Screening for Colorectal Cancer with CT Colonography

Perry J. Pickhardt, MD

KEYWORDS

• Colorectal cancer • Colorectal polyps • Screening • CT colonography • Virtual colonoscopy

KEY POINTS

- Colorectal cancer (CRC) is readily preventable via screen detection of clinically relevant polyps using either virtual or optical colonoscopy.
- In addition to primary cancer prevention, detection of early-stage cancer is another important goal of CRC screening.
- Computed tomographic colonography (CTC) is a validated screening test that is equivalent to invasive colonoscopy for detection of advanced neoplasia, but is safer, more cost-effective, and more convenient for patients.
- High-quality results can be achieved with CTC screening in clinical practice when proven methods are applied.
- This review provides an updated blueprint for setting up a successful CTC screening program.

INTRODUCTION

Colorectal cancer (CRC) remains the second-leading cause of cancer death, despite the fact that it is readily preventable via screen detection (and removal) of clinically relevant polyps.[1] This disconnect is primarily due to the fact that many adults are not screened, whereas others undergo only stool-based testing, which does not confer effective cancer prevention.[2] Given the critical importance of cancer prevention beyond cancer detection alone, the American Cancer Society expressed a strong preference for the endoscopist and radiologic tests that provide for visualization of benign but potentially precancerous polyps in its landmark 2008 screening guidelines.[3] Although the double-contrast barium enema was included in these guidelines, it was made clear that this screening test was quickly becoming obsolete because of both the emergence of computed tomographic colonography (CTC) and the vanishing expertise for performing this examination. The demoted status of the barium enema was further reinforced by its exclusion in the recent US Preventive Services Task Force screening guidelines.[4] Therefore, CTC represents the radiologic test of choice for CRC screening going forward.[5] CTC is a well-validated screening test that is equivalent to optical colonoscopy (OC) for the detection of advanced adenomas,[6–8] but is also safer, more cost-effective, and preferred by patients.[9–13] Beyond primary cancer prevention, detection of early-stage cancer is another important goal of CRC screening, for which CTC is also ideally suited.[14] In comparison, the

Disclosures: Dr P.J. Pickhardt is co-founder of VirtuoCTC; consultant to Check-Cap and Bracco; and shareholder in SHINE, Elucent, and Cellectar Biosciences.

Gastrointestinal Imaging, Department of Radiology, University of Wisconsin School of Medicine and Public Health, 600 Highland Avenue, Madison, WI 53792, USA

E-mail address: ppickhardt2@uwhealth.org

Radiol Clin N Am 55 (2017) 1183–1196
http://dx.doi.org/10.1016/j.rcl.2017.06.009

accuracy of routine computed tomography (CT) without preparation or distention for detecting cancer is greatly diminished.[15]

The University of Wisconsin Hospital and Clinics (UWHC) has enjoyed relatively broad third-party coverage for CTC screening since 2004.[16,17] This program has shown that high-quality results can be achieved with CTC screening in clinical practice when their proven methods are used. This practical review endeavors to provide an updated roadmap for programmatic CTC screening, essentially "how we do it" at UWHC.[18,19] The program has evolved from its origins that trace back to the National Naval Medical Center in Bethesda, Maryland, where the Department of Defense (DoD) screening trial was conducted.[6] With well over a decade of continuous experience, this program gained unique insights into the various challenges involved in setting up a clinical screening program, with many lessons learned along the way. With expanded coverage for CTC screening now on the horizon, the time is ripe for a practical overview. The intent is not to provide an exhaustive literature review or compare with other CTC techniques in use elsewhere, but rather to provide a blueprint for an established approach to high-quality CRC screening, focusing herein primarily on CTC technique and interpretation. Other considerations such as CTC program personnel, patient scheduling, and database management are covered elsewhere.[20]

CT COLONOGRAPHY TECHNIQUE

If all facets of the CTC examination are adequately addressed (namely, colonic preparation, luminal distention, multidetector CT [MDCT] scanning, and CTC image interpretation), effective detection of clinically relevant lesions is readily achievable. As each technical component is individually discussed, it is important to recognize the interconnected nature of these factors, such that any weak link in the chain may upset the outcome. For example, even the most robust CTC software system is destined to fail in the setting of inadequate colonic preparation or distention. Similarly, optimal preparation and distention may not compensate for an ineffective interpretive approach.

Bowel Preparation

Robust bowel preparation for screening CTC is important for accurate lesion detection and generally involves a combination of catharsis and contrast tagging. UWHC's standard low-volume CTC bowel preparation has evolved over the years, but has always combined 3 basic

components: a laxative for catharsis, dilute 2% barium for tagging of solid residual stool, and iodinated water-soluble contrast for opacification of luminal fluid and secondary cleansing. Overall, the bowel regimen has been simplified, reduced, and improved since the multicenter DoD trial.[21–25] UWHC receives few complaints from patients about their current standard low-volume preparation, which consists mainly of magnesium citrate, 2% barium, and iohexol (Table 1). The streamlined nature of this preparation was designed with working adults in mind, because it does not require taking a day off to complete. Perhaps more importantly, UWHC has not yet encountered any significant preparation-related complications in more than 10,000 patients dating back to the screening trial. In addition to the main preparation components, which are taken the evening before the examination, the patient also maintains a clear liquid diet throughout the day and takes bisacodyl tablets around noon. Bisacodyl will generally not cause diarrhea but serves to "prime the pump" for later on. Because the preparation combines over-the-counter laxatives and prescription oral contrast agents, UWHC's pharmacy packages the constituents into one convenient kit, which can either be mailed out or dispensed at one of several satellite pharmacies.[19] In addition to the specific preparation instructions, they also provide a pamphlet containing general information about CTC screening within the kit. Ultimately, a commercialized version of their bowel preparation kit

Table 1 University of Wisconsin Hospital and Clinics standard computed tomographic colonographic bowel preparation	
Time Window	Oral Dosage Instructions
2–6 PM	1st 296-mL bottle of magnesium citrate
4–9 PM	2nd bottle of magnesium citrate & 225 mL of 2% barium
6–11 PM	50 mL iohexol (350 mgI/mL)

Note: 1. The above preparation is performed in conjunction with a clear liquid diet the day before CTC. 2. Two 5-mg bisacodyl tablets are also taken before 11 AM with 1 cup of clear liquid. 3. Each step above should be separated by 2 to 3 h; exact timing is flexible for patient convenience. 4. Before commencing with steps 2 and 3, patients are instructed to drink 4 to 8 cups of clear liquid. 5. For 4-L PEG alternative, the patient begins the laxative around noon to allow for the larger volume. See text for more specific details.

would be more practical for other CTC programs that are starting up.

The specific choice of laxative depends on the health status of the individual. When UWHC first started the CTC screening program, a single 45-mL dose of sodium phosphate served as the laxative for their standard bowel preparation and was used in about 90% of screening studies. Although this regimen was well tolerated and UWHC encountered no serious complications, sodium phosphate was discontinued over a concern for acute phosphate nephropathy, a very rare but serious side effect. For cases where sodium phosphate was best avoided, they had previously substituted magnesium citrate, given in liquid form as two 296-mL bottles. Formal retrospective studies have demonstrated equivalence between these 2 regimens,[23,24] and magnesium citrate has served as UWHC's standard cathartic for many years now. Use of magnesium citrate has greatly streamlined patient scheduling because it eliminated the need to screen for renal or cardiac insufficiency, or other contraindications for sodium phosphate. For the rare brittle or tenuous patients who cannot tolerate even moderate fluid or electrolyte shifts, they continue to use polyethylene glycol (PEG), which is given as a standard 4-L solution. Although the safety profile of this lavage is most favorable, this preparation is also associated with the poorest compliance. Fortunately, this preparation is only rarely necessary, accounting for less than 1% of UWHC's cases. They generally have patients begin drinking the PEG solution around noon the day before CTC to allow more time for the oral contrast agents later on, with the goal of about one 8-ounce glass of PEG every 10 to 15 minutes until finished.

Regardless of the laxative used, the dual oral contrast regimen remains the same, consisting of 2% barium followed by iohexol (see **Table 1**). The author surmises that the complementary actions of these 2 contrast agents, in conjunction with catharsis, provide for the optimal CTC preparation.[18] The total volume of each oral contrast agent has been cut in half from the original trial and reduced to a single dose of each, without any discernible drop-off in the fidelity of the preparation. The rationale behind the specific order of the 3 preparation components is that the laxative provides catharsis for the bulk removal of fecal material; the barium tags any residual solid stool that remains, and the iodinated water-soluble agent serves the dual purpose of uniform fluid tagging and secondary catharsis.[18] To administer the barium before the primary catharsis would require a much greater volume because it would need to tag the entire stool bulk, nearly all of which

will then be eliminated by the laxative. UWHC strongly prefers the dilute 2% "CT grade" barium products over the 40% weight/volume high-density barium products, which are unnecessarily dense and may lead to difficulty at same-day OC.

The author suspects that the water-soluble iodinated contrast is the real secret to the success of this preparation. Not only does this agent uniformly opacify the residual luminal fluid, but it also provides for a mild secondary catharsis that acts to decrease the amount of adherent solid debris. This last feature is critical, because adherent stool can be a major source of false positives and often precludes the preferred primary 3-dimensional (3D) polyp detection approach. Although those at UWHC were initially wary that the nonionic iodinated contrast agents, such as iohexol, might not provide the same cathartic "kick" or slippery nature, a head-to-head trial showed that iohexol was essentially equivalent to diatrizoate.[25] Because of the additional advantages of iohexol over diatrizoate, including improved safety profile, more palatable taste, and now lower cost, the decision to switch to the nonionic agent was straightforward.

The dual contrast tagging regimen likely improves the accuracy of CTC in several ways: (1) it increases specificity by tagging residual stool (barium effect) and decreases the amount of adherent stool (iohexol effect), (2) it increases sensitivity by allowing for detection in polyps submerged under fluid (iohexol effect), and (3) it improves detection of serrated and other flat lesions via surface coating of adherent contrast.[26–29] This focal contrast coating can serve as a vital beacon for detection for flat lesions that may otherwise be relatively inconspicuous against the adjacent bowel mucosa (**Fig. 1**) and is also seen frequently in tubulovillous adenomas and other advanced neoplasms (**Fig. 2**).[30–32] Once considered optional, these advantages demonstrate why the use of oral contrast tagging is now considered standard practice for CTC.

The prospect for minimal or noncathartic bowel preparation for CTC screening warrants consideration. For starters, it should be made clear that the term "prepless CTC" is a generally a misnomer for minimal preparation or noncathartic CTC approaches and therefore should be avoided. In fact, some noncathartic preparations can be more onerous than UWHC's low-volume cathartic standard preparation when they entail complicated and prolonged oral contrast regimens and dietary modifications, which extend for several days. The main theoretic advantage to noncathartic CTC is the avoidance of laxatives, presumably leading to increased patient compliance.

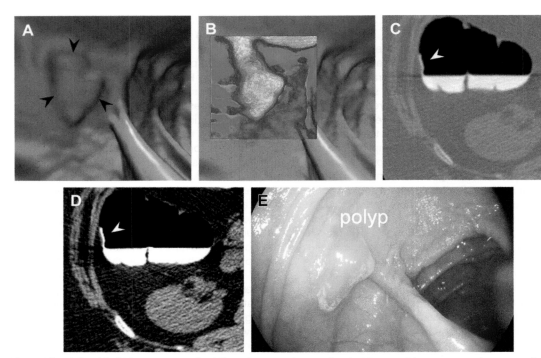

Fig. 1. Flat right-sided 14-mm serrated sessile polyp at CTC screening in 55-year-old asymptomatic woman (missed at prospective evaluation). 3D endoluminal image (*A*) shows a flat plaquelike lesion (*arrowheads*) in the right colon near the hepatic flexure. 3D image with translucency rendering (*B*) shows prominent white overlay from surface coating of oral contrast, which was initially mistaken for tagged adherent stool. Corresponding 2D images with polyp (*C*) and soft tissue (*D*) windowing show the subtle flat soft tissue lesion with overlying dense contrast cap (*arrowheads*). This flat lesion was found at same-day OC (*E*). Note the mucus cap, which is the OC correlate for contrast coating. The OC was performed for a CTC-detected cecal polyp (not shown), which was confirmed and proved to be a tubular adenoma. Recognition of contrast coating of flat lesions will prevent such lesions from being missed at CTC.

However, there are several disadvantages that preclude this approach from being a singular solution.[33] For one, primary 3D polyp detection is often not feasible because of the amount of residual adherent stool. Furthermore, patients would not be able to undergo same-day polypectomy, something that is highly valued by patients because it avoids the need for additional full preparation for colonoscopy on a subsequent day. The penalty for a false-positive call at noncathartic CTC is amplified because it leads to an unnecessary invasive colonoscopy (and second preparation) that likely could have been avoided with the standard cathartic CTC approach. Finally, the accuracy will be lower, because both false negatives (polyps obscured by stool) and false positives (stool masquerading as polyps) would almost certainly increase in a low-prevalence setting. Nonetheless, because it may bring in otherwise resistant patients, a noncathartic CTC option might be a useful alternative for those unwilling to take laxatives.

Certain diagnostic scenarios require a different approach to bowel preparation compared with the screening setting. Same-day CTC following incomplete OC has provided challenges in terms of adequate contrast tagging.[34] In general, deferring the CTC examination to allow for a standard bowel preparation yields a much higher-quality study relative to a same-day CTC with salvage oral contrast.[34] Other factors that affect the decision to perform same-day CTC after failed OC include the perceived fidelity of the preparation, the colonic segment reached, and whether a "deep" biopsy was performed. When same-day CTC is pursued, a 30-mL oral dose of iohexol or diatrizoate is administered after the patient has recovered from sedation, and CTC is performed about 2 hours later. The decision to perform CTC with intravenous (IV) contrast should be considered in symptomatic elderly or frail patients for whom excluding cancer (colonic or extracolonic) is a primary goal. In such cases, a less aggressive bowel preparation will generally suffice.

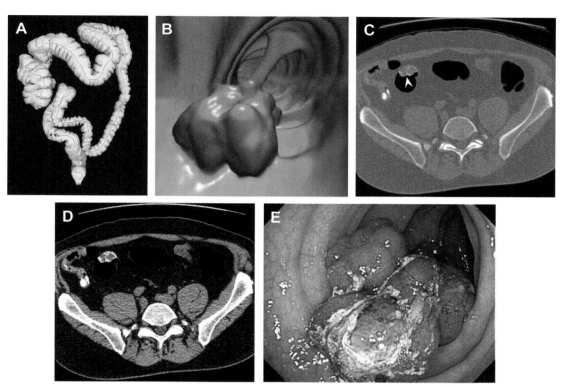

Fig. 2. Large pedunculated tubulovillous adenoma (with high-grade dysplasia) at CTC screening in 54-year-old asymptomatic man. 3D colon map (*A*) shows the sigmoid location of a large 2.8-cm pedunculated polyp, which is demonstrated at 3D (*B*) and 2D (*C*, *D*) CTC images (*arrowhead*). Note the prominent surface coating of oral contrast, which corresponds to the mucus cap seen at same-day OC (*E*).

For patients on warfarin or clopidogrel, the author suggests that patients continue these medications unless their referring provider specifically instructs them otherwise. The relatively low prevalence of large polyps or masses that would necessitate invasive colonoscopy generally does not warrant stopping these medications to allow for same-day polypectomy. For diabetic patients, they are asked that they discuss medication management and frequency of blood sugar testing before CTC with their doctor. UWHC also asks that patients who are otherwise eligible for same-day colonoscopy stop all nonsteroidal anti-inflammatory (NSAID) medications 5 days before their CTC examination. Although these medications will not affect the CTC study, it could impact subsequent colonoscopy. Unlike anticoagulation therapy, short-term stoppage of NSAIDs is generally safe and does not require physician oversight. All of these considerations are included in the printed instructions that are found within the patient's preparation kit.

Colonic Distention

As with bowel preparation, adequate luminal distension of the colon is critical to a successful CTC study. UWHC's distention protocol has evolved and improved over time, resulting in inadequate segmental distention in less than 1% of cases.[35] The use of automated low-pressure carbon dioxide (CO_2) delivery is clearly preferred over manual room air insufflation.[18,36,37] Nearly all early reports of perforation at CTC involved the use of manual staff-controlled room air insufflation in symptomatic patients, whereas the risk of perforation with automated CO_2 delivery likely approaches zero for asymptomatic screening.[13] With regard to both study quality (ie, degree of distention) and after-procedural discomfort, the author has shown that automated CO_2 is superior to the manual room air technique.[36,37] The continuous low-pressure delivery provided with automated CO_2 reduces spasm and discomfort and provides better distention in segments with advanced diverticular disease. The much more rapid resorption of CO_2 through the colon wall (up to 150 times faster than room air) accounts for the improved comfort immediately following the procedure. Furthermore, UWHC's CT technologists unanimously prefer automated CO_2 over staff- or patient-controlled room air insufflation.[37] The decreased operator dependence with automated CO_2 results in better and more consistent distention with less variability among technologists. For these reasons, the CO_2 device is recommended, albeit the additional cost may be somewhat prohibitive for practices with a very low CTC volume. Rarely, manual room air insufflation may be needed to adequately distend the colon in morbidly obese patients when low-pressure CO_2 fails, although bilateral decubitus positioning is another option.

There are several reasons spasmolytics are not used in the author's practice.[37] Several studies evaluating the effect of glucagon on colonic distension at CTC have found mixed but largely negative results, likely due in part to relaxation of the ileocecal valve. The need for needle administration of a drug adds invasiveness and patient discomfort, creates an opportunity for additional side effects, increases examination duration, and increases overall study costs. As mentioned above, nondiagnostic segmental distention is so uncommon with UWHC's current distention protocol that the need for spasmolytics is quite limited regardless. Finally, even if a net benefit exists for using hyoscine-N-butylbromide, this agent is not available for use in the United States.

UWHC has refined their protocol for colonic distention through years of observational experiences and valuable input from their CT technologists. To maintain efficiency, they have trained their CT technologists to independently acquire the entire CTC examination, including placement of the rectal catheter, assessment of distention quality, and decision as to whether an additional decubitus series is needed. The CTC radiologist is only consulted for difficult or unusual situations, allowing more time for image interpretation. The technologist first inquires about the patient's perspective regarding the fidelity of the preparation. However, regardless of this perception, the preparation is generally adequate as long as the instructions were followed (and even in most cases where deviations occurred). Immediately before the examination, the patient is encouraged to use the restroom to minimize rectal fluid.

UWHC's distention protocol is summarized in **Box 1**. Following rectal catheter placement, the patient remains in the left lateral decubitus position for the initial 1.5 L of CO_2 delivered by the automated device. To reduce the transient discomfort related to early rectal spasm, the equilibrium pressure is decreased from the maximum setting (25 mm Hg) down to 17 to 20 mm Hg. The patient is then placed in the right lateral decubitus position until about 3 L has been delivered in total, followed by supine positioning until a steady-state equilibrium has been reached, at which time the initial

---

Box 1
University of Wisconsin Hospital and Clinics colonic distention protocol with automated CO_2

- Catheter inserted with patient in left lateral decubitus (LLD) position and balloon inflated
- Installation pressure initiated at 17 to 20 mm Hg (can slowly increase to 25 mm Hg)
- Fill to 1.5 L in LLD position, then turn to right lateral decubitus (RLD) position
- Fill to 3.0 L in RLD position
- Turn supine and acquire scout (at equilibrium pressure)
- If adequate, initiate supine MDCT scan in end-expiration
- Turn prone, repeat scout, (deflate balloon), and scan prone series
- Assess need for additional decubitus series (by online review of 2D images)

---

scout view is obtained. The positional changes help minimize under-distention related to a fluid block or bowel kink. Before scanning in the prone position, the technologist deflates the catheter balloon to provide better evaluation of the low rectum, where interpretive pitfalls are common.[38,39] The supine and prone scans are acquired at end-expiration to raise the diaphragm and allow more room for the splenic flexure and transverse colon. It is also important to acquire the CT images at equilibrium pressure to ensure active replacement of CO_2. Of note, the total volume of CO_2 "dispensed" varies widely because of actual anatomic differences,[40] but also from variable degrees of ileocecal valve reflux, loss around the catheter, and continuous colonic resorption. Therefore, the final volume reading has relatively little meaning and can range from 2 to 3 L to more than 10 L.

Although the CT scout view provides a rough indication of colonic distention, it is unreliable for excluding focal areas of inadequate distention, especially in the sigmoid and descending colon. Rather, the 2-dimensional (2D) cross-sectional images must be reviewed online at the console to ensure that there are no areas of focal collapse or near-collapse involving the same point on both the supine and the prone images, which would necessitate a lateral decubitus series. UWHC's CT technologists are trained to recognize inadequate distention by review of the cross-sectional images while the patient remains on the scanner gantry. Because inadequate distention nearly always affects the left colon, an additional right lateral decubitus position is generally obtained, which usually provides the best distention.[41,42] In the rare cases where distention remains inadequate after the decubitus series, the group at UWHC may offer the patient same-day unsedated flexible sigmoidoscopy, versus shorter-term interval follow-up.

Multidetector Computed Tomographic Scanning

Given the forgiving nondynamic nature of CTC, state-of-the-art imaging can be achieved with nearly any MDCT scanner. UWHC's CTC scanning protocol is shown in **Table 2**. Given the nature of the soft tissue–air interface for polyp detection at CTC, the radiation dose can be significantly lowered from the usual diagnostic levels. With the use of more advanced iterative reconstruction algorithms, sub-milliSievert CTC has become a reality.[43] However, dose reduction should not be pushed to a level where diagnostic ability is impacted, because the very small theoretic risk of low-dose radiation exposure is clearly outweighed by the actual risk of not being screened for CRC.[44,45] Because of the high diagnostic accuracy of CTC screening when oral contrast tagging and 3D polyp detection are used, routine use of IV contrast is not indicated for asymptomatic screening. In addition to the thin-section (1.25 mm) source data used for polyp detection, the author also reconstructs a separate supine series of 5-mm-thick images at 3-mm intervals to decrease image noise and simplify review for extracolonic findings.[46–49]

CT COLONOGRAPHY INTERPRETATION

Lesion detection, confirmation, and reporting are important components of CTC interpretation. In addition to reporting all potentially relevant colorectal findings, it is imperative to understand what not to report (ie, isolated diminutive lesions). From a programmatic perspective, it is also important to track screening results, to include having a mechanism in place to review discordant cases. Interpretation of extracolonic findings at CTC is another key topic but beyond the scope of this review.[11,35,46–53]

Lesion Detection and Confirmation

UWHC has tested a broad variety of CTC workstations from different vendors over the years, but the Viatronix V3D is the only system that the author's group has ever used for patient

Table 2 University of Wisconsin Hospital and Clinics multidetector computed tomographic protocol for screening computed tomographic colonography		
Patient Position	Supine	Prone
Detector coverage (mm)	40	40
Detector rows	64	64
Detector configuration	64 × 0.625	64 × 0.625
Scan FOV	Large body	Large body
Pitch	1.375	1.375
Speed (mm/rot)	55.0	55.0
Rotation time (s)	0.5	0.5
kV	120	120
Smart mA range	30–340	30–340
Noise index	25	60
Reconstruction 1		
Reconstruction type	Standard	Standard
Window/Level	2000/0	2000/0
Recon option	Plus	Plus
Recon option	IQ Enhance	IQ Enhance
Slice thickness (mm)	1.25	1.25
Interval (mm)	0.625	0.625
Recon 2 (Extracolonic)		
Reconstruction type	Standard	—
Window/Level	400/50	—
Recon option	Plus	—
Slice thickness (mm)	5.0	—
Interval (mm)	3.0	—

For typical 64-detector-row GE scanner; scout protocol not shown.

care.[54] This 3D system was the first to be clinically validated for colorectal screening and to receive US Food and Drug Administration (FDA) approval for screening. It allows for a highly effective and time-efficient primary 3D polyp search, in addition to several other diagnostic advantages. The CT source images are sent to the V3D system, which then segments out the gas-filled intestine and generates an automated centerline for navigation (**Figs. 2** and **3**). Ever since the DoD trial, UWHC has used a biphasic 3D-2D interpretive approach, including both a primary 2D and a 3D evaluation. The 2D survey can assess the quality of colonic preparation

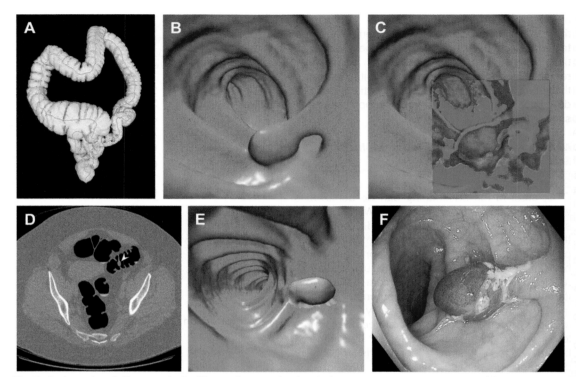

Fig. 3. Pedunculated 12-mm tubulovillous adenoma (with HGD) at CTC screening in 59-year-old asymptomatic woman. 3D colon map (*A*) shows the sigmoid location of a pedunculated 12-mm polyp, which is demonstrated at 3D endoluminal CTC without (*B*) and with (*C*) translucency rendering. 2D CTC (*D*) confirms a pedunculated soft tissue lesion (*arrowhead*). CAD detected the lesion (*E*), which was confirmed and removed at same-day CTC (*F*).

and distention as well as identify obvious masses and submerged polyps. However, most polyp detection occurs on the 3D endoluminal evaluation, where the increased conspicuity renders most polyps readily identifiable.[55] For the minority of cases where abundant adherent residual stool or luminal fluid is present, primary 2D evaluation serves a more vital role. For all suspected 3D-detected lesions, the 2D view is essential for confirmation.

The 3D endoluminal fly-through provides a highly effective detection mechanism for focal colorectal lesions (see **Figs. 1–3**). The lack of easy, automated centerline navigation has been a major drawback with most other CTC systems, but continued improvement has been shown by some. UWHC's primary 3D review for the DoD trial initially entailed bidirectional fly-through using a 90° field-of-view (FOV) angle on both supine and prone series. However, they have since found that widening the FOV angle to 120° allows greatly improved mucosal visualization, generally allowing for one-way fly-through of each series (rectum-to-cecum on supine and

cecum-to-rectum on prone) without sacrificing polyp detection.[56] Bidirectional fly-through at 120° on at least one series remains prudent, however, for cases with suboptimal distention. The V3D system continually monitors and updates what portion of the endoluminal surface covered, which not only increases reader confidence but also marks where one left off if interrupted during interpretation. On average, 77% and 94% of the luminal surface are seen with unidirectional flight and bidirectional flight, respectively, with 90° FOV.[57] With 120° FOV, the unidirectional coverage increases to approximately 90%. In addition, the "missed region tool" on V3D allows the reader to rapidly click through the mucosal patches not seen during routine navigation, generally increasing luminal coverage to 98% to 99%. The typical flight time from rectum to cecum (or vice versa) along the centerline is approximately 1 minute, not including the additional time needed to interrogate suspected lesions.

Rapid interrogation of potential lesions detected on 3D can be rapidly accomplished with translucency rendering, which provides information on the internal density of a lesion.[58] When used properly, the translucency rendering tool can decrease interpretation time by reducing the need for 2D confirmation for obvious false positives, particularly tagged stool. However, pitfalls exist and 2D correlation is ultimately how any suspicious 3D lesion is confirmed (see Figs. 1–3).[38] Although the V3D system has always allowed for digital fluid subtraction of opacified luminal fluid,[59] the author's group has disabled this function ever since the DoD trial ended.[18,60] In their opinion, the artifacts created by electronic cleansing outweigh the benefits, greatly complicating and prolonging the 3D evaluation. With their current preparation, combined supine-prone 3D endoluminal evaluation of the gas-filled colon without electronic cleansing reliably covers the entire mucosal surface through positional fluid shifts. For most screening CTC cases, the entire study can be read in less than 10 minutes, but difficult or frankly positive cases will of course take longer.

When a suspicious lesion measuring 5 to 6 mm or greater is detected on 3D (or 2D) and confirmed to be composed of soft tissue on 2D, an electronic bookmark is placed on the colon map (see Figs. 2 and 3). The vast majority of actual polyps can also be identified on the alternate supine or prone view, which greatly increases overall diagnostic confidence. Those at UWHC have found computer-aided detection (CAD) to be useful in both the research[61–66] and clinical settings,[67] because it can provide further assurance and diagnostic confidence (see Fig. 3). CAD demonstrates excellent sensitivity for detecting relevant polyps, but the extremely low specificity, which essentially approached zero, requires that experienced CTC readers sift through the CAD marks, not novice readers. Unknown to many is that some third-party payers will reimburse for CAD at CTC.[67] The overall positive predictive value or concordance rate for CTC-detected lesions at subsequent colonoscopy is greater than 90%, and even greater when the reader confidence is high.[32,68] Accurate linear measurement of polyps is an important task that requires some thought. The 2D measurement tends to underestimate polyp size if not perfectly aligned with the long axis, whereas the 3D view can overestimate size in some cases. As such, the author has found it useful to take both 2D and 3D measurements into account before arriving at a final value.[69] In the future, polyp volume assessment may play a more prominent role because it is a more accurate indicator of actual soft tissue mass present and more sensitive for detecting interval change.[70,71]

Lesion Reporting and Management Algorithm

A screening CTC study is considered positive when any lesion $\geq$6 mm is detected, although the findings of greatest clinical significance are large polyps ($\geq$10 mm) and masses ($\geq$3 cm). UWHC offers same-day OC to all eligible patients with a positive CTC study, which avoids the need for separate bowel preparation.[7,16,33] However, because the inherent neoplastic risk of 1 or 2 small polyps (6–9 mm) detected at CTC are likely outweighed by the procedural risks associated with colonoscopic polypectomy,[72] they also offer the option of CTC surveillance at 3 years for this C-RADS C2 category.[73,74] They work in close collaboration with their gastroenterology colleagues, particularly with regard to same-day polypectomies, providing them with the relevant images on PACS, including the polyp location on the 3D map, 3D endoluminal projections, and corresponding 2D images.

The CTC dictation lends itself well to structured reporting. UWHC's dictation template includes subheadings for study indication, examination technique, colorectal findings, extracolonic findings, and final impression (Box 2). They do not explicitly report C-RADS categories in the report to clinicians, because they feel it unnecessarily complicates the communication, but they do record them in their internal database. For each colorectal lesion detected at CTC, they record the linear size, segmental location, polyp morphology (pedunculated, sessile, or flat), and diagnostic confidence score (3-point scale) for each polyp. Diagnostic confidence correlates well with the likelihood of finding a corresponding lesion at CTC and is useful for program quality assurance.[68] Specific note is also made of polyps located on the backside of folds, which are more easily missed at OC.[75,76] Special attention for relatively flat or nonpolypoid colorectal lesions has led to improved detection at CTC.[27,29–31,77] Careful review is particularly important for right-sided serrated lesions, because these indolent yet subtle lesions often demonstrate surface coating of oral contrast at CTC.[28,78,79]

Approximately 85% to 90% of screening CTC 2examinations are negative for polyps $\geq$6 mm,[7,16,35] and repeat routine colorectal screening is recommended in 5 years. Nonreporting of potential isolated diminutive lesions is justified to prevent unnecessary interventions, and this practice has been clinically validated.[77,79,80] This practice is explicitly described in the dictation template (see Box 2). For individuals who are found to be negative at follow-up screening CTC at 5 or more years, subsequent screening can likely be extended out to 10 years.[79]

Box 2
University of Wisconsin Hospital and Clinics dictation template for screening computed tomographic colonography

Indication

Routine CRC screening. [Modify as needed][a]

Technique

The patient underwent standard virtual colonoscopy bowel preparation the day before the examination, consisting of oral magnesium citrate, CT barium, and water-soluble iodinated contrast (iohexol). Following automated CO_2 insufflation per rectum, supine and prone CT images were obtained without IV contrast. Images were sent to the Viatronix V3D workstation for combined 2D–3D evaluation of the colon for polyps. Interpretation was supplemented by the use of an FDA-approved version of CAD. CT-derived dual-energy X-ray absorptiometry (DXA)-equivalent bone mineral density evaluation of the left femoral neck was also performed.

Findings
Colon

[Describe quality or adequacy of bowel preparation and distention.]

[Comment of presence of colonic redundancy, diverticular disease, and so forth.]

[Report all colorectal polyps ≥6 mm, including size, morphology, and segmental location; consider adding additional information, such as diagnostic confidence, location behind a fold. Emphasize large polyps and masses.]

Note: CT colonography is not intended for the detection of isolated diminutive colonic polyps (ie, tiny polyps ≤5 mm), the presence or absence of which will not change management of the patient. In addition, digital rectal examination is recommended in conjunction with CTC to complete evaluation of the anorectal region.

Extracolonic

Abdominal aortic aneurysm (AAA) screening: No aortoiliac aneurysms are present [Modify as needed].

Osteoporosis screening: DXA-equivalent T score of the left femoral neck is [X.X].

Note: Extracolonic evaluation is limited by the low-dose CT technique and lack of IV contrast.

Impression

[1. Summarize relevant colorectal findings and recommendations.]

[2. Note any significant extracolonic findings and recommendations.]

  [a] Bracketed portions are either comments or require more patient-specific language.

Quality assurance is a critical component of any successful screening program. Those at UWHC closely track their performance at CTC screening, including overall positive rate, nondiagnostic rate, OC referral rate, and CTC-OC concordance rate for polypectomy.[35] For all discordant cases where a nondiminutive lesion called at CTC is not confirmed at subsequent OC, they formally review the case (with 2 CTC radiologists not involved in the original interpretation). After prolonged follow-up, a substantial proportion of discordant cases concerning for possible OC false negatives (as opposed to CTC false-positives) is ultimately proven to be real.[76] Therefore, the term "concordance rate" is more appropriate than "positive predictive value" in this setting. Those at UWHC also track their complication rate but, to date, have yet to encounter a significant complication at CTC.

It is also important to have an appreciation for the sensitivity of CTC for detecting relevant lesions, especially CRC and advanced adenomas, relative to other available screening tests (Table 3). In general, CTC rivals OC in terms of detection sensitivity and is generally higher than the various stool- and serum-based tests, especially for advanced adenomas. Detection of advanced adenomas is critical because it is this preventive

Table 3
Sensitivity of colorectal cancer screening tests for advanced neoplasia

Screening Test	Sensitivity	
	CRC, %	Advanced Adenoma, %
CTC	96[14]	67–94[81] (≥10 mm) 73–98[81] (≥6 mm)
OC	95[14]	89–98[81] (≥10 mm) 75–93[81] (≥6 mm)
FSIG	58–75[82,83]	77–86[83,84]
FIT	73–96[81]	22–40[81]
FIT-DNA	92[81]	42[81]
mSEPT9 DNA	48[85]	11[85]

Abbreviations: FIT, fecal immunohistochemical test; FIT-DNA, multitarget stool DNA (Cologuard); FSIG, flexible sigmoidoscopy; mSEPT9 DNA, serology test (epi ProColon).
   Adapted from the UW Health Preventive Care Guidelines. © 2017 University of Wisconsin Hospitals and Clinics Authority. All rights reserved. Printed with permission; and *Data from* Refs.[14,80–85]

aspect of CRC screening that provides much of its value at the population level. Specificity of OC and CTC for advanced neoplasia is also considerably higher than the other tests, but direct comparison is more difficult as the stool- and serum-based tests generally report specificity according to cancer, whereas OC and CTC generally report according to both polyps and cancer.

SUMMARY

Despite being readily preventable, CRC remains the second-leading cause of cancer deaths. If preventive screening tests that effectively detect advanced adenomas and early cancers were broadly applied, this situation could be easily reversed. CT colonography reflects an ideal balance of minimal invasiveness with high-level performance, assuming all facets of the examination are appropriately addressed. Nonetheless, this promising screening test remains grossly underused. This review of the technical and interpretive approaches used by one successful CTC screening program may serve as a roadmap to other groups looking to get involved.

REFERENCES

1. Siegel R, DeSantis C, Jemal A. Colorectal cancer statistics, 2014. CA Cancer J Clin 2014;64:104–17.
2. Pickhardt PJ. Emerging stool-based and blood-based non-invasive DNA tests for colorectal cancer screening: the importance of cancer prevention in addition to cancer detection. Abdom Radiol (NY) 2016;41:1441–4.
3. Levin B, Lieberman DA, McFarland B, et al, American Cancer Society Colorectal Cancer Advisory Group, US Multi-Society Task Force, American College of Radiology Colon Cancer Committee. Screening and surveillance for the early detection of colorectal cancer and adenomatous polyps, 2008: a joint guideline from the American Cancer Society, the US Multi-Society Task Force on Colorectal Cancer, and the American College of Radiology. CA Cancer J Clin 2008;58:130–60.
4. Bibbins-Domingo K, Grossman DC, Curry SJ, et al. Screening for colorectal cancer: US preventive services task force recommendation statement. JAMA 2016;315:2564–75.
5. Pickhardt PJ. CT colonography for population screening: ready for prime time? Dig Dis Sci 2015;60:647–59.
6. Pickhardt PJ, Choi JR, Hwang I, et al. Computed tomographic virtual colonoscopy to screen for colorectal neoplasia in asymptomatic adults. N Engl J Med 2003;349:2191–200.
7. Kim DH, Pickhardt PJ, Taylor AJ, et al. CT colonography versus colonoscopy for the detection of advanced neoplasia. N Engl J Med 2007;357:1403–12.
8. Johnson CD, Chen MH, Toledano AY, et al. Accuracy of CT colonography for detection of large adenomas and cancers. N Engl J Med 2008;359:1207–17.
9. Pyenson B, Pickhardt PJ, Sawhney TG, et al. Medicare cost of colorectal cancer screening: CT colonography vs. optical colonoscopy. Abdom Imaging 2015;40:2966–76.
10. Pooler BD, Baumel MJ, Cash BD, et al. Screening CT colonography: multicenter survey of patient experience, preference, and potential impact on adherence. Am J Roentgenol 2012;198:1361–6.
11. Hassan C, Pickhardt PJ, Laghi A, et al. Computed tomographic colonography to screen for colorectal cancer, extracolonic cancer, and aortic aneurysm: model simulation with cost-effectiveness analysis. Arch Intern Med 2008;168:696–705.
12. Pickhardt PJ, Hassan C, Laghi A, et al. Cost-effectiveness of colorectal cancer screening with computed tomography colonography: the impact of not reporting diminutive lesions. Cancer 2007;109:2213–21.
13. Pickhardt PJ. Incidence of colonic perforation at CT colonography: review of existing data and implications for screening of asymptomatic adults. Radiology 2006;239:313–6.
14. Pickhardt PJ, Hassan C, Halligan S, et al. Colorectal cancer: CT colonography and colonoscopy for detection—systematic review and meta-analysis. Radiology 2011;259:393–405.
15. Ozel B, Pickhardt PJ, Kim DH, et al. Accuracy of routine nontargeted CT without colonography

technique for the detection of large colorectal polyps and cancer. Dis Colon Rectum 2010;53: 911–8.

16. Pickhardt PJ, Taylor AJ, Kim DH, et al. Screening for colorectal neoplasia with CT colonography: initial experience from the 1st year of coverage by third-party payers. Radiology 2006;241:417–25.

17. Smith MA, Weiss JM, Potvien A, et al. Insurance coverage for CT colonography screening: impact on overall colorectal cancer screening rates. Radiology 2017;284(3):717–24.

18. Pickhardt PJ. Screening CT colonography: how I do it. AJR Am J Roentgenol 2007;189:290–8.

19. Pickhardt PJ, Taylor AJ, Johnson GL, et al. Building a CT colonography program: necessary ingredients for reimbursement and clinical success. Radiology 2005;235:17–20.

20. Pickhardt PJ, Kim DH. CT colonography: principles and practice of virtual colonoscopy. Philadelphia: Saunders; 2010.

21. Kim DH, Pickhardt PJ, Hinshaw JL, et al. Prospective blinded trial comparing 45-mL and 90-mL doses of oral sodium phosphate for bowel preparation before computed tomographic colonography. J Comput Assist Tomogr 2007;31:53–8.

22. Van Uitert RL, Summers RM, White JM, et al. Temporal and multiinstitutional quality assessment of CT colonography. AJR Am J Roentgenol 2008;191: 1503–8.

23. Borden ZS, Pickhardt PJ, Kim DH, et al. Bowel preparation for CT colonography: blinded comparison of magnesium citrate and sodium phosphate for catharsis. Radiology 2010;254:138–44.

24. Bannas P, Bakke J, del Rio AM, et al. Intra-individual comparison of magnesium citrate and sodium phosphate for bowel preparation at CT colonography: automated volumetric analysis of residual fluid for quality assessment. Clin Radiol 2014;69:1171–7.

25. Johnson B, Hinshaw JL, Robbins JB, et al. Objective and subjective intrapatient comparison of iohexol versus diatrizoate for bowel preparation quality at CT colonography. Am J Roentgenol 2016;206:1202–7.

26. O'Connor SD, Summers RM, Choi JR, et al. Oral contrast adherence to polyps on CT colonography. J Comput Assist Tomogr 2006;30:51–7.

27. Kim DH, Hinshaw JL, Lubner MG, et al. Contrast coating for the surface of flat polyps at CT colonography: a marker for detection. Eur Radiol 2014;24: 940–6.

28. Kim DH, Matkowskyj KA, Lubner MG, et al. Serrated polyps at CT colonography: prevalence and characteristics of the serrated polyp spectrum. Radiology 2016;280(2):455–63.

29. Pickhardt PJ, Lam VP, Weiss JM, et al. Carpet lesions detected at CT colonography: clinical, imaging, and pathologic features. Radiology 2014;270: 435–43.

30. Pickhardt PJ, Kim DH, Robbins JB. Flat (nonpolypoid) colorectal lesions identified at CT colonography in a US screening population. Acad Radiol 2010;17:784–90.

31. Pickhardt PJ, Nugent PA, Choi JR, et al. Flat colorectal lesions in asymptomatic adults: implications for screening with CT virtual colonoscopy. Am J Roentgenol 2004;183:1343–7.

32. Pickhardt PJ, Wise SM, Kim DH. Positive predictive value for polyps detected at screening CT colonography. Eur Radiol 2010;20:1651–6.

33. Pickhardt PJ. Colonic preparation for computed tomographic colonography: understanding the relative advantages and disadvantages of a noncathartic approach. Mayo Clin Proc 2007;82:659–61.

34. Theis J, Kim DH, Lubner MG, et al. CT colonography after incomplete optical colonoscopy: bowel preparation quality at same-day vs. deferred examination. Abdom Radiol (NY) 2016;41:10–8.

35. Pooler BD, Kim DH, Lam VP, et al. CT colonography reporting and data system (C-RADS): benchmark values from a clinical screening program. AJR Am J Roentgenol 2014;202:1232–7.

36. Patrick JL, Bakke JR, Bannas P, et al. Objective volumetric comparison of room air versus carbon dioxide for colonic distention at screening CT colonography. Abdom Imaging 2015;40:231–6.

37. Shinners TJ, Pickhardt PJ, Taylor AJ, et al. Patient-controlled room air insufflation versus automated carbon dioxide delivery for CT colonography. Am J Roentgenol 2006;186:1491–6.

38. Pickhardt PJ, Kim DH. CT colonography: pitfalls in interpretation. Radiol Clin North Am 2013;51:69–88.

39. Pickhardt PJ, Choi JR. Adenomatous polyp obscured by small-caliber rectal catheter at low-dose CT colonography: a rare diagnostic pitfall. Am J Roentgenol 2005;184:1581–3.

40. Khashab MA, Pickhardt PJ, Kim DH, et al. Colorectal anatomy in adults at computed tomography colonography: normal distribution and the effect of age, sex, and body mass index. Endoscopy 2009;41:674–8.

41. Pickhardt PJ, Bakke J, Kuo J, et al. Volumetric analysis of colonic distention according to patient position at ct colonography: diagnostic value of the right lateral decubitus series. Am J Roentgenol 2014;203:W623–8.

42. Buchach CM, Kim DH, Pickhardt PJ. Performing an additional decubitus series at CT colonography. Abdom Imaging 2011;36:538–44.

43. Lubner MG, Pooler BD, Kitchin DR, et al. Sub-milli-Sievert (sub-mSv) CT colonography: a prospective comparison of image quality and polyp conspicuity at reduced-dose versus standard-dose imaging. Eur Radiol 2015;25:2089–102.

44. Brenner DJ, Elliston CD. Estimated radiation risks potentially associated with full-body CT screening. Radiology 2004;232:735–8.

45. Radiation risk in perspective: position statement of the Health Physics Society. Health Physics Society; 2010.

46. Pickhardt PJ, Hanson ME, Vanness DJ, et al. Unsuspected extracolonic findings at screening CT colonography: clinical and economic impact. Radiology 2008;249:151–9.

47. Pickhardt PJ, Taylor AJ. Extracolonic findings identified in asymptomatic adults at screening CT colonography. Am J Roentgenol 2006;186:718–28.

48. Pooler BD, Kim DH, Pickhardt PJ. Potentially important extracolonic findings at screening CT colonography: incidence and outcomes data from a clinical screening program. AJR Am J Roentgenol 2016;206(2):313–8.

49. Pooler BD, Kim DH, Pickhardt PJ. Indeterminate but likely unimportant extracolonic findings at screening CT colonography (C-RADS category E3): incidence and outcomes data from a clinical screening program. AJR Am J Roentgenol 2016; 207:996–1001.

50. Pickhardt PJ, Hassan C, Laghi A, et al. CT colonography to screen for colorectal cancer and aortic aneurysm in the Medicare population: cost-effectiveness analysis. AJR Am J Roentgenol 2009; 192:1332–40.

51. Kim DH, Pickhardt PJ, Hanson ME, et al. CT colonography: performance and program outcome measures in an older screening population. Radiology 2010;254:493–500.

52. Pickhardt PJ, Kim DH, Meiners RJ, et al. Colorectal and extracolonic cancers detected at screening CT colonography in 10,286 asymptomatic adults. Radiology 2010;255:83–8.

53. Ziemlewicz TJ, Binkley N, Pickhardt PJ. Opportunistic osteoporosis screening: addition of quantitative CT bone mineral density evaluation to CT colonography. J Am Coll Radiol 2015;12:1036–41.

54. Pickhardt PJ. Three-dimensional endoluminal CT colonography (virtual colonoscopy): comparison of three commercially available systems. Am J Roentgenol 2003;181:1599–606.

55. Pickhardt PJ, Lee AD, Taylor AJ, et al. Primary 2D versus primary 3D polyp detection at screening CT Colonography. Am J Roentgenol 2007;189:1451–6.

56. Pickhardt PJ, Schumacher C, Kim DH. Polyp detection at 3-dimensional endoluminal computed tomography colonography: sensitivity of one-way fly-through at 120 degrees field-of-view angle. J Comput Assist Tomogr 2009;33:631–5.

57. Pickhardt PJ, Taylor AJ, Gopal DV. Surface visualization at 3D endoluminal CT colonography: degree of coverage and implications for polyp detection. Gastroenterology 2006;130:1582–7.

58. Pickhardt PJ. Translucency rendering in 3D endoluminal CT colonography: a useful tool for increasing polyp specificity and decreasing interpretation time. Am J Roentgenol 2004;183:429–36.

59. Pickhardt PJ, Choi JHR. Electronic cleansing and stool tagging in CT colonography: advantages and pitfalls with primary three-dimensional evaluation. Am J Roentgenol 2003;181:799–805.

60. Pickhardt PJ. Differential diagnosis of polypoid lesions seen at CT colonography (virtual colonoscopy) - author's response. Radiographics 2004; 24:1558–9.

61. Summers RM, Franaszek M, Miller MT, et al. Computer-aided detection of polyps on oral contrast-enhanced CT colonography. Am J Roentgenol 2005;184:105–8.

62. Summers RM, Yao JH, Pickhardt PJ, et al. Computed tomographic virtual colonoscopy computer-aided polyp detection in a screening population. Gastroenterology 2005;129:1832–44.

63. Petrick N, Haider M, Summers RM, et al. CT colonography with computer-aided detection as a second reader: observer performance study. Radiology 2008;246:148–56.

64. Summers RM, Handwerker LR, Pickhardt PJ, et al. Performance of a previously validated CT colonography computer-aided detection system in a new patient population. AJR Am J Roentgenol 2008; 191:168–74.

65. Lawrence EM, Pickhardt PJ, Kim DH, et al. Colorectal polyps: stand-alone performance of computer-aided detection in a large asymptomatic screening population. Radiology 2010;256:791–8.

66. Mang T, Bogoni L, Salganicoff M, et al. Computer-aided detection of colorectal polyps in CT colonography with and without fecal tagging a stand-alone evaluation. Invest Radiol 2012;47:99–108.

67. Ziemlewicz TJ, Kim DH, Hinshaw JL, et al. Computer-aided detection of colorectal polyps at CTC: prospective clinical performance and third-party reimbursement. AJR Am J Roentgenol 2017; 208(6):1244–8.

68. Pickhardt PJ, Choi JR, Nugent PA, et al. The effect of diagnostic confidence on the probability of optical colonoscopic confirmation of potential polyps detected on CT colonography: prospective assessment in 1,339 asymptomatic adults. Am J Roentgenol 2004;183:1661–5.

69. Pickhardt PJ, Lee AD, McFarland EG, et al. Linear polyp measurement at CT colonography: in vitro and in vivo comparison of two-dimensional and three-dimensional displays. Radiology 2005;236:872–8.

70. Pickhardt PJ, Lehman VT, Winter TC, et al. Polyp volume versus linear size measurements at CT colonography: implications for noninvasive surveillance of unresected colorectal lesions. Am J Roentgenol 2006;186:1605–10.

71. Pickhardt PJ, Kim DH, Pooler BD, et al. Assessment of volumetric growth rates of small colorectal polyps

with CT colonography: a longitudinal study of natural history. Lancet Oncol 2013;14:711–20.

72. Pickhardt PJ, Kim DH. Colorectal cancer screening with CT colonography: key concepts regarding polyp prevalence, size, histology, morphology, and natural history. Am J Roentgenol 2009;193:40–6.

73. Pickhardt PJ, Hassan C, Laghi A, et al. Clinical management of small (6- to 9-mm) polyps detected at screening CT colonography: a cost-effectiveness analysis. AJR Am J Roentgenol 2008;191:1509–16.

74. Pickhardt PJ, Hassan C, Laghi A, et al. Small and diminutive polyps detected at screening CT colonography: a decision analysis for referral to colonoscopy. Am J Roentgenol 2008;190:136–44.

75. Pickhardt PJ, Nugent PA, Mysliwiec PA, et al. Location of adenomas missed by optical colonoscopy. Ann Intern Med 2004;141:352–9.

76. Pooler BD, Kim DH, Weiss JM, et al. Colorectal polyps missed with optical colonoscopy despite previous detection and localization with CT colonography. Radiology 2016;278(2):422–9.

77. Pickhardt PJ, Kim DH. Performance of CT colonography for detecting small, diminutive, and flat polyps. Gastrointest Endosc Clin N Am 2010;20:209–26.

78. Kim DH, Matkowskyj KA, Pickhardt PJ. Serrated polyps are detected at CT colonography: clinical observations over the past decade and results from CTC-based screening of average risk adults. Abdom Radiol (NY) 2016;41:1445–7.

79. Pickhardt PJ, Pooler BD, Mbah I, et al. Colorectal findings at repeat CT colonography screening after initial CT colonography screening negative for polyps larger than 5 mm. Radiology 2017;282(1):139–48.

80. Kim DH, Pooler BD, Weiss JM, et al. Five year colorectal cancer outcomes in a large negative CT colonography screening cohort. Eur Radiol 2012;22:1488–94.

81. Lin JS, Piper MA, Perdue LA, et al. Screening for colorectal cancer: updated evidence report and systematic review for the US preventive services task force. JAMA 2016;315(23):2576–94.

82. Imperiale TF, Wagner DR, Lin CY, et al. Risk of advanced proximal neoplasms in asymptomatic adults according to the distal colorectal findings. N Engl J Med 2000;343(3):169–74.

83. Whitlock E, Lin J, Liles E, et al. Screening for colorectal cancer: an updated systematic review. Rockville (MD): Agency for Healthcare Research and Quality; 2008.

84. Lieberman DA, Weiss DG, Bond JH, et al. Use of colonoscopy to screen asymptomatic adults for colorectal cancer. Veterans Affairs Cooperative Study Group 380. N Engl J Med 2000;343(3):162–8.

85. Church TR, Wandell M, Lofton-Day C, et al. Prospective evaluation of methylated SEPT9 in plasma for detection of asymptomatic colorectal cancer. Gut 2014;63(2):317–25.

Screening and Surveillance of Hepatocellular Carcinoma

An Introduction to Ultrasound Liver Imaging Reporting and Data System

David T. Fetzer, MD[a], Shuchi K. Rodgers, MD[b],
Alison C. Harris, MBChB, FRCR, FRCPC[c],
Yuko Kono, MD, PhD[d,e], Ashish P. Wasnik, MD[f],
Aya Kamaya, MD[g,1], Claude Sirlin, MD[h,*,1]

KEYWORDS

- Hepatocellular carcinoma • HCC • Screening • Surveillance • Ultrasound • Reporting

KEY POINTS

- Hepatocellular carcinoma has a high prevalence among populations with cirrhosis, is increasing in incidence, and is associated with significant morbidity and mortality. Therefore, a robust screening and surveillance program is needed.
- Most societies advocate ultrasound as the first-line screening and surveillance modality for at-risk populations, despite variability in sensitivity, which may in part be caused by the inherent user dependence and variability in performance between individuals and sites. A standardized imaging protocol, reporting language, and set of management recommendations may significantly improve patient care; this is the basis behind the American College of Radiology (ACR) Ultrasound Liver Imaging Reporting and Data System (US LI-RADS) for screening and surveillance.
- This article provides an introduction to US LI-RADS, discusses the applicable target population and impact on clinical work flow and patient management, and offers example cases and images.

Disclosures: No author reports relevant commercial or financial conflicts of interest related to the content of this article. The authors disclose the following: speaking and research agreements with Philips Healthcare (D.T. Fetzer); receives royalties from Elsevier (A. Kamaya); industry research grants from Bayer, Guerbet, Siemens, GE, Supersonic, Arterys; research laboratory service agreements with Alexion, AstraZeneca, Bioclinica, BMS, Bracco, Celgene, Fibrogen, Galmed, Genentech, Genzyme, Gilead, Icon, Intercept, Isis, Janssen, NuSirt, Perspectum, Pfizer, Profil, Sanofi, Shire, Synageva, Tobira, Takeda, Virtual Scopics (C. Sirlin).

[a] Department of Radiology, UT Southwestern Medical Center, 5323 Harry Hines Boulevard, Dallas, TX 75390-8896, USA; [b] Department of Radiology, Sidney Kimmel Medical College at Thomas Jefferson University, Einstein Medical Center, 5501 Old York Road, Philadelphia, PA 19141, USA; [c] Department of Radiology, Vancouver General Hospital, 899 West 12th Avenue, Vancouver, British Columbia V5Z 1M9, Canada; [d] Department of Medicine, University of California, San Diego, 200 West Arbor Drive, San Diego, CA 92103, USA; [e] Department of Radiology, University of California, San Diego, 200 West Arbor Drive, San Diego CA 92103, USA; [f] Department of Radiology, University of Michigan Health System, 1500 East Medical Center Drive, Ann Arbor, MI 48109, USA; [g] Department of Radiology, Stanford University, 300 Pasteur Drive, H1307, Stanford, CA 94305, USA; [h] Liver Imaging Group, Department of Radiology, University of California, San Diego, 9500 Gilman Drive, MC 0888, San Diego, CA 92093-0888, USA

[1] Cosenior authors.
* Corresponding author.
E-mail address: csirlin@ucsd.edu

Radiol Clin N Am 55 (2017) 1197–1209
http://dx.doi.org/10.1016/j.rcl.2017.06.012

INTRODUCTION

Hepatocellular carcinoma (HCC) is the fifth most common cancer, and the second most common cause of cancer-related death in the world.[1] More than 80% of HCC cases worldwide are attributed to liver disease related to hepatitis B virus (HBV) and hepatitis C virus (HCV).[2] SEER (Surveillance, Epidemiology, and End Results) registries showed a 3-fold increase in incidence of HCC from 1975 to 2007 in the United States.[3] HCC is the fastest increasing cause of cancer-related death among Americans and in other parts of the world. In 2012, there were 782,000 new cases of HCC worldwide, with 746,000 deaths, resulting in a ratio of mortality to incidence of 0.95.[4]

Survival is poor in most cases because patients are typically diagnosed at a late stage. However, if detected early, HCC potentially may be cured by surgical resection, liver transplant, or local ablation.[5] Advancements in locoregional treatments, such as radiofrequency ablation, microwave ablation, and transcatheter arterial chemoembolization (TACE), have also extended survival of patients with HCC.[5,6] Therefore, a robust screening program is needed for high-risk populations to identify early-stage disease amenable to curative treatment.[7]

SCREENING AND SURVEILLANCE

Screening is an application of a diagnostic test in patients at risk for a disease but in whom there is no a priori reason to specifically suspect that disease is present. Surveillance is the repeated application of the screening test in the population at risk.[8] As described later, the goal of screening/surveillance is to detect suspected disease in at-risk populations, not necessarily to establish a diagnosis; the latter typically requires additional diagnostic testing.

Screening and surveillance is recommended for populations at high risk for HCC to detect suspected HCC at an early stage, thereby improving health outcomes and survival. A risk assessment is required to determine whether screening and surveillance is cost-effective, and in what target population screening and surveillance provides a benefit. Surveillance for HCC is deemed cost-effective if the expected HCC risk exceeds 1.5% per year in patients with cirrhosis, and 0.2% per year in patients with chronic HBV without cirrhosis.[8] The difference in thresholds reflects differences in underlying life expectancy: patients with HBV without cirrhosis are otherwise healthy and are expected to have long lives in the absence of HCC; by comparison, patients with cirrhosis are at risk of dying from liver disease even if HCC does not develop.

Target Population

HCC screening and surveillance is recommended in any patient with cirrhosis irrespective of cause, and in subsets of patients with HBV irrespective of cirrhosis (Box 1).[7–9] Some medical societies also include noncirrhotic chronic HCV carriers with stage 3 fibrosis in their target populations for screening and surveillance. Some populations, such as those with chronic right heart failure, hemochromatosis, or suspected nonalcoholic steatohepatitis, are not officially endorsed as a target population, although may be included in a screening and surveillance population depending on institutional and regional practices and policies. Minor risk factors such as older age, male sex, heavy alcohol use, and smoking do not increase the HCC incidence above the threshold needed to warrant HCC screening or surveillance.

Screening and Surveillance Strategies for Hepatocellular Carcinoma

Many retrospective studies have shown that surveillance resulted in smaller HCC tumor size and an earlier disease stage at initial diagnosis, as well as a survival benefit, compared with nonsurveillance populations.[10–12] Most major hepatology and cancer societies endorse ultrasound (US) for HCC screening and surveillance, based on a single randomized controlled trial[13] and multiple cost-effectiveness studies.[7–10,14,15] Alpha-fetoprotein (AFP) is a commonly used serum test and some societies endorse its use for HCC screening, typically in combination with US.[8,15] However, because of the suboptimal performance, as detailed later, the American Association for the Study of Liver Diseases (AASLD) and European

---

Box 1

Populations for whom hepatocellular carcinoma screening/surveillance is recommended

- Patients with cirrhosis, irrespective of cause
- Chronic HBV carriers in:
  - Asian men more than 40 years of age
  - Asian women more than 50 years of age
  - Africans and North American black people
  - HBV and cirrhosis
  - Family history of HCC

From Bruix J, Sherman M, American Association for the Study of Liver Diseases. Management of hepatocellular carcinoma: an update. Hepatology 2011;53(3):1020–2; with permission.

Association for the Study of the Liver (EASL) stopped endorsing the use of AFP in their most recently published guidelines in 2011 and 2012, respectively.[8,10] New guidelines from these societies are anticipated in the next 1 to 2 years, and the use of AFP may be reconsidered. Rather than US, some centers perform contrast-enhanced computed tomography (CT) or MR imaging for screening and surveillance, although the use of these modalities for this purpose is not considered to be cost-effective and therefore is not endorsed by most societies.

Surveillance Interval

At-risk patients should undergo HCC screening/surveillance every 6 months.[8] When a screening/surveillance US examination reveals a focal observation of less than 1 cm, a short-term follow-up examination (generally 3 months) is recommended.[9] If there is no growth for 2 years, the patient may return to routine surveillance. If the focal observation grows, or measures greater than 1 cm, the screening/surveillance US examination is considered positive, which triggers a diagnostic test to confirm or rule out HCC or other malignancy.

Diagnostic Examinations

Multiphasic contrast-enhanced MR imaging, multiphasic contrast-enhanced CT, and contrast-enhanced US (CEUS) may be used to characterize a detected lesion and establish a noninvasive, definitive diagnosis of HCC. At present, AASLD and EASL do not include CEUS as a diagnostic test,[8,10] whereas other societies, including the Liver Imaging Reporting and Data System (LI-RADS), support the use of CEUS for HCC diagnosis.[11,15,16] Further discussion of these diagnostic tests is beyond the scope of this article.

CURRENT EVIDENCE FOR COMMON SCREENING TESTS

As mentioned earlier, screening and surveillance of patients at risk for HCC is recommended by all major international hepatology societies.[8,10,15,17,18] US is advocated as the primary imaging modality because it is widely available, reportedly cost-effective, noninvasive, well tolerated by patients, and safe. Moreover, US has an acceptable diagnostic accuracy when used as a surveillance test, with a sensitivity ranging from 58% to 89% and a specificity of greater than 90%.[19,20]

The finding of a focal observation larger than 1 cm, new venous thrombus, or suspicious parenchymal distortion detected sonographically in a patient at risk for developing HCC should prompt further investigation with a diagnostic multiphasic contrast-enhanced examination.[8] The ability of US to detect focal hepatic observations depends on operator experience as well as patient factors. The modality may be less accurate in obese patients[21,22] and in nodular cirrhotic livers; however, additional research is required to determine how these patient factors may affect management guidelines.[22,23]

Only a small number of studies have addressed the efficacy of US in HCC surveillance. One randomized controlled trial from China involving nearly 19,000 patients with hepatitis B, with and without cirrhosis, showed that HCC-related mortality was reduced by 37% in the surveillance arm with US and AFP obtained every 6 months, compared with the control arm without surveillance, despite suboptimal (60%) surveillance adherence.[13] In a large meta-analysis, US surveillance identified most HCC tumors before clinical presentation, with a pooled sensitivity of 94%, but was less effective in detecting early-stage HCC, with a sensitivity of only 63%.[12] In a Japanese cohort of 1432 patients, US surveillance detected more than 90% of HCC tumors, with mean size of 1.6 ± 0.6 cm, and less than 2% of cases exceeding 3 cm.[24]

Of the serologic tests available, serum AFP has been the most extensively evaluated.[7,25] When used as a diagnostic test with a cutoff value of 20 ng/mL, serum AFP has a moderate sensitivity of 60%, but a low specificity. At a cutoff value of 200 ng/mL (the cutoff currently advocated by the Asian Pacific Association for the Study of Liver [APASL]),[15] sensitivity decreases to 22%. Reducing the cutoff value improves sensitivity but leads to a concurrent increase in false-positive results, potentially causing psychological harms to patients (anxiety) and leading to unnecessary diagnostic testing. Moreover, serum AFP levels can be increased in hepatic processes such as an acute viral infection or significant alcohol consumption, in intrahepatic cholangiocarcinoma, and non-HCC malignancies such as gastric and pancreaticobiliary cancers, and nonseminomatous germ cell tumors.[26]

Some studies have investigated the efficacy of serum AFP in combination with other serum markers. As part of the HALT-C (Hepatitis C Antiviral Long-term Treatment against Cirrhosis) trial, serum AFP and another marker, des-gamma carboxyprothrombin (DCP; also known as prothrombin induced by vitamin K absence II [PIVKA II]) were measured at intervals in a group of patients with hepatitis C cirrhosis on maintenance interferon and ribavirin therapy resistant to an initial course of standard antiviral therapy.[27] In the 39 subjects who developed HCC, neither serologic marker was adequate for surveillance

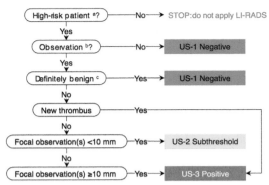

Fig. 1. US LI-RADS decision tree for assigning an observation category. US-1, negative; US-2, subthreshold; US-3, positive. [a] In general, cirrhosis of any cause; hepatitis B in absence of cirrhosis; [b] Distinctive area compared with background liver; [c] Examples: simple cyst, focal fat sparing, or fat deposition; previously confirmed hemangioma. (Reprinted from American College of Radiology, Reston, VA; with permission.)

purposes, even when results were combined. Other serologic tests, such as the ratio of glycosylated AFP (L3 fraction) to total AFP, alphafucosidase, glypican 3, and HSP-70 have been tested as diagnostic markers but have not yet been adequately investigated as screening tools.[28,29]

INTRODUCTION TO US LI-RADS IN SCREENING AND SURVEILLANCE

Although all major international hepatology societies recommend US as the preferred screening and surveillance imaging test in patients at risk for HCC, until now, a unified system for implementation and interpretation has not existed. To address this gap, a multidisciplinary team of experts was convened by the ACR to develop the US LI-RADS. US LI-RADS provides a unified

language, precise criteria for interpretation, and standardized reporting and follow-up recommendations in hepatic US evaluation of patients at risk for developing HCC. Recommended US technique, imaging protocols, and correlative image examples are provided later. As experience and data accrue, refinements will be made. A unified system has the benefit of facilitating multi-institutional data collection in screening and surveillance strategies and potentially altering future recommendations and management algorithms. In addition, robust cost-effective analyses and outcomes analyses may be more easily performed with such a system.

US LI-RADS Algorithm

LI-RADS provides recommendations on how to apply an algorithmic approach to screening and surveillance US studies and assigning a US LI-RADS category and a visualization score. The US LI-RADS category is based on liver observations. An observation is defined as any distinctive area compared with background liver. Fig. 1 provides a decision tree for assigning the US LI-RADS category, the details of which are discussed later. The visualization score is an assessment of study quality. The US LI-RADS category and visualization scores are two key elements that should be included in the radiology report, along with specific recommendations, to clearly communicate findings and to guide patient management.

US LI-RADS Categories

There are 3 different categories that serve to summarize the study results and determine the most appropriate follow-up: US-1, negative; US-2, subthreshold; and US-3, positive. Table 1 summarizes the US LI-RADS observation categories.

Table 1
US LI-RADS Screening and Surveillance observation categories

Category	Concept	Definition	Recommendation
US-1 Negative	No US evidence of HCC	No observation, or only definitely benign observations	6-mo follow-up US
US-2 Subthreshold	Observation that may warrant short-term US surveillance	Observations <10 mm in diameter, not definitely benign	US follow-up at 3–6 mo
US-3 Positive	Observation that may warrant multiphasic contrast-enhanced imaging	Observations ≥10 mm in diameter, not definitely benign, or new thrombus in vein	Multiphasic contrast-enhanced CT or MR imaging, or CEUS

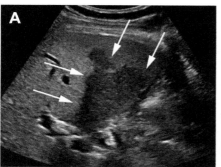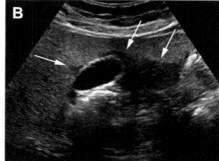

Fig. 2. LI-RADS US-1, negative. In a 54-year-old woman with nonalcoholic fatty liver disease (*A, B*), US images show geographic, wedge-shaped area of relative hypoechogenicity near gallbladder fossa (*arrows*), characteristic of focal fatty sparing.

LI-RADS US-1, negative

LI-RADS US-1, negative, indicates no evidence of HCC. These patients may have no focal observations or only definitely benign observations. Definitely benign observations may include simple cysts, focal fat sparing or deposition, or an observation previously proved to be benign, such as a hemangioma diagnosed on a prior contrast-enhanced imaging test (**Figs. 2** and **3**). For US-1, negative examinations, continued routine surveillance with a 6-month US scan is recommended, as supported by clinical practice guidelines endorsed by several societies.[8,10,15]

LI-RADS US-2, subthreshold

LI-RADS US-2, subthreshold, indicates an observation that may require short-term US follow-up. This follow-up may include an observation less than 10 mm in diameter that is not definitely benign. An example of a US-2 subthreshold observation is a solid nodule of any echogenicity measuring less than 10 mm (**Fig. 4**). Based mainly on expert opinion, current AASLD guidelines recommend follow-up in 3 months for such nodules. Because there is no high-level scientific evidence to inform the optimal follow-up interval, US LI-RADS permits greater flexibility, allowing repeat surveillance US to be performed between 3 and 6 months to assess for stability, change, or resolution. If the observation regresses, the patient may return to a routine surveillance interval (6 months).[8] An area of controversy is the duration of close (3-month to 6-month) follow-up for observations that remain stable, neither regressing nor growing. Based on expert opinion, current AASLD guidelines recommend close follow-up for 18 to 24 months before returning to routine surveillance.[8]

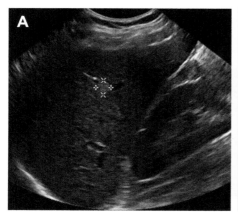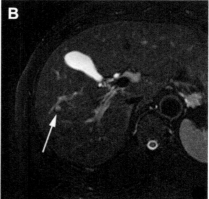

Fig. 3. LI-RADS US-1, negative. A 61-year-old man with cirrhosis. US image through right lobe (*A*) shows a small, hyperechoic nodule measuring 10 mm (*caliper markers*). T2-weighted MR image (*B*) from examination performed previously shows a markedly hyperintense nodule (*arrow*); dynamic postcontrast MR imaging (not shown) revealed peripheral puddling with progressive centripetal fill-in, confirming diagnosis of hemangioma.

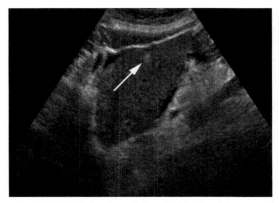

Fig. 4. LI-RADS US-2, subthreshold. An 80-year-old woman with cryptogenic cirrhosis. US image shows small, hyperechoic nodule in anterior left lobe (*arrow*), measuring only 8 mm. US follow-up at 3 to 6 months was recommended.

LI-RADS US-3, positive

LI-RADS US-3, positive, is an observation that warrants further evaluation with a diagnostic contrast-enhanced test. A US-3 positive study is defined by a solid focal observation greater than or equal to 10 mm in diameter and not definitely benign; new thrombus in vein, regardless of whether it is suspected to be a tumor in vein or bland thrombus; and parenchymal distortion distinct from the background liver, not previously confirmed to be benign (**Figs. 5–8**). Parenchymal distortion is defined by a parenchymal area greater than 10 mm showing 1 or more of the following features: ill-defined area of heterogeneity, refractive edge shadows, and/or loss of normal hepatic architecture.

US LI-RADS Visualization Scores

One of 3 visualization scores is assigned to the US study based on perceived (or potential) limitations

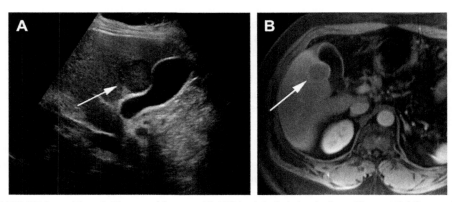

Fig. 5. LI-RADS US-3, positive. A 61-year-old man with HCV-related cirrhosis. Surveillance US (*A*) reveals rounded, hypoechoic mass adjacent to gallbladder fossa (*arrow*) measuring more than 1 cm. Postcontrast, T1-weighted image from follow-up MR imaging, obtained in portal venous phase (*B*) shows washout from nodule along with capsule appearance (*arrow*); nodule also showed arterial-phase hyperenhancement (not shown), diagnostic for HCC. At resection, poorly differentiated HCC was confirmed.

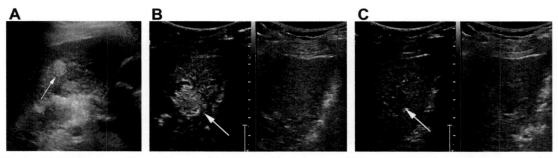

Fig. 6. LI-RADS US-3, positive. A 68-year-old woman with cirrhosis and history of HCC after radiofrequency ablation. Image from surveillance US 2 years later (*A*) shows hypoechoic nodule (*caliper markers*) adjacent to ablation zone (*arrow*). Images from contrast-enhanced US study (*B*, *C*) revealed arterial-phase hyperenhancement (*arrow*) at 25 seconds postinjection (*B*) with subsequent mild, late washout (*arrow*) visualized at 98 seconds (*C*), diagnostic for HCC.

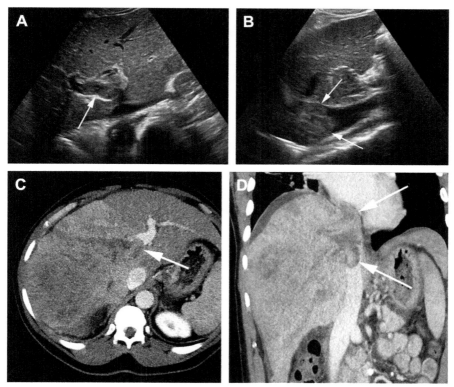

Fig. 7. LI-RADS US-3, positive. A 58-year-old man with cirrhosis and AFP of 44 ng/mL. US images through right portal vein (*A*) and retrohepatic inferior vena cava (*B*) show heterogeneous intraluminal thrombus within vein (*arrows*). Contrast-enhanced CT images show large area of parenchymal heterogeneity replacing much of the right lobe, suspicious for infiltrative subtype of HCC, with tumor in vein (*arrows*) at portal bifurcation (*C*) and into the right hepatic vein and inferior vena cava (*D*), a finding often seen with this subtype.

in liver visualization during the US examination. These compromising factors may include, but are not limited to, obscuration of portions of the liver by lung, rib shadow, and/or bowel gas; marked hepatic parenchymal heterogeneity or nodularity that would compromise the detection of a focal observation distinct from the background liver; or poor acoustic penetration caused

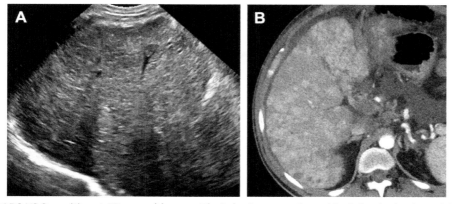

Fig. 8. LI-RADS US-3, positive. A 53-year-old man with cirrhosis, presenting with abdominal pain and AFP greater than 60,500 ng/mL. US image through right lobe (*A*) reveals marked parenchymal heterogeneity with vessel distortion, refractive edge shadowing, and loss of normal portal triads. Image from subsequent CT (*B*) reveals innumerable foci of arterial-phase hyperenhancement throughout liver, interpreted as diffuse infiltrative HCC.

Table 2
US LI-RADS Screening and Surveillance visualization scores

Score	Concept	Examples
A. No or minimal limitations	Sensitivity of test unlikely to be affected	• Homogeneous or minimally heterogeneous liver • Minimal beam attenuation or shadowing • Nearly entire liver visualized
B. Moderate limitations	Small masses may be obscured	• Moderately heterogeneous liver • Moderate beam attenuation or shadowing • Some areas of liver or diaphragm not visualized
C. Severe limitations	Significantly decreased sensitivity for focal liver lesions	• Severely heterogeneous liver • Severe beam attenuation or shadowing • Most (>50%) of the liver not visualized • Most (>50%) of the diaphragm not visualized

by marked hepatic and/or abdominal wall attenuation. **Table 2** summarizes the visualization scores.

Visualization score A
Visualization score A indicates that there were no limitations that are expected to significantly affect the sensitivity of the test for detecting HCC. Examples include a homogeneous or minimally heterogeneous liver which can be visualized in its entirety or near entirety, with no or only minimal beam attenuation (**Fig. 9**).

Visualization score B
Visualization score B indicates that limitations were encountered that may obscure small masses. These limitations may result from rib shadow or obscuration by bowel gas or lung, moderately heterogeneous liver parenchyma, or moderate acoustic beam attenuation. Small portions of the liver or diaphragm may not have been visualized (**Figs. 10 and 11**).

Visualization score C
Visualization score C refers to studies that may have significantly decreased sensitivity for detecting focal liver lesions. The liver may be severely heterogeneous because of cirrhosis, or be affected by marked beam attenuation, such as in severe fatty liver, or when an estimated greater than 50% of the liver may not be visualized because of obscuration by bowel gas, rib

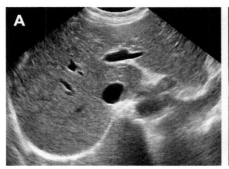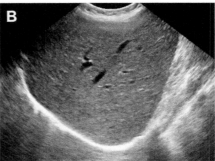

Fig. 9. Visualization score A. A 56-year-old man with HCV-related cirrhosis. Representative US images of the liver show good acoustic penetration, adequate fine detail, and lack of significant artifact or obscuring elements (*A, B*), allowing confident evaluation of the entire liver.

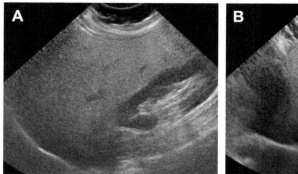

Fig. 10. Visualization score B. A 44-year-old woman with increased liver function tests, found to have nonalcoholic steatohepatitis. Representative US images through liver (*A*, *B*) show moderate loss of acoustic power in the far field (pronounced beam attenuation) and acoustic scatter, compromising visibility of deep liver.

shadow, and so forth (**Figs. 12** and **13**). Note that US LI-RADS does not make specific recommendations as to the appropriate management of patients assigned a visualization score C because it has not been established that alternative imaging modalities for screening and surveillance are cost-effective in this population; however, as performance and outcomes data are collected, specific recommendations, such as alternative screening strategies, may be provided in the future.

Technical Recommendations

The screening US examination should be performed in accordance with the ACR Practice Parameter and Technical Standard for Performance of Ultrasound of the Abdomen and Retroperitoneum.[30] The study should be compared with prior examinations whenever possible, and it is strongly recommended that a standard imaging protocol be adopted to improve reproducibility and facilitate comparison between technologists and imaging sites.

To improve evaluation of the liver for cirrhosis and for focal or diffuse observations, images through the entire liver should be obtained. To achieve adequate liver visualization, US LI-RADS recommends the following: instructing the patient to be fasting 4 to 6 hours before examination; adjusting patient positioning, inspiration level, and acoustic window to identify optimal acoustic windows; applying adequate probe pressure against the abdominal wall; and adjusting image settings (eg, transducer presets, pulse frequency, harmonics) to optimize penetration and fine detail

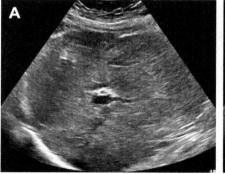
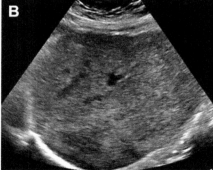

Fig. 11. Visualization score B. A 54-year-old woman with cirrhosis. Representative US images through liver (*A*, *B*) show moderate parenchymal heterogeneity, reducing confidence that a small focal lesion could be distinguished from background parenchyma.

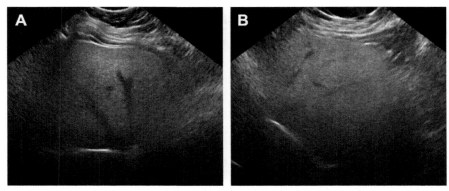

Fig. 12. Visualization score C. A 46-year-old woman with nonalcoholic steatohepatitis. Representative US images through liver (*A, B*) show severe loss of acoustic power in far field (marked beam attenuation) and acoustic scatter, compromising visibility of at least 50% of liver.

depending on intrinsic patient factors. A standardized protocol specifying the required views is another necessity. Cine sweeps through the liver may assist with documentation and longitudinal comparison of surveillance examinations. Documentation of patency of the main portal vein with gray-scale and color Doppler is also generally recommended. If thrombus is identified, spectral Doppler to assess for arterialized flow in the thrombus would favor tumor in vein and is important to report. Color Doppler of right and left portal veins, and hepatic veins, and spectral Doppler of the main portal vein to assess waveform, velocity, and flow direction, may also be considered. A linear transducer may be used to depict surface nodularity and assess the subcapsular parenchyma. Imaging of the gallbladder and bile ducts

is also considered part of the routine liver examination. A complete list of suggested views can be found in **Box 2**.

Liver observations should be documented in transverse and longitudinal views in gray scale and with color/power Doppler. Optional cine sweeps through observations may be considered to aid in characterization. The size of each liver observation in 3 dimensions; the involved liver lobe and Couinaud segment, if known; and relationship to vessels, liver capsule, or bile ducts should be recorded.

Findings of portal hypertension that may be important to patient management may be included as a part of a liver US examination: spleen size, with or without volume, and documenting the presence and degree of ascites.

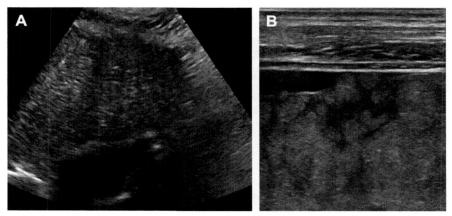

Fig. 13. Visualization score C. A 44-year-old man with alcohol-related cirrhosis. Representative US images through liver (*A, B*) show severe parenchymal heterogeneity, likely precluding the ability to distinguish focal lesion from background parenchyma.

Box 2
US LI-RADS list of recommended views

Longitudinal images

Recommended

Left lobe

- Left of midline
- At midline; include proximal abdominal aorta, celiac artery, and superior mesenteric artery
- With inferior vena cava; include caudate lobe, main portal vein, and pancreatic head
- With left portal vein

Right lobe

- With gallbladder
- With right kidney
- Including right hemidiaphragm and adjacent pleural space
- Far lateral

 Main portal vein; include gray-scale and color Doppler

 Common bile duct at porta hepatis; include diameter measurement

Optional

Color Doppler of the right and left portal veins, and hepatic veins

Spectral Doppler of main portal vein to assess waveform, velocity, and flow direction

Transverse images

Recommended

Dome with hepatic veins; include entire right and left lobes with medial and lateral liver edges (on separate images as needed)

Left lobe

- With left portal vein
- Falciform ligament to evaluate for the presence of patent paraumbilical vein

 Main portal vein bifurcation

Right lobe

- With right portal vein
- With main portal vein
- With gallbladder
- With right kidney
- Near liver tip

Optional

Color Doppler view of additional vascular structures

Cine loops

Optional

Longitudinal and transverse cine sweeps of left and right lobes, including as much hepatic parenchyma as possible.

Recommended views can be obtained in any order per institutional protocol. Additional views of focal observations should be obtained as needed. Additional anatomic and Doppler measurements may be included per institutional preferences and needs.

SUMMARY

Given the high prevalence, increasing incidence, and significant morbidity and mortality associated with HCC, an accurate and cost-effective screening and surveillance program is needed. Although most societies advocate US for HCC screening and surveillance, until now, a standardized system for the use of US in this context has not been established. US LI-RADS provides recommendations and an algorithmic framework designed to improve the performance of US and unify follow-up and management recommendations. This unified system may also facilitate multi-institutional data collection for future studies. This system is expected to evolve as correlative performance and outcomes data become available.

REFERENCES

1. Mittal S, El-Serag HB. Epidemiology of hepatocellular carcinoma: consider the population. J Clin Gastroenterol 2013;47(Suppl):S2–6.
2. Bosch FX, Ribes J, Cleries R, et al. Epidemiology of hepatocellular carcinoma. Clin Liver Dis 2005;9(2): 191–211, v.
3. Howlader N, Noone AM, Krapcho M, et al, editors. SEER cancer statistics review, 1975-2013. Bethesda (MD): National Cancer Institute; 2016. Available at: https://seer.cancer.gov/csr/1975_2013/.
4. Ferlay J, Soerjomataram I, Ervik M, et al. GLOBO-CAN 2012 v1.0, cancer incidence and mortality worldwide, International Agency for research on cancer. Lyon, France. Available from: http:// globocan.iarc.fr.
5. Njei B, Rotman Y, Ditah I, et al. Emerging trends in hepatocellular carcinoma incidence and mortality. Hepatology 2015;61(1):191–9.
6. Lencioni R. Loco-regional treatment of hepatocellular carcinoma. Hepatology 2010;52(2):762–73.
7. Marrero JA. Screening tests for hepatocellular carcinoma. Clin Liver Dis 2005;9(2):235–51, vi.
8. Bruix J, Sherman M, American Association for the Study of Liver Diseases. Management of hepatocellular carcinoma: an update. Hepatology 2011;53(3): 1020–2.
9. El-Serag HB, Davila JA. Surveillance for hepatocellular carcinoma: in whom and how? Therap Adv Gastroenterol 2011;4(1):5–10.
10. European Association for the Study of the Liver, European Organisation for Research and Treatment of Cancer. EASL-EORTC clinical practice guidelines: management of hepatocellular carcinoma. J Hepatol 2012;56(4):908–43.
11. Kokudo N, Hasegawa K, Akahane M, et al. Evidence-based Clinical Practice Guidelines for Hepatocellular Carcinoma: the Japan Society of Hepatology 2013 update (3rd JSH-HCC guidelines). Hepatol Res 2015;45(2):123–7.
12. Singal AG, Pillai A, Tiro J. Early detection, curative treatment, and survival rates for hepatocellular carcinoma surveillance in patients with cirrhosis: a meta-analysis. PLoS Med 2014;11(4): e1001624.
13. Zhang BH, Yang BH, Tang ZY. Randomized controlled trial of screening for hepatocellular carcinoma. J Cancer Res Clin Oncol 2004;130(7): 417–22.
14. Benson AB 3rd, Abrams TA, Ben-Josef E, et al. NCCN clinical practice guidelines in oncology: hepatobiliary cancers. J Natl Compr Cancer Netw 2009; 7(4):350–91.
15. Omata M, Lesmana LA, Tateishi R, et al. Asian Pacific Association for the study of the liver consensus recommendations on hepatocellular carcinoma. Hepatol Int 2010;4(2):439–74.
16. Claudon M, Dietrich CF, Choi BI, et al. Guidelines and good clinical practice recommendations for contrast enhanced ultrasound (CEUS) in the liver - update 2012: A WFUMB-EFSUMB initiative in cooperation with representatives of AFSUMB, AIUM, ASUM, FLAUS and ICUS. Ultrasound Med Biol 2013;39(2):187–210.
17. Korean Liver Cancer Study Group (KLCSG), National Cancer Center, Korea (NCC). 2014 Korean Liver Cancer Study Group–National Cancer Center Korea practice guideline for the management of hepatocellular carcinoma. Korean J Radiol 2015;16(3): 465–522.
18. Kudo M, Izumi N, Koskudo N, et al. Management of hepatocellular carcinoma in Japan: consensus-based clinical practice guidelines proposed by the Japan Society of Hepatology (JSH) 2010 updated version. Dig Dis 2011;29(3):339–64.
19. Bolondi L. Screening for hepatocellular carcinoma in cirrhosis. J Hepatol 2003;39(6):1076–84.
20. Kim CK, Lim JH, Lee WJ. Detection of hepatocellular carcinomas and dysplastic nodules in cirrhotic liver: accuracy of ultrasonography in transplant patients. J Ultrasound Med 2001;20(2): 99–104.
21. Tong MJ, Blatt LM, Kao VW. Surveillance for hepatocellular carcinoma in patients with chronic viral hepatitis in the United States of America. J Gastroenterol Hepatol 2001;16(5):553–9.
22. Simmons O, Fetzer DT, Yokoo T, et al. Predictors of adequate ultrasound quality for hepatocellular carcinoma surveillance in patients with cirrhosis. Aliment Pharmacol Ther 2017;45(1):169–77.
23. Larcos G, Sorokopud H, Berry G, et al. Sonographic screening for hepatocellular carcinoma in patients with chronic hepatitis or cirrhosis: an evaluation. AJR Am J Roentgenol 1998;171(2): 433–5.

24. Sato T, Tateishi R, Yoshida H, et al. Ultrasound surveillance for early detection of hepatocellular carcinoma among patients with chronic hepatitis C. Hepatol Int 2009;3(4):544–50.

25. Trevisani F, D'Intino PE, Morselli-Labate AM, et al. Serum alpha-fetoprotein for diagnosis of hepatocellular carcinoma in patients with chronic liver disease: influence of HBsAg and anti-HCV status. J Hepatol 2001; 34(4):570–5.

26. Bialecki ES, Di Bisceglie AM. Diagnosis of hepatocellular carcinoma. HPB (Oxford) 2005; 7(1):26–34.

27. Lok AS, Sterling RK, Everhart JE, et al. Des-gamma-carboxy prothrombin and alpha-fetoprotein as biomarkers for the early detection of hepatocellular carcinoma. Gastroenterology 2010;138(2):493–502.

28. Lok AS, Seeff LB, Morgan TR, et al. Incidence of hepatocellular carcinoma and associated risk factors in hepatitis C-related advanced liver disease. Gastroenterology 2009;136(1):138–48.

29. Marrero JA, Su GL, Wei W, et al. Des-gamma carboxyprothrombin can differentiate hepatocellular carcinoma from nonmalignant chronic liver disease in American patients. Hepatology 2003;37(5):1114–21.

30. ACR–AIUM–SPR–SRU Practice parameter for the performance of an ultrasound examination of the abdomen and/or retroperitoneum. Practice parameter online resource, 2012; Reston (VA): American College of Radiology; 2017. Available at: https://www.acr.org/Quality-Safety/Standards-Guidelines/Practice-Guidelines-by-Modality/Ultrasound. Accessed May 1, 2017.

Imaging and Screening of Cancer of the Gallbladder and Bile Ducts

Kumar Sandrasegaran, MD[a],*, Christine O. Menias, MD[b]

KEYWORDS

• Gallbladder cancer • Cholangiocarcinoma • Sclerosing cholangitis • CT • MR imaging

KEY POINTS

• Gallbladder cancer (GBC), may appear as a mass replacing the gallbladder, irregular gallbladder wall thickening, or a polypoid lesion in the gallbladder.
• The diagnosis of a biliary stricture as benign or malignant may be difficult and requires imaging and endoscopy-related tests.
• In staging perihilar cholangiocarcinoma (CCA), a combination of PET-computed tomography scans and MR imaging may be required.
• Invasion of bilateral secondary biliary radicals or hepatic vessels usually precludes surgical resection of perihilar CCA.
• Intrahepatic CCA is increasingly identified in cirrhotic patients, and may have atypical computed tomography or MR imaging appearances in this cohort.

BILIARY CANCER SCREENING

Biliary cancers include gallbladder cancer (GBC) and cholangiocarcinoma (CCA). These tumors are associated with a poor prognosis, and much literature has been devoted to early detection of these cancers. Some gallbladder polyps at low risk of GCA may be screened with ultrasound imaging. Bile duct strictures that may be CCA, particularly in patients with primary sclerosing cholangitis (PSC) may need to be investigated, sometimes repeatedly. The imaging features of biliary tumors are well-established. This review discusses the current state of screening and diagnosis of GBC and CCA.

GALLBLADDER CANCER

GBC has a high incidence in Chile and India. In the United States, this cancer is uncommon but is more prevalent in Hispanic and American Indian populations. As with most gallbladder diseases, GBC is more common in females than males (3:1 ratio). Risk factors for GBC include gallstones, which are seen in 60% to 90% of GBC cases.[1] Stones larger than 2 cm are associated with a greater risk of GBC.[2] Porcelain gallbladder used to be thought of as a strong risk factor for GBC; however, current literature does not support this notion.[3,4] Anomalous pancreaticobiliary junction is also a recognized risk factor for GBC, particularly in young Asian females without gallstones.[1] GBC occurs in 10% to 15% of Asian patients with this anomaly.[2] Patients with PSC have a 2% incidence of GBC.[5] Hence, patients with PSC without gallbladder disease may benefit from annual right upper quadrant ultrasound screening.[5–8]

Unlike the case with colon cancer, GBC is not thought to undergo an adenoma–carcinoma sequence. It is more likely that, over several years,

Disclosures: Consultant to Guerbet Pharmaceuticals (K. Sandrasegaran). None (C.O. Menias).
[a] Department of Radiology, Indiana University School of Medicine, UH 0279, 550 North University Boulevard, Indianapolis, IN 46202, USA; [b] Mayo Clinic, 5777 East Mayo Boulevard, Phoenix, AZ 85054, USA
* Corresponding author.
E-mail address: ksandras@iupui.edu

radiologic.theclinics.com

dysplasia progresses to cancer.[2,9] The sites of GBC are the gallbladder fundus (60%), body (30%), and neck (10%). More than 90% of GBC are adenocarcinomas.[2] Squamous cell, small cell, neuroendocrine-type, melanoma, and lymphoma account for the remainder of GBC. The staging of GBC is given in **Table 1**.[2,10] The overall prognosis of GBC is poor with a 5-year survival[11,12] rate of 10% for advanced cancer (T3 or T4).

Screening for Gallbladder Cancer

We consider the role of screening for cancer in those with increased risk of this disease.

Gallstones
Gallstones are present in about 60% to 90% of patients with GBC,[13] and a history of gallstones seems to be one of the strongest risk factors for the development of GBC.[1] However, the incidence of GBC in patients with gallstones is only 0.5% to 3.0%.[14] The risk is greater with larger gallstones, particularly larger than 3 cm (relative risk is 10:1)[10] and with a longer duration of gallstone disease. At present, screening for GBC in patients with gallstones is not recommended.

Porcelain gallbladder
This entity is an uncommon manifestation of chronic cholecystitis with calcification of the gallbladder wall. More than 95% of patients with porcelain gallbladder have gallstones. Earlier studies reported a high incidence of GBC in patients with porcelain gallbladder ($\leq$60%).[15] More recent studies indicate that the increase in GBC risk is minimal with an incidence of 2% to 3%[3,4,16] (**Fig. 1**). A metaanalysis of the association between porcelain gallbladder and GBC concluded that there was no need for cholecystectomy in porcelain gallbladder, unless there were other indications for surgery. There were no recommendations for screening these patients for GBC.[16]

Gallbladder polyps
Gallbladder polyps are seen in up to 12% of cholecystectomy specimens and in about 5% to 7% of right upper quadrant sonography studies.[11,17,18] Most small gallbladder polyps are asymptomatic, benign lesions that do not progress to GBC. A metaanalysis of 12 studies, reporting on more than 5000 polyps, estimated that only 0.6% of all gallbladder polyps were malignant.[19] Thus, it is important to stratify the risk of cancer in gallbladder polyps. Polyps larger than 10 mm have a higher risk (45%–65% likelihood) of malignancy.[18,19] Other factors that increase the risk of cancer include patient age greater than 50 years,[18] presence of gallstones, solitary sessile polyps, and presence of PSC.[2,18–20]

Table 1	
TNM staging of gallbladder cancer	

T staging		
	T0	No evidence of primary tumor
	T1	Tumor invades lamina propria or muscular layer
	T1a	Tumor invades lamina propria
	T1b	Tumor invades muscular layer
	T2	Tumor invades perimuscular connective tissue; no extension beyond serosa or into liver
	T3	Tumor perforates the serosa and/or directly invades liver and/or one other adjacent organ, for example, stomach, duodenum, colon, pancreas, omentum, or extrahepatic bile ducts
	T4	Tumor invades main portal vein or hepatic artery or invades 2 or more extrahepatic organs
N staging		
	N0	No regional lymph node metastasis
	N1	Metastases to nodes along cystic duct, common bile duct, hepatic artery, and/or portal vein
	N2	Metastases to periaortic, pericaval, superior mesenteric artery, or celiac artery lymph nodes
M staging		
	M0	No distant metastasis
	M1	Distant metastasis

Stage I is T1, N0, M0. Stage II is T2, N0, M0. Stage IIIA is T3, N0, M0. Stage IIIB is T1-3, N1, M0. Stage IVA is T4, N0, M0. Stage IVB is any T, N2, M0 or any T, any N, M1.

Data from Reid KM, Ramos-De la Medina A, Donohue JH. Diagnosis and surgical management of gallbladder cancer: a review. J Gastrointest Surg 2007;11(5):671–81; and Misra S, Chaturvedi A, Misra NC, et al. Carcinoma of the gallbladder. Lancet Oncol 2003;4(3):167–76.

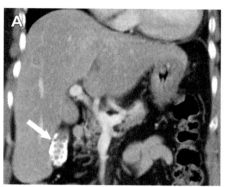
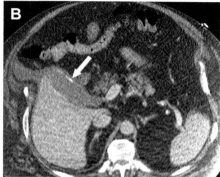

Fig. 1. (*A*) A 71-year-old woman with dense calcification of gallbladder wall (*arrow*) consistent with porcelain gallbladder. Such dense calcification is now considered to be a low risk for gallbladder cancer (GBC). (*B*) A 64-year-old man with mild mucosal calcification of gallbladder (*arrow*). Such stippled calcification is reported to be a higher risk factor for GBC than the findings in A.

Polyps are divided into nontumorous lesions, and benign and malignant tumors[20,21] (**Fig. 2** and **Table 2**). Imaging tests are not reliable in distinguishing between the benign and malignant causes of polypoid gallbladder lesions. There are varying opinions on how gallbladder polyps should be managed. The recommendations of the American Society for Gastrointestinal Endoscopy[21] are often quoted. We have given a modified algorithm for managing gallbladder polyps (**Fig. 3**) based on these recommendations, and using the literature that has been accumulated since the publication of these recommendations.[18–20] Follow-up screening is performed using transabdominal ultrasonography, which is inexpensive and has a high accuracy for gallbladder polyps. CT and MR imaging are not superior to ultrasonography in detecting polyps and are not part of the screening algorithm. The duration of follow-up in patients with apparently stable gallbladder polyps has not been established. One study suggested that it took about 7 years for the development of neoplasia in gallbladder polyps that were followed.[22] Thus, a follow-up of at least 10 years has been suggested.[23]

Polypoid gallbladder lesions occur in 4% to 7% of patients with PSC,[24] about the same incidence as in the general population. A high proportion of

Table 2	
Histology of gallbladder polyps	
Tumor Polyps	**Nontumor Polyps**
Benign tumors	
Adenoma (5%)	Cholesterol polyps (70%, <5 mm)
Mesenchymal: leiomyoma, lipoma	Adenomyomatosis (15%, predominantly fundal)
Granular cell tumor	Xanthogranulomatous polyps
Malignant tumor	
Primary gallbladder cancer (7%) Metastases	Inflammatory polyps (10%, associated with chronic cholecystitis)

Data from Mellnick VM, Menias CO, Sandrasegaran K, et al. Polypoid lesions of the gallbladder: disease spectrum with pathologic correlation. Radiographics 2015;35(2):387–99; and Anderson MA, Appalaneni V, Ben-Menachem T, et al. The role of endoscopy in the evaluation and treatment of patients with biliary neoplasia. Gastrointest Endosc 2013;77(2):167–74.

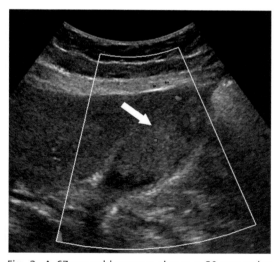

Fig. 2. A 67-year-old woman shows a 20-mm polyp (*arrow*) in the gallbladder. Given its size the patient underwent cholecystectomy. Final pathology was a benign adenomatous polyp.

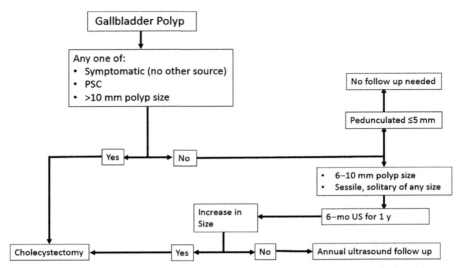

Fig. 3. Algorithm for managing gallbladder polyp (see text). PSC, primary sclerosing cholangitis; US, ultrasound imaging.

these lesions (about 60%) show high-grade dysplasia or cancer.[24,25] There is some support for performing cholecystectomy in patients with PSC, regardless of the size of gallbladder polyps.[8] Nevertheless, patients with advanced liver disease, especially Child class C, have an increased risk of morbidity and mortality after cholecystectomy and the risks and benefits of operative intervention need to be considered.[7]

Imaging Features of Gallbladder Cancer

Imaging findings of GBC include a mass replacing part or all of the gallbladder (seen in 45%–60%), wall thickening (seen in 20%–30%), and an intraluminal polypoid lesion (seen in 15%–25%).[26]

Mass-forming gallbladder cancer

A large mass arising from the gallbladder is considered GBC until proved otherwise. It is important to determine local spread, such as into the liver, duodenum, hepatic flexure of the colon, diaphragm, portal vein and branches, and hepatic arteries. In addition, it is important to distinguish between hepatic hilar lymph nodes and more distant nodes at celiac, mesenteric, and retroperitoneal sites. GBC has a tendency to spread along the hepatoduodenal ligament to become closely applied to the main portal vein or hepatic artery. Such infiltration precludes R0 resection (ie, tumor-free resection margins). The staging of GBC is given in **Table 1**.

Gallbladder cancer with wall thickening

GBC may present with irregular or nodular gallbladder wall thickening (**Fig. 4**). The main differential diagnosis are benign entities such as adenomyomatosis and various types of cholecystitis (see **Fig. 4**; **Table 3**).[27,28] It is difficult to distinguish early GBC from adenomyomatosis. Adenomyomatosis typically causes fundal thickening and, in some cases, cystic spaces may be seen in the thickened wall in keeping with intramural diverticula seen in this condition. Adenomyomatosis may also show uptake on PET with 2-flurodexoyglucose (FDG; **Fig. 5**). Well-differentiated GBC may also show intratumoral cystic components. Endoscopic ultrasound (EUS) imaging may help to stratify the gallbladder wall into mucosa, muscle, and serosa. Discontinuity or irregular thickening of the innermost hyperechoic layer (mucosa), irregular thickening of the outermost hyperechoic layer (serosa), or loss of the multilayer pattern are clues to GBC.[26] Short-term follow-up MR imaging (1–2 months) may also help.

Polypoid gallbladder cancer

Imaging tests, including FDG PET and diffusion-weighted MR imaging, do not reliably differentiate benign and malignant polyps.[26] EUS imaging may be used as a modality for local staging of GBC, because it is accurate in assessing the depth of tumor.[29] Nevertheless, there is no firm data on the usefulness of EUS to separate benign and malignant gallbladder polyps or if it is superior to transabdominal sonography in this respect.[21] Contrast-enhanced ultrasound imaging has been investigated to determine if it may provide additional information to conventional ultrasonography in differentiating benign and malignant gallbladder

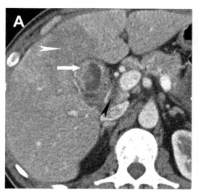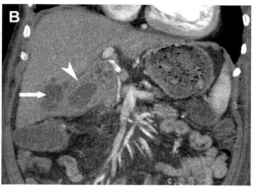

Fig. 4. (*A*) A 74-year-old woman with thickened gallbladder wall (*white arrow*) confirmed to be gallbladder cancer (GBC). The tumor infiltrates into adjacent liver (*arrowhead*), which per se is not a contraindication to surgery. However, the tumor also infiltrates along the hepatic hilum (*black arrowhead*) close to major hepatic vessels. This finding precludes resection of tumor. (*B*) A 44-year-old woman a with 2-week history of right upper quadrant pain. The gallbladder is thick walled (*arrowhead*) with a fluid collection (*arrow*) adjacent to it. The imaging appearances are suggestive of GBC with local invasion and perforation. Surgical pathology was xanthogranulomatous cholecystitis.

lesions. Both types of lesions show increased arterial enhancement.[30] Most cancers and a minority of benign lesions showed washout or rapid fading of enhancement within 60 seconds of injection.[31] Destruction of the gallbladder mucosa was also a feature of malignant lesions. At present, contrast-enhanced ultrasound imaging may be used to increase confidence of a benign lesion, but is not yet part of the algorithm for the management of gallbladder polyps (see **Fig. 3**).

CHOLANGIOCARCINOMA

CCA is a malignant tumor arising from cholangiocytes, which are the epithelial cells lining the biliary tree. CCA is the second most common primary hepatic malignancy and is increasing in incidence in Western countries.[32] CCA demonstrates a poor prognosis, with a median survival of less than 24 months.[33,34]

Risk Factors for Cholangiocarcinoma

There are many known risk factors for CCA (**Box 1**).[35–37] In the United States, the most important risk factor for perihilar or distal CCA is PSC, which is an idiopathic, cholestatic liver disease characterized by inflammation and subsequent fibrosis of the biliary tract. PSC is more common in males (70%–80%) and affects the young and

Table 3
Causes of gallbladder wall thickening mimicking GBC

Diagnosis	Comments
Adenomyomatosis	Predominantly fundal, may show cystic spaces in wall (MR imaging > CT). Moderately FDG avid on PET. EUS may help (see text).
Acute cholecystitis and its variants	Clinically different presentation but GBC found in of 6%–9% of cholecystectomy pathology for acute cholecystitis. Look for focally enhancing mass in wall.
Xanthogranulomatous cholecystitis	Predominantly middle-aged women. Can cause marked wall thickening with intramural abscess mimicking necrosis. May have adjacent hepatic abscess.
Nonspecific wall thickening	Heart failure, cirrhosis, hepatitis, hypoalbuminemia, renal failure usually cause mild diffuse thickening. No nodularity or focal mass invading liver.

Abbreviations: CT, computed tomography; EUS, endoscopic ultrasound; FDG, fluorodeoxyglucose; GBC, gallbladder cancer.

Data from Clemente G, Nuzzo G, De Rose AM, et al. Unexpected gallbladder cancer after laparoscopic cholecystectomy for acute cholecystitis: a worrisome picture. J Gastrointest Surg 2012;16(8):1462–8; and Levy AD, Murakata LA, Abbott RM, et al. From the archives of the AFIP. Benign tumors and tumorlike lesions of the gallbladder and extrahepatic bile ducts: radiologic-pathologic correlation. Armed Forces Institute of Pathology. Radiographics 2002;22(2):387–413.

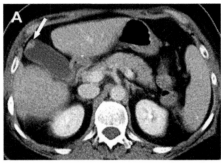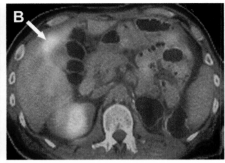

Fig. 5. A 52-year-old man with right upper quadrant pain. (*A*) Computed tomography (CT) scanning shows a mass in the gallbladder fundus with a focal cystic area (*arrow*). (*B*) PET-CT shows increased uptake of fluorodeoxyglucose by the lesion (*arrow*). Cholecystectomy was performed and the preoperative diagnosis of adenomyomatosis was confirmed.

middle-aged population with the peak onset at ages 30 to 50 years. The rate progression of biliary disease is variable, but is continually progressive leading to biliary cirrhosis within 20 years in most patients. The incidence of CCA in PSC is estimated to be 5% to 10%, which is up to 1500 times that of the general population.[38–40] The risk of developing CCA is greatest highest shortly after PSC is diagnosed, with up to one-third to one-half of patients developing cancer within the first year of diagnosis. The subsequent risk of CCA is estimated to be 1% per year. Screening for CCA

in patients with PSC is not recommended in the national guidelines from the United States, Europe, Japan, or China.[34,41,42] The guidelines from the British Society of Gastroenterologists[37] recommends screening for CCA in patients with PSC, and so do other articles.[7] The cost effectiveness of this screening is not clear. In the absence of good data, some physicians screen for CCA in patients with PSC with annual or semi-annual carbohydrate antigen 19-9 (CA19-9) and imaging studies.[43]

Congenital choledochal cysts and recognized anomalous biliopancreatic malformations are independent risk factors for CCA. Japanese guidelines recommend resection of extrahepatic bile ducts and the gallbladder in patients diagnosed with these entities.[34]

Imaging of Cholangiocarcinoma

Most CCA (90%) arise from the extrahepatic bile ducts, and are further divided into perihilar (previously called Klatskin type) or distal duct types. Intrahepatic CCA is less common. CCA may also be classified according to its growth pattern as infiltrating periductal lesion, papillary or intraductal lesion, or mass forming.

Intrahepatic Cholangiocarcinoma

Intrahepatic CCA presents as a mass that has characteristic imaging features (**Fig. 6** and **Table 4**[44]). There may or may not be adjacent biliary obstruction. The main differential diagnosis for a large heterogeneous mass in the liver, particularly in a cirrhotic liver, is HCC. The typical contrast enhancement pattern of HCC is hypervascular in the arterial phase with washout on subsequent phases, and possibly a delayed enhancing capsule. Thus, the enhancement of HCC and CCA are very different. CCA is

---

Box 1
Risk factors for CCA

Strong Association

Primary sclerosing cholangitis

Choledochal cyst

Caroli disease

Liver parasites: *Opisthorchis viverrini, Clonorchis sinensis*

Biliary-enteric anastomosis

Anomalous pancreaticobiliary junction

Primary biliary cirrhosis (for intrahepatic CCA)

Viral hepatitis B and C (for intrahepatic CCA)

Week association

Asbestos

Nitrosamines

Isoniazid

Oral contraceptives

Cigarette smoking

Abbreviation: CCA, cholangiocarcinoma.
   Data from Refs.[35–37]

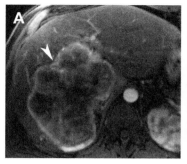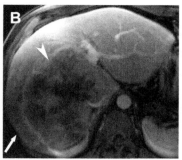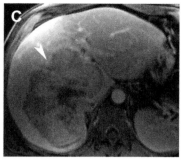

Fig. 6. A 67-year-old man with abnormal liver function tests. There is a 12-cm mass (*arrowhead*) with shows (*A*) rim enhancement on arterial phase, (*B*) patchy central enhancement on venous phase and some capsular retraction (*arrow*), and (*C*) increased enhancement on 5-minute delayed phase imaging. These findings are typical of intrahepatic cholangiocarcinoma.

increasingly identified in cirrhotic patients (see **Box 1**). Lesions in such patients tend to be atypical and may be small (owing to early detection), hypervascular, and show peripheral capsule (which is not usually seen in CCA arising in a non-cirrhotic liver). Rarely, a tumor in a cirrhotic patient may have both HCC and CCA components, the so-called biphenotypic HCC–CCA. The enhancement of these lesions depends on the proportion of HCC and CCA and may vary in different parts of the tumor (**Fig. 7**).

Perihilar and Distal Duct Cholangiocarcinoma

These are the most common types of CCA and typically present with jaundice. There are many causes of perihilar biliary strictures (**Table 5**).[45] Most of these entities are obvious from the clinical picture. IgG4 sclerosing cholangitis is an important mimic of malignant biliary stricture (**Fig. 8**). The American Gastroenterology Association makes a conditional recommendation for checking IgG4 serum levels in patients with PSC with biliary strictures.[8,40]

Perihilar CCA is one of the more challenging cancers to stage on imaging. It is important for the radiologist to comment on the degree of local spread and vascular invasion. The staging of perihilar CCA is performed using the Bismuth-Collette classification (**Fig. 9**). The criteria for unresectability of tumor are given in **Box 2**[46] and **Fig. 10**. Multislice CT is useful for determining invasion of adjacent tissue and vascular invasion, with sensitivity and specificity in the 90% range.[46] However, CT is limited in the assessment of spread along the length of bile ducts, particularly in determining whether secondary biliary radicals are involved. In this respect, MR imaging with magnetic resonance cholangiopancreatography is superior (see **Fig. 7**) and we use both modalities in preoperative staging. Both CT and MR imaging underestimate nodal and peritoneal metastases, with accuracy ranging from 30% to 70%.[46] FDG PET with CT is often used to improve preoperative evaluation of more distant metastases. A limitation for CT and MR imaging is the presence of biliary stents, even plastic stents, which cause streak artifacts

Table 4 Imaging features of intrahepatic cholangiocarcinoma	
Technique	**Features**
Ultrasound	Heterogeneous echogenicity Peripheral dilated bile ducts
CT	Hypodense mass ± satellite lesions Capsular retraction (seen in 20%)
MR	T1-weighted: Isointense or hypointense to liver T2-weighted: Periphery more intense than center MRCP may show bile duct invasion
Postcontrast[a]	Arterial phase: Rim enhancement Venous phase: Patchy central enhancement Delayed phase: Increased central enhancement (desmoplastic stroma)

Abbreviations: CT, computed tomography; MR, magnetic resonance; MRCP, magnetic resonance cholangiopancreatography.

[a] The typical pattern of enhancement is described. The delayed central enhancement may not occur or not be seen until at least 20 minutes after contrast injection.

Data from Lim JH. Cholangiocarcinoma: morphologic classification according to growth pattern and imaging findings. AJR Am J Roentgenol 2003;181(3):819–27.

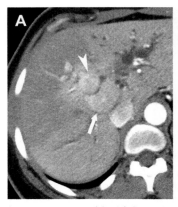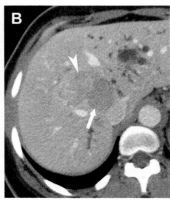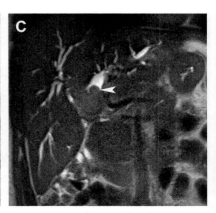

Fig. 7. A 45-year-old with hepatitis C and cirrhosis shows a mass that has a component (*arrow*) that shows hypervascularity in the arterial phase (*A*) and washout on the venous phase (*B*). Another part of the tumor shows persistent enhancement on the venous phase (*arrowhead*). Coronal T2-weighted MR imaging (*C*) shows intraductal invasion by tumor (*arrowhead*). The appearances are atypical for conventional hepatocellular carcinoma (HCC). Biopsy revealed HCC and cholangiocarcinoma elements in keeping with a biphenotypic tumor.

and secondary inflammation that may be confused for cancer. The following gives an approach to investigating biliary strictures.

INVESTIGATION OF BILIARY STRICTURE

There is no single study that has high sensitivity and specificity for diagnosing a biliary stricture as benign or malignant. Hence, a series of imaging and endoscopic tests are used. A potential

Table 5	
Causes of perihilar biliary stricture	
Benign	Iatrogenic (liver transplant, cholecystectomy)[a]
	Primary sclerosing cholangitis
	IgG4 sclerosing cholangiopathy
	Mirizzi syndrome[a]
	Infections (tuberculosis, viral, parasitic, human immunodeficiency virus cholangiopathy)[a]
	Ischemia: hepatic arterial thrombosis, chemotherapy induced[a]
	Vasculitis[a]
	Eosinophilic cholangitis[a]
	Radiation therapy[a]
Malignant	Cholangiocarcinoma
	Extrinsic compression by metastatic nodal disease[a]

[a] Imaging findings or clinical history may distinguish from cholangiocarcinoma.
Data from Singh A, Gelrud A, Agarwal B. Biliary strictures: diagnostic considerations and approach. Gastroenterol Rep (Oxf) 2015;3(1):22–31.

algorithm[7] for screening and diagnosing CCA in patients with PSC is shown in **Fig. 11**.

Imaging Studies

A dominant stricture is a stenosis with a diameter of less than 1.5 mm in the common bile duct or less than 1 mm in the hepatic duct.[8] This finding is seen in 50% to 60% of patients with PSC. It is thought that the accuracy of MR imaging in diagnosing a biliary stricture is at least as good as endoscopic retrograde cholangiopancreatography. Nevertheless, a dominant stricture in the extrahepatic ducts diagnosed by MR imaging with magnetic resonance cholangiopancreatography or endoscopic retrograde cholangiopancreatography has only a sensitivity of 66% and specificity of 50% for cancer. Benign causes of strictures include inflammation and ischemia.

Tumor Markers

Tumor markers play a limited role in early detection of CCA, especially in patients with PSC.[47] CA19-9 is a glycolipid expressed by cancer cells that may be used as a marker to detect hepatic and extrahepatic malignancies. Elevated CA19-9 marker has only an average sensitivity (50%–60%) for CCA. False-positive results may occur with inflammatory bowel disease or infective cholangitis. CA19-9 also requires the Lewis blood group antigen to be expressed, and up to 10% of the population lack the enzyme to produce the marker.[5] Carcinoembryonic antigen is a glycoprotein involved in cellular adhesions and is expressed by many gastrointestinal malignancies. The marker was found to have a low sensitivity of 33% for CCA in patients with PSC.

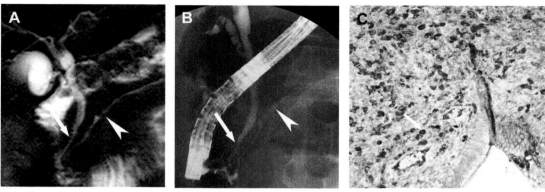

Fig. 8. A 46-year-old man with jaundice. (*A*) Magnetic resonance cholangiopancreatography and (*B*) endoscopic retrograde cholangiopancreatography show a stricture of the distal common bile duct (*arrows*). The main pancreatic duct (*arrowheads*) is not dilated. Brushings and fluorescence in situ hybridization analysis were equivocal. The patient underwent a radical pancreaticoduodenectomy. (*C*) Surgical pathology showed plasma cells (*arrow*) staining positive for IgG4, consistent with IgG4 sclerosing cholangitis.

Endoscopic Techniques

Endoscopic retrograde cholangiopancreatography has the advantage of not only performing a cholangiogram, but also concomitant brushing, biopsies for chromosomal analysis, and cholangioscopy of the main bile ducts. The sensitivity of brush cytology in diagnosing CCA is low, ranging from 20% to 40%.[8] It is usual to perform fluorescence in situ hybridization analysis,[5,38] which increases the detection of malignancy by looking for chromosomal aneuploidy or polysomy in cytologic specimen. Multifocal fluorescence in situ hybridization polysomy is a strong predictor of

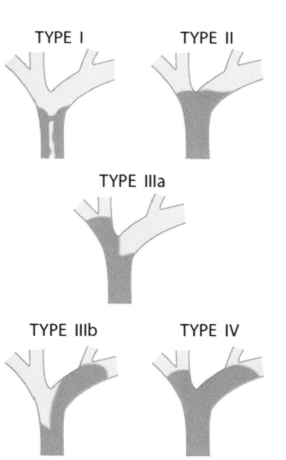

Fig. 9. Bismuth Colette classification of perihilar cholangiocarcinoma.

Box 2
Diagnostic criteria for unresectability of perihilar CCA

1. Tumor extension to secondary bile ducts bilaterally

2. Bilateral invasion of the hepatic artery branches

3. Bilateral invasion of the portal vein branches

4. Invasion of long segment of main hepatic artery or main portal vein

5. Atrophy of one lobe with contralateral vascular invasion

6. Metastases to mesenteric, celiac or para-aortic nodes (N2 disease)

7. Distant metastases (M1 disease)

Data from Choi JY, Kim MJ, Lee JM, et al. Hilar cholangiocarcinoma: role of preoperative imaging with sonography, MDCT, MRI, and direct cholangiography. AJR Am J Roentgenol 2008;191(5):1448–57.

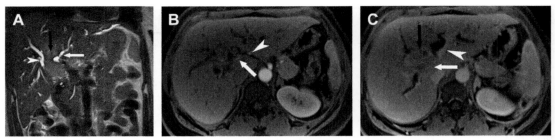

Fig. 10. A 75-year-old with jaundice proven to have perihilar cholangiocarcinoma (CCA). (*A*) Coronal T2-weighted MR imaging shows obstruction of the distal left (*white arrow*) and right (*arrowhead*) hepatic ducts by a mildly hyperintense mass (*black arrow*). The tumor does not invade along the wall of the right and left hepatic ducts into secondary branches. (*B*) Arterial phase image shows that the tumor involves the right hepatic artery (*arrow*) but not the left hepatic artery (*arrowhead*). (*C*) Venous phase image shows that the tumor (*black arrow*) enhances more in this phase. The lesion causes thrombosis of the right portal vein branch (*white arrow*) but not the left portal vein branch (*arrowhead*). These features, in the absence of distant adenopathy or metastasis, suggest that the CCA may be resectable with partial right hepatectomy to leave a viable left liver lobe. The patient underwent surgery with negative surgical margins.

CCA.[48] Fluorescence in situ hybridization is proven to be a valuable additional step in determining malignancy, by diagnosing cancer with sensitivity of about 60% and specificity of 90% when brush cytology was negative.[5,49]

Immunohistochemical examination for molecular markers, for example, p53 and K-ras mutation, have not been shown to improve cancer detection when compared with the results of brush cytology. Cholangioscopy is a newer technique for directly visualizing the mucosa of biliary ductal irregularities to detect superficial spreading cancer. Cholangioscopy may show a polypoid or villous intraductal mass in malignant strictures, whereas the mucosa of benign strictures are typically ulcerated or smooth. Small reports have suggested

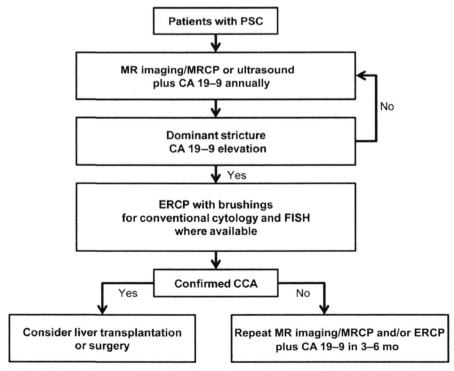

Fig. 11. Algorithm for bile structure. CA 19-9, carbohydrate antigen 19-9; CCA, cholangiocarcinoma; ERCP, endoscopic retrograde cholangiopancreatography; FISH, fluorescence in situ hybridization; MRCP, magnetic resonance cholangiopancreatography; PSC, primary sclerosing cholangitis.

sensitivity and specificity of about 90% for a diagnosis of CCA.[21]

EUS imaging may be used in some cases of patients with PSC with indeterminate dominant biliary strictures, or adenopathy. In a small study, EUS-guided fine needle aspiration was positive in 70% of patients who had cancer on surgical pathology.[50] Another study showed that EUS imaging changed management in more than 80% of patients by avoiding surgery in those with inoperable malignant disease or benign disease and enabling surgery in those with operable malignant disease.[47] However, EUS-guided fine needle aspiration has a low negative predictive value, in common with most cytologic assessments.

SUMMARY

The location of CCA may be classified as intrahepatic, perihilar, or distal duct. On imaging, CCA may appear as mass-forming, periductal infiltrating lesion or an intraductal papillary lesion. On imaging, GBC may be a mass, thickened gallbladder wall, or polypoid lesion in the gallbladder.

Both CCA and GBC have poor outcomes once clinically evident. Some high-risk groups may benefit from screening. Patients with gallbladder polyps that are at low risk for GBC, that is, 6 to 10 mm in size without concomitant risk factors such as solitary sessile polyp or PSC, may be screened with ultrasonography. Those with moderate and high risk for GBC would benefit from empiric cholecystectomy. Patients with PSC would benefit from annual gallbladder ultrasonography to assess for polyps.

For perihilar and distal ductal CCA, the main risk factor is PSC. There are no consensus guidelines for the cost effectiveness of screening for CCA in these patients. Nevertheless, many physicians perform annual sonography and/or MR imaging with magnetic resonance cholangiopancreatography together with semiannual CA19-9 measurements. If suspicion for CCA is raised, such as increasing CA19-9 levels or dominant biliary stricture on imaging, further testing would be required. In some cases, repeat endoscopic procedures may be required at 3 and 6 months. Many causes of cirrhosis increase the risk of intrahepatic CCA. Fortunately, many of these patients are screened for HCC, and additional screening for CCA is not required.

REFERENCES

1. Goldin RD, Roa JC. Gallbladder cancer: a morphological and molecular update. Histopathology 2009;55(2):218–29.

2. Reid KM, Ramos-De la Medina A, Donohue JH. Diagnosis and surgical management of gallbladder cancer: a review. J Gastrointest Surg 2007;11(5):671–81.

3. Stephen AE, Berger DL. Carcinoma in the porcelain gallbladder: a relationship revisited. Surgery 2001;129(6):699–703.

4. Towfigh S, McFadden DW, Cortina GR, et al. Porcelain gallbladder is not associated with gallbladder carcinoma. Am Surg 2001;67(1):7–10.

5. Horsley-Silva JL, Rodriguez EA, Franco DL, et al. An update on cancer risk and surveillance in primary sclerosing cholangitis. Liver Int 2017;37(8):1103–9.

6. Eaton JE, Thackeray EW, Lindor KD. Likelihood of malignancy in gallbladder polyps and outcomes following cholecystectomy in primary sclerosing cholangitis. Am J Gastroenterol 2012;107(3):431–9.

7. Razumilava N, Gores GJ, Lindor KD. Cancer surveillance in patients with primary sclerosing cholangitis. Hepatology 2011;54(5):1842–52.

8. Chapman R, Fevery J, Kalloo A, et al. Diagnosis and management of primary sclerosing cholangitis. Hepatology 2010;51(2):660–78.

9. Trivedi V, Gumaste VV, Liu S, et al. Gallbladder cancer: adenoma-carcinoma or dysplasia-carcinoma sequence? Gastroenterol Hepatol 2008;4(10):735–7.

10. Misra S, Chaturvedi A, Misra NC, et al. Carcinoma of the gallbladder. Lancet Oncol 2003;4(3):167–76.

11. Corwin MT, Siewert B, Sheiman RG, et al. Incidentally detected gallbladder polyps: is follow-up necessary?–Long-term clinical and US analysis of 346 patients. Radiology 2011;258(1):277–82.

12. Donald G, Sunjaya D, Donahue T, et al. Polyp on ultrasound: now what? The association between gallbladder polyps and cancer. Am Surg 2013;79(10):1005–8.

13. Paraskevopoulos JA, Dennison AR, Johnson AG. Primary carcinoma of the gallbladder. HPB Surg 1991;4(4):277–89.

14. Carriaga MT, Henson DE. Liver, gallbladder, extrahepatic bile ducts, and pancreas. Cancer 1995;75(1 Suppl):171–90.

15. Cornell CM, Clarke R. Vicarious calcification involving the gallbladder. Ann Surg 1959;149(2):267–72.

16. Khan ZS, Livingston EH, Huerta S. Reassessing the need for prophylactic surgery in patients with porcelain gallbladder: case series and systematic review of the literature. Arch Surg 2011;146(10):1143–7.

17. Andren-Sandberg A. Diagnosis and management of gallbladder polyps. N Am J Med Sci 2012;4(5):203–11.

18. Bhatt NR, Gillis A, Smoothey CO, et al. Evidence based management of polyps of the gall bladder: a systematic review of the risk factors of malignancy. Surgeon 2016;14(5):278–86.

19. Elmasry M, Lindop D, Dunne DF, et al. The risk of malignancy in ultrasound detected gallbladder polyps: a systematic review. Int J Surg 2016;33(Pt A):28–35.

20. Mellnick VM, Menias CO, Sandrasegaran K, et al. Polypoid lesions of the gallbladder: disease spectrum with pathologic correlation. Radiographics 2015;35(2):387–99.

21. Anderson MA, Appalaneni V, Ben-Menachem T, et al. The role of endoscopy in the evaluation and treatment of patients with biliary neoplasia. Gastrointest Endosc 2013;77(2):167–74.

22. Park JY, Hong SP, Kim YJ, et al. Long-term follow up of gallbladder polyps. J Gastroenterol Hepatol 2009; 24(2):219–22.

23. Gallahan WC, Conway JD. Diagnosis and management of gallbladder polyps. Gastroenterol Clin North Am 2010;39(2):359–67, x.

24. Karlsen TH, Schrumpf E, Boberg KM. Gallbladder polyps in primary sclerosing cholangitis: not so benign. Curr Opin Gastroenterol 2008;24(3):395–9.

25. Buckles DC, Lindor KD, Larusso NF, et al. In primary sclerosing cholangitis, gallbladder polyps are frequently malignant. Am J Gastroenterol 2002; 97(5):1138–42.

26. Kim SW, Kim HC, Yang DM, et al. Gallbladder carcinoma: causes of misdiagnosis at CT. Clin Radiol 2016;71(1):e96–109.

27. Clemente G, Nuzzo G, De Rose AM, et al. Unexpected gallbladder cancer after laparoscopic cholecystectomy for acute cholecystitis: a worrisome picture. J Gastrointest Surg 2012;16(8):1462–8.

28. Levy AD, Murakata LA, Abbott RM, et al. From the archives of the AFIP. Benign tumors and tumorlike lesions of the gallbladder and extrahepatic bile ducts: radiologic-pathologic correlation. Armed Forces Institute of Pathology. Radiographics 2002;22(2): 387–413.

29. Sadamoto Y, Kubo H, Harada N, et al. Preoperative diagnosis and staging of gallbladder carcinoma by EUS. Gastrointest Endosc 2003;58(4):536–41.

30. Xu HX. Contrast-enhanced ultrasound in the biliary system: potential uses and indications. World J Radiol 2009;1(1):37–44.

31. Xie XH, Xu HX, Xie XY, et al. Differential diagnosis between benign and malignant gallbladder diseases with real-time contrast-enhanced ultrasound. Eur Radiol 2010;20(1):239–48.

32. Gatto M, Alvaro D. New insights on cholangiocarcinoma. World J Gastrointest Oncol 2010;2(3): 136–45.

33. Olnes MJ, Erlich R. A review and update on cholangiocarcinoma. Oncology 2004;66(3):167–79.

34. Cai Y, Cheng N, Ye H, et al. The current management of cholangiocarcinoma: a comparison of current guidelines. Biosci Trends 2016;10(2):92–102.

35. Benavides M, Anton A, Gallego J, et al. Biliary tract cancers: SEOM clinical guidelines. Clin Transl Oncol 2015;17(12):982–7.

36. Gatto M, Bragazzi MC, Semeraro R, et al. Cholangiocarcinoma: update and future perspectives. Dig Liver Dis 2010;42(4):253–60.

37. Khan SA, Davidson BR, Goldin RD, et al. Guidelines for the diagnosis and treatment of cholangiocarcinoma: an update. Gut 2012;61(12):1657–69.

38. Burak K, Angulo P, Pasha TM, et al. Incidence and risk factors for cholangiocarcinoma in primary sclerosing cholangitis. Am J Gastroenterol 2004;99(3):523–6.

39. Cullen SN, Chapman RW. Review article: current management of primary sclerosing cholangitis. Aliment Pharmacol Ther 2005;21(8):933–48.

40. Lindor KD, Kowdley KV, Harrison ME. ACG clinical guideline: primary sclerosing cholangitis. Am J Gastroenterol 2015;110(5):646–59 [quiz: 660].

41. Benson AB 3rd, Abrams TA, Ben-Josef E, et al. NCCN clinical practice guidelines in oncology: hepatobiliary cancers. J Natl Compr Canc Netw 2009; 7(4):350–91.

42. Bridgewater J, Galle PR, Khan SA, et al. Guidelines for the diagnosis and management of intrahepatic cholangiocarcinoma. J Hepatol 2014;60(6):1268–89.

43. Charatcharoenwitthaya P, Enders FB, Halling KC, et al. Utility of serum tumor markers, imaging, and biliary cytology for detecting cholangiocarcinoma in primary sclerosing cholangitis. Hepatology 2008; 48(4):1106–17.

44. Lim JH. Cholangiocarcinoma: morphologic classification according to growth pattern and imaging findings. AJR Am J Roentgenol 2003;181(3):819–27.

45. Singh A, Gelrud A, Agarwal B. Biliary strictures: diagnostic considerations and approach. Gastroenterol Rep (Oxf) 2015;3(1):22–31.

46. Choi JY, Kim MJ, Lee JM, et al. Hilar cholangiocarcinoma: role of preoperative imaging with sonography, MDCT, MRI, and direct cholangiography. AJR Am J Roentgenol 2008;191(5):1448–57.

47. El Fouly A, Dechene A, Gerken G. Surveillance and screening of primary sclerosing cholangitis. Dig Dis 2009;27(4):526–35.

48. Eaton JE, Barr Fritcher EG, Gores GJ, et al. Biliary multifocal chromosomal polysomy and cholangiocarcinoma in primary sclerosing cholangitis. Am J Gastroenterol 2015;110(2):299–309.

49. Salomao M, Gonda TA, Margolskee E, et al. Strategies for improving diagnostic accuracy of biliary strictures. Cancer Cytopathol 2015;123(4):244–52.

50. DeWitt J, Misra VL, Leblanc JK, et al. EUS-guided FNA of proximal biliary strictures after negative ERCP brush cytology results. Gastrointest Endosc 2006;64(3):325–33.

Imaging and Screening of Pancreatic Cancer

Kristine S. Burk, MD*, Grace C. Lo, MD, Michael S. Gee, MD, PhD, Dushyant V. Sahani, MD

KEYWORDS

- Pancreatic cancer • Pancreatic neuroendocrine tumor • Pancreatic ductal adenocarcinoma
- Cancer screening • Hereditary tumor predisposition syndromes • Precursor lesions
- Familial pancreatic cancer syndrome

KEY POINTS

- Pancreatic cancer screening is not recommended for the general population; the low disease prevalence drives down the positive predictive value of even the best imaging examinations.
- Screening for pancreatic ductal adenocarcinoma is recommended for patients with an increased lifetime risk.
- Screening for pancreatic neuroendocrine tumors is recommended for those patients with multiple endocrine neoplasia type 1, tuberous sclerosis complex, and Von Hippel Lindau disease.
- MR imaging, magnetic resonance cholangiopancreatography (MRCP), endoscopic ultrasound, and multidetector computed tomography (MDCT) can all be used for pancreatic cancer screening.

INTRODUCTION

Pancreatic neoplasms can be split into 2 broad categories—neoplasms of the exocrine cells and ductal system, and neoplasms of the endocrine islet cells. Pancreatic ductal adenocarcinoma (PDAC) is by far the most common type of exocrine neoplasm, and indeed the most common type of neoplasm of the pancreas overall. The American Cancer Society estimates there were 53,070 new cases of PDAC in 2016. Unfortunately, PDAC carries a poor prognosis; it is estimated to be the third leading cause of cancer deaths in 2017, after lung and colorectal cancers. Risk factors for PDAC seen in the general population are nonspecific and include advancing age, fatty infiltration associated with obesity, cigarette smoking, new-onset diabetes, and chronic pancreatitis. Although these risk factors are common, the average lifetime risk of developing pancreatic cancer remains low at 1.5%.[1] Even though the disease caries high morbidity and mortality, screening for PDAC is not recommended for the general population because the low incidence of the disease drives down the positive predictive value of even high sensitivity assays.[2] In the general population, screening may even result in a small loss of net life expectancy related to unnecessary surgical mortality risks from false-positive diagnoses.[3,4]

Certain populations are at higher than normal risk for the development of PDAC, including those with precursor lesions such as intraductal papillary mucinous neoplasms (IPMN) of the pancreas, and those with predisposing genetic conditions including familial atypical multiple mole melanoma, Peutz-Jeghers syndrome, and hereditary breast–ovarian cancer, to name a few. In these high-risk populations with a higher prevalence of the disease, screening is recommended because PDAC that is discovered earlier may be potentially curable. Successful screening has been defined

Disclosure Statement: The authors have nothing to disclose.
Department of Radiology, Massachusetts General Hospital, 55 Fruit Street, Boston, MA 02114, USA
* Corresponding author.
E-mail address: ksburk@partners.org

radiologic.theclinics.com

by the International Cancer of the Pancreas Screening Consortium as the detection and treatment of T1N0M0 margin negative PDAC or high-grade dysplastic precursor lesions including pancreatic intraepithelial neoplasia, IPMN with high-grade dysplasia, and mucinous cystic neoplasm with high-grade dysplasia.[4]

Pancreatic neuroendocrine tumors are a diverse group of tumors originating from the endocrine cells of the pancreas, with subtypes including insulinomas, gastrinomas, glucagonomas, somatostatinomas, and VIPomas. These tumors can be symptomatic causing hormonal phenomena like hypoglycemia or Zollinger-Ellison syndrome and, when they are symptomatic, are often found with imaging when they are very small. Asymptomatic tumors, in contrast, are most often found incidentally and are commonly large at presentation. As a group, neuroendocrine tumors are rare, making up less than 3% of all pancreatic tumors. The current overall incidence is 5.86 per 100,000 cases per year.[5] Given their low incidence, screening for neuroendocrine tumors is also not recommended for the general population. However, as with exocrine neoplasms, there are certain genetic conditions that predispose to neuroendocrine tumors, including multiple endocrine neoplasia type 1 (MEN1), Von Hippel Lindau syndrome, and others, for which screening is recommended to minimize morbidity and mortality.[6]

IMAGING MODALITIES

Multiple imaging modalities can be used to detect pancreatic masses including multidetector computed tomography (MDCT) and MR imaging, magnetic resonance cholangiopancreatography (MRCP), and endoscopic ultrasound (EUS). A summary of the relative performance of these modalities for detection of particular imaging features is found in **Table 1**.

Multidetector Computed Tomography

The most sensitive MDCT examination is a triple phase, pancreatic protocol examination. Three phases of contrast are obtained: the arterial phase at 30 seconds, the pancreatic parenchymal phase at 45 seconds, and the portal venous phase at 60 to 70 seconds. Overall, for the detection of solid pancreatic masses, the pancreatic protocol MDCT is greater than 90% sensitive and 99% specific.[7] However, for the detection of small tumors less than 2 cm sensitivity decreases to approximately 77%,[8] possibly because of the tendency for small tumors to be isodense rather than hypodense to the surrounding pancreatic parenchyma.[9] For the detection of small cystic pancreatic masses, MDCT has inferior performance compared with MR imaging, MRCP, or EUS.[10] In the evaluation for malignant features of larger cystic masses, pancreatic protocol MDCT detects septae with 94% sensitivity, mural nodules with 71% sensitivity, and main duct communication with 86% sensitivity.[11] An additional feature of MDCT is the ability to detect calcification within a lesion, which can be more difficult with MR imaging, MRCP, or EUS.

One drawback of pancreatic protocol MDCT is radiation dose exposure, driven largely by the multiple phases of contrast enhancement required for the evaluation. As a result, screening with MR imaging–MRCP rather than MDCT has generally been recommended.[4] More recently, however advances in dual energy CT (DECT) technology have reestablished CT as a reasonable screening option. DECT allows for a 2-fold decrease in radiation dose through use of virtual non–contrast-enhanced sequences and low kilovolt images that enhance the soft tissue contrast between hypoattenuating PDAC and the surrounding pancreatic parenchyma (**Fig. 1**).[12–15] DECT also allows for the possibility of decreased doses of intravenous contrast while maintaining or even possibly improving diagnostic interpretability.[16,17]

Table 1
Performance of screening modalities for detection of specific features

Detection of Feature	MDCT	MR Imaging and MRCP	EUS
Small solid lesion	++	++	+++
Cyst septa	+++	+++	+++
Cyst mural nodules	++	+++	+++
Cyst MPD communication	++	+++	+++
Other	+ Calcification	+ No radiation	− Invasive

Abbreviations: EUS, endoscopic ultrasound; MDCT, multidetector computed tomography; MPD, main pancreatic duct; MRCP, magnetic resonance cholangiopancreatography.

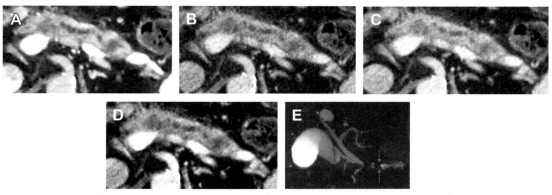

Fig. 1. A 66-year-old with recent onset diabetes was found to have a pancreatic ductal adenocarcinoma in the pancreatic neck with upstream pancreatic ductal dilatation. This mass is best seen on the pancreatic phase monoenergetic 50 keV images (A), although it is also well seen on monoenergetic 55 keV (B) and 65 keV (C) images obtained in the portal venous phase, and on the iodine map (D). These demonstrate how dual energy computed tomography (CT) scanning can increase lesion conspicuity, potentially eliminating the need for multiphasic CT examinations. Magnetic resonance cholangiopancreatography performed in the same patient (E) demonstrates distal pancreatic duct dilatation and irregularity with an abrupt cutoff at the level of the pancreatic neck mass (red arrows).

For patients with cancer with a high likelihood of comorbidities and possible use of renal toxic medications, reduction of iodine administration may be crucial in maintaining renal function.

MR Imaging and Magnetic Resonance Cholangiopancreatography

MR imaging of the pancreas with MRCP is a second screening option, and is the preferred method of screening in young patients for whom minimization of radiation is paramount.[18] Commonly used sequences in this evaluation are listed in **Box 1**.[19,20]

Box 1
Example MR imaging/MRCP protocol

Axial T2 FSE with or without fat suppression

Coronal T2 FSE with or without fat suppression

Axial T1 in-phase and opposed-phase GRE

Axial diffusion-weighted imaging

Axial 3D T1 fat-suppressed spoiled GRE

Axial T1 post-pancreatic phase

Axial T1 post-portal venous phase

Axial T1 post-equilibrium phase or delayed phase

Coronal thick slab T2-weighted MRCP

Coronal 3D space T2-weighted MRCP

Abbreviations: 3D, 3-dimensional; GRE, gradient recalled echo; FSE, fast spin echo; MRCP, magnetic resonance cholangiopancreatography; MRP, magnetic resonance pancreatography.

MR imaging with MRCP compares favorably with MDCT for the conspicuity of solid lesions less than 3 cm with greater than 98% sensitivity.[21] MR imaging with MRCP also has improved sensitivity compared with MDCT for evaluation of cystic lesions, with higher sensitivities for features including septa (91%) and main duct communication (100%). Overall, MR imaging with MRCP performs on par with MDCT for detection of solid lesions given the presence of secondary features, and for accuracy of distinguishing benign from malignant cystic lesions (73%–95%).[22,23]

A more recent development has been the use of whole body screening MR imaging for children with multiorgan hereditary cancer predisposition syndromes such as Li-Fraumeni syndrome. Protocols described in the literature include coronal short T1 inversion recovery (STIR) and T1-weighted sequences, axial short T1 inversion recovery, T2-weighted fast spin sequences, and triplanar single shot fast spin echo half Fourier acquisition single shot turbo spin echo (SSFSE HASTE) sequences.[24] This technique may play a role in the future for screening for pancreatic neuroendocrine tumors in young patients.

Endoscopic Ultrasound Imaging

The final modality that has been used for pancreatic cancer screening is EUS. EUS examination has been shown to be superior to MDCT scanning for the detection of small solid pancreatic lesions, with one study citing 98% sensitivity.[25] It performs similarly to MR imaging for the evaluation of cystic lesions, with similar performance detecting septa, solid nodules, main pancreatic duct communication, and main pancreatic duct dilatation.[26] A major drawback of this examination is its invasive nature, which has discouraged some from using this modality for screening. However, EUS examination plays a large role in the further characterization of suspicious findings found on MDCT or MR imaging, particularly when aspiration or biopsy is required.

EXOCRINE TUMORS
Precursor Lesions of Pancreatic Ductal Adenocarcinoma

The most common PDAC precursor lesion encountered in the general population is the IPMN. These are seen more often in men than women (60%/40%), are typically found in the 6th and 7th decades, and come in 2 types: main duct IPMNs and side branch IMPNs.[27] Main duct IPMNs are characterized by a mucin-filled, diffusely dilated main pancreatic duct. Side branch IPMNs, in contrast, predominantly involve side-branch pancreatic ducts and affect the main pancreatic duct only minimally if at all. Side branch IPMNs are macrocystic and sometimes multiloculated in appearance with a visible connection to the main pancreatic duct, distinct walls, and septae.[27]

The presence of an IPMN is increases the risk of pancreatic cancer through 2 mechanisms: the development of high-grade dysplasia or malignancy within the IPMN itself, and the development of a separate PDAC. The risk of degeneration to high-grade dysplasia or malignancy is far greater for main duct IPMNs than for side branch IPMNs: a 57% to 92% chance within 5 years versus a 6% to 46% chance within 5 years.[28] As a result, patients with main duct IPMNs are typically recommended to undergo immediate surgical excision.[29] Those with side branch IPMNs may be followed with imaging and be screened over time for the development of worrisome features within the IPMN or the development of a new PDAC.

The appropriate screening algorithm has been a topic of much debate over the last decade. In 2017, the ACR Incidental Findings Committee published guidelines for follow up of cystic pancreatic lesions in JACR.[30] These guidelines updated those recommendations made by the Sendai International Consensus Group in 2012[31], and are summarized in **Fig. 2**.

Pancreatic intraepithelial neoplasia is a more recently recognized precursor lesion that has been associated with increasing age, diffuse inflammatory conditions such as chronic pancreatitis, and pancreatic lipomatosis.[32,33] It is a microscopic lesion consisting of noninvasive epithelial neoplasia, which is graded (1–3) based on the degree of nuclear atypia. Given that they are microscopic, these are radiographically occult and typically found incidentally in pancreatic cyst resection specimens.[32] Additional precursor lesions include mucinous cystadenomas, which degenerate to cystadenocarcinomas in 6% to 36% if left untreated,[34] and solid pseudopapillary tumors of the pancreas, which carry a 15% to 16% chance of malignancy.[35–37] These lesions are commonly encountered in middle-aged and young adult patients, respectively, and owing to their high malignancy risk are surgically excised after diagnosis rather than followed. Thus, a discussion of screening does not apply to these cancers.

Genetically High-Risk Populations

It has been estimated that approximately 10% of PDAC has a familial basis. Pancreatic cancer with a familial link can be divided into 3 groups: those that are hereditary tumor predisposition syndromes, syndromes with chronic inflammation of the pancreas, and familial pancreatic cancer (FPC) syndrome.

Hereditary tumor predisposition syndromes include Peutz-Jeghers syndrome, familial atypical multiple mole melanoma, hereditary breast-ovarian cancer, hereditary nonpolyposis colorectal carcinoma, and familial adenomatous polyposis.[38] Associated gene mutations, risk of PDAC development, and screening recommendations are summarized in **Table 2**.[4,39–46] Syndromes with chronic inflammation of the pancreas includes hereditary pancreatitis and cystic fibrosis. As a chronic inflammatory process, these diseases have a secondarily increased risk of developing pancreatic cancer. FPC syndrome applies to families with 2 or more first-degree relatives with pancreatic cancer that does not fall into the first 2 categories. Although no single gene is clearly associated with FPC syndrome, it likely is caused by at least 1 major gene and is commonly associated with gene mutations such as BRCA2.[47] In each of these populations of patients, who have a relative risk greater than 2.4 in men and 2.7 in women, screening results in a net gain in life expectancy attributed to increased detection of precursor lesions and early PDAC.[3] Indeed, screening for patients with 2 relatives and at least 1 first-degree relative with PDAC from an FPC syndrome, Peutz-Jeghers syndrome, or p16, BRCA2, and hereditary nonpolyposis colorectal carcinoma mutations and at least 1 first-degree relative with PDAC

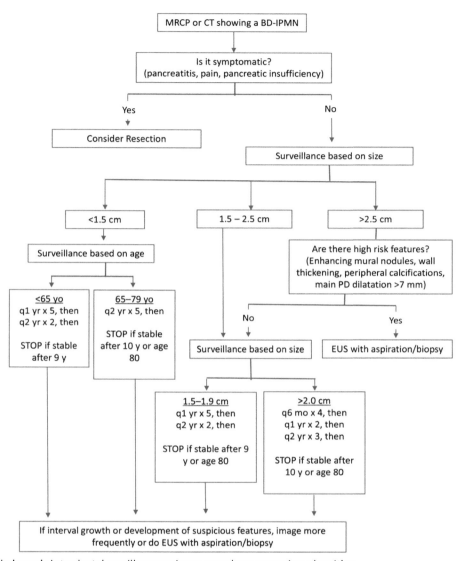

Fig. 2. Side branch intraductal papillary mucinous neoplasm screening algorithm.

has been recommended by the International Cancer of the Pancreas Screening Consortium.[10]

There is no consensus on the optimal time to begin screening for PDAC, which has an average age at diagnosis of 68 years in FPC syndrome.[48] A recent study suggested that screening at the age of 50 would avert the greatest number of deaths associated with PDAC.[3] A notable exception are patients with *PRSS1* mutations and hereditary pancreatitis, who should be screened beginning at age 40 because the average age of PDAC diagnosis was much younger.[46] There is similarly no consensus in the literature regarding the frequency of interval screening examinations or the appropriate age

to stop screening. However, many support a 12-month interval between screening examinations, although this is not largely substantiated with support in the literature.

Imaging Features of Pancreatic Ductal Adenocarcinoma

When screening for the development of a new PDAC, one will typically be looking for small, subtle tumors. Classically, PDACs seem to be hypodense relative to the surrounding pancreas, but in 5.4% of cases they can seem to be isodense, especially when less than 2 cm in size.[26] These isoattenuating lesions are sometimes best seen

Table 2
Pancreatic ductal adenocarcinoma predisposition syndromes

Genetic Syndrome	Gene Mutations	Relative Risk	Screening Recommendation	References
Peutz-Jeghers syndrome	STK11	132x	Screen regardless of family history	Canto 2013, Giardiello 1998
Hereditary breast-ovarian cancer	BRCA1 BRCA2	3.6x 3.5–10x	Screen BRCA2 carriers with one affected FDR or with 2 affected family members (no FDR)	Canto 2013, Grover 2010, Templeton 2013, Peterson 2016
	PALB2	Unknown	Screen PALB2 carriers with one affected FDR	
Familial atypical multiple mole melanoma	p16/CDKN2A	13–22x	Screen p16 carriers with 1 affected FDR	Canto 2013, Lynch 2008
HNPCC	MLH1, MSH2, MSH6, PMS2	8.6x	Screen HNPCC patients with on affected FDR	Canto 2013, Kastrinos 2009
Hereditary pancreatitis	PRSS1, SPINK1	50–80x	Screen starting at age 40	Canto 2013, Grover 2010, Chang 2014, Ulrich 2001
Familial pancreatic cancer	Unknown	32x with 3+ FDR 6.4x with 2 FDR	Screen FPC patients with 2 affected family members with at least 1 FDR	Canto 2013, Chang 2014

Abbreviations: FDR, first-degree relative; HNPCC, hereditary nonpolyposis colorectal carcinoma.

on the pancreatic phase, and other times the portal venous phase, making vigilance on all series paramount.[9] On MR imaging, PDACs are T1 hypointense relative to the surrounding inherently T1 bright pancreatic parenchyma.

Secondary signs are seen in 88% of isodense pancreatic cancers that are less than 2 cm, increasing overall conspicuity; these are especially common when the cancer is in the head or body (Fig. 3). These include pancreatic duct cutoff, pancreatic duct or common bile duct dilatation, parenchymal atrophy, and a new contour abnormality (Fig. 4). Less common appearances of new pancreatic cancers include cystic lesions and acute pancreatitis. Frequencies of each of these appearances are summarized in Table 3.[9,49] In cases mimicking acute pancreatitis, the duct-penetrating sign, in which the main pancreatic duct clearly courses through and becomes stenotic in the mass, can increase concern for neoplasm over inflammation with a sensitivity of 85% and specificity of 96%.[50]

Changes within an existing IPMN that should raise concern include growth to greater than 3 cm, the development of solid mural nodules,

the development of thickened or enhancing cyst walls, and dilatation of the main pancreatic duct to greater than 6 mm. These features and their odds ratio of malignant degeneration are listed in Table 4 and illustrated in Fig. 5.[51,52] A clinical example of malignant degeneration in a side branch IPMN is provided in Fig. 6.

ENDOCRINE TUMORS
Genetically High-Risk Populations

There are 3 genetic syndromes that predispose to the development of pancreatic neuroendocrine tumors, namely, MEN1, Von Hippel Lindau disease, and tuberous sclerosis complex.

It is estimated that 30% to 80% of patients with MEN1 will develop a PNET in their lifetime, with gastrinomas, insulinomas, and nonfunctioning PNETs being the most common subtypes of PNETs found. The average size of MEN1 related PNETs found on imaging varies from 2.4 to 4 cm; however, most studies also cite an average of 2.9 to 4.8 PNETs discovered in surgical specimens so contribution from microscopic disease is likely underestimated.[6] Current

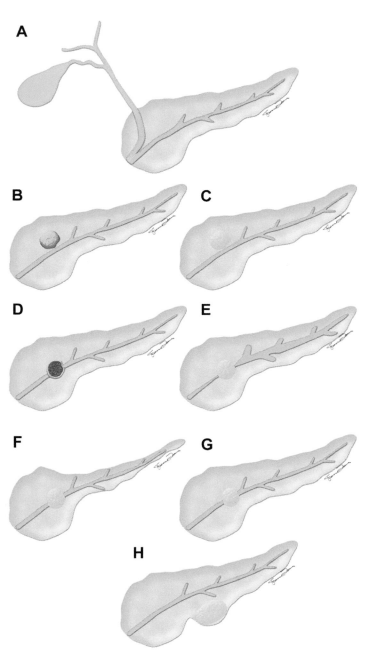

Fig. 3. Imaging features of subtle pancreatic ductal adenocarcinoma. Normal appearance of the pancreas, pancreatic duct, and distal common bile duct (A). A hypodense pancreatic cancer is conspicuous in the pancreatic phase of contrast enhancement (B), whereas an isodense pancreatic cancer can be difficult to detect (C). Secondary signs, which can aid in the detection of an isodense lesion, include cystic degeneration (D), distal pancreatic duct dilatation (E), distal pancreatic parenchymal atrophy (F), a focal pancreatic duct cutoff (G), or parenchymal contour abnormality (H).

guidelines recommend annual imaging screening (by MR imaging, EUS, or CT) in MEN1 patients beginning at younger than 10 years of age, in addition to biochemical screening for insulinomas and gastrinomas beginning at ages 5 and 20, respectively.[53]

Von Hippel Lindau disease is an autosomal dominant condition that predisposes to the development of pancreatic cysts, cystadenomas (in 12%), hemangioblastomas (in <1%), adenocarcinomas (in <1%), and nonfunctioning neuroendocrine tumors, seen in 10% to 17%. In contrast with MEN1, PNETs seen in Von Hippel Lindau disease are typically singular, although their average size is similar at 2.6 to 4.3 cm.[6] Current guidelines recommend annual imaging screening for tumors

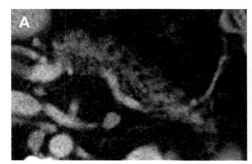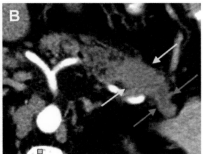

Fig. 4. A 76-year-old with a baseline scan (A) showing a normal pancreatic tail. Follow-up examination 11 months later (B) demonstrates a new contour abnormality and focal increased density of the pancreatic parenchyma (*yellow arrows*), as well as upstream pancreatic ductal dilatation and tail parenchymal atrophy (*red arrows*).

of the pancreas, adrenals, and kidneys beginning at age 8.[54] Given the indolent nature of most of these tumors, imaging follow-up rather than upfront surgery is recommended for small, nonfunctioning PNETs; furthermore, natural history studies have emerged suggesting these do not require annual surveillance, but rather can be followed less frequently.[55]

Tuberous sclerosis complex is the third condition that predisposes to the development of PNETs, with both functional and nonfunctional PNETs diagnosed in these patients. The mechanism of increased risk is thought to be related to the contribution of the mammalian target of rapamycin signaling pathways to PNET development. Overall the frequency of PNET development in tuberous sclerosis complex is small, although some studies cite a frequency of pancreatic tumors of up to 9%.[56] As a result, dedicated pancreatic imaging is not recommended. However, attention to the pancreatic parenchyma on annual renal MR imaging screening

examinations is advised, and is typically how these tumors are diagnosed.[57]

Imaging Features

Typical neuroendocrine tumors are well-defined, rounded and encapsulated, hypodense to isodense to the surrounding pancreatic parenchyma on nonenhanced MDCT, and avidly enhance. They are intrinsically T1 hypointense and T2 bright, and avidly enhance on MR imaging (**Fig. 7**). Asymptomatic tumors that are found incidentally can be quite large and heterogeneous in appearance.[58] More rarely, asymptomatic tumors can by hypoenhancing rather than hyperenhancing; they can also demonstrate intravascular growth, cystic degeneration in up to 10% of cases, and calcifications in up to 16% of cases.[59]

Table 3
Secondary signs of early PDAC

Secondary Sign of PDAC	Frequency (%)	Citation
Total	88	Yoon, 2011
PD or CBD dilatation	63	Yoon, 2011
Pancreatic duct cutoff	59	Yoon, 2011
Parenchymal atrophy	21	Yoon, 2011
Contour abnormality	14	Yoon, 2011
Cystic appearance	8	Kim, 2010
Acute pancreatitis	3	Kim, 2010

Abbreviations: CBD, common bile duct; PD, pancreatic duct; PDAC, pancreatic ductal adenocarcinoma.

Table 4
Signs of malignant degeneration of an Intraductal papillary mucinous neoplasm

Change in Intraductal Papillary Mucinous Neoplasms Appearance	OR	Citation
Growth to >3 cm	2.3–62.4	Kim, 2014; Anand, 2013
Solid mural nodule	6.0–9.3	Kim, 2014; Anand, 2013
Thickened enhancing cyst walls	2.3	Kim, 2014
Dilation of the main pancreatic duct >6 mm	3.4–7.3	Kim, 2014; Anand, 2013

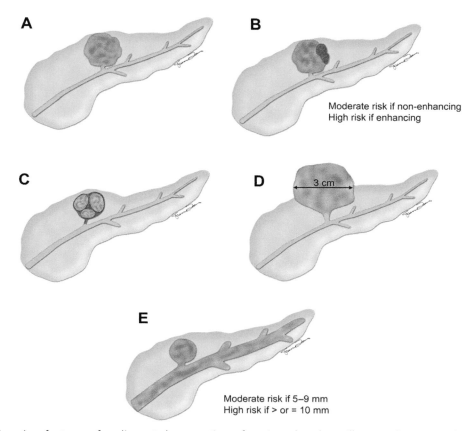

Fig. 5. Imaging features of malignant degeneration of an intraductal papillary mucinous neoplasm. Typical appearance of a side branch intraductal papillary mutinous neoplasm (A). Moderate risk features include a non-enhancing mural nodule (B), thickened or enhancing cyst walls (C), size greater than 3 cm (D), and main pancreatic ductal dilatation of 5 to 9 mm (E). High-risk features include an enhancing mural nodule (B) and main pancreatic ductal dilatation of greater than or equal to 10 mm (E).

Recent work has focused on the differentiation of neuroendocrine tumor grade by MR imaging features. Imaging findings that suggest a high-grade PNET include ill-defined borders, hypoenhancement relative to the normal pancreatic parenchyma on venous and delayed phases, and restricted diffusion.[60,61] Although this works well for larger tumors, diffusion-weighted imaging

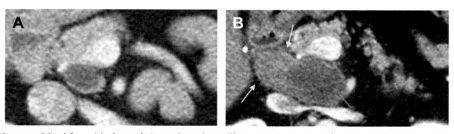

Fig. 6. A 60-year-old with a side branch intraductal papillary mucinous neoplasm. Initial examination showed a unilocular cystic lesion in the head of the pancreas (A). The patient was lost to follow-up. A repeat examination 3 years later (B) showed the development of enhancing septae (red arrow) and a large, enhancing, solid nodular component (yellow arrows), consistent on endoscopic ultrasound-guided biopsy with malignant degeneration into pancreatic adenocarcinoma.

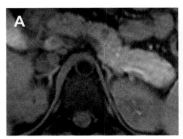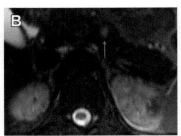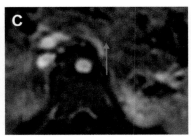

Fig. 7. An 18-year-old with tuberous sclerosis complex. On this MR imaging examination of the kidneys, an incidental pancreatic body lesion was found (*red arrows*). The lesion is T1 hypointense to the normal pancreatic parenchyma (*A*), T2 hyperintense (*B*), and demonstrates arterial enhancement on subtraction images (*C*). On distal pancreatectomy, it was found to be a well-differentiated neuroendocrine tumor.

is less accurate for lesions less than 1 cm, making determination of histologic grade more difficult.

SUMMARY

Pancreatic cancer screening in select populations of patients can significantly impact patient outcomes through the detection and subsequent treatment of pancreatic cancers at an early stage. With advances in noninvasive imaging modalities such as DECT and whole body MR imaging, radiologic studies are replacing invasive endoscopy-based imaging methods for screening evaluation. An understanding of associated cancer types and their imaging features is necessary for a successful screening program. Collaboration with gastroenterology, oncology, and hepatobiliary surgery is critical because the imaging guidelines are still evolving for many pancreatic cancer predisposition syndromes.

REFERENCES

1. Key statistics for pancreatic cancer. Available at: http://www.cancer.org/cancer/pancreaticcancer/detailedguide/pancreatic-cancer-key-statistics. Accessed January 5, 2017.

2. Poruk KE, Firpo MA, Adler DG, et al. Screening for pancreatic cancer why, how, and who? Ann Surg 2013;257(1):17–26.

3. Pandharipande PV, Heberle C, Dowling EC, et al. Targeted screening of individuals at high risk for pancreatic cancer: results of a simulation model. Radiology 2015;275(1):177–87.

4. Canto MI, Harinck F, Hruban RH, et al. International Cancer of the Pancreas Screening (CAPS) Consortium summit on the management of patients with increased risk for familial pancreatic cancer. Gut 2013;62:339–47.

5. Hallet J, Law CH, Cukier M, et al. Exploring the rising incidence of neuroendocrine tumors: a population-based analysis of epidemiology, metastatic presentation, and outcomes. Cancer 2015; 121:589–97.

6. Jensen R, Berna MJ, Vingham DB, et al. Inherited pancreatic endocrine tumor syndrome: advances in molecular pathogenesis, diagnosis, management, and controversies. Cancer 2008;113(7): 1807–43.

7. Long EE, Van Dam J, Weinstein S, et al. Computed tomography, endoscopic, laparoscopic, and intraoperative sonography for assessing resectability of pancreatic cancer. Surg Oncol 2005;14(2): 105–13.

8. Bronstein YL, Loyer EM, Kaur H, et al. Detection of small pancreatic tumors with multiphasic helical CT. AJR Am J Roentgenol 2004;182:619.

9. Yoon SH, Lee JM, Cho JY, et al. Small pancreatic adenocarcinomas: analysis of enhancement patterns and secondary signs with multiphasic multidetector CT. Radiology 2011;259(2):442–52.

10. Canto MI, Hruban RH, Fishman EK. Frequent detection of pancreatic lesions in asymptomatic high-risk individuals (CAPS 3 study). Gastroenterology 2012; 142:796–804.

11. Sahani DV, Sainani NI, Blake MA, et al. Prospective evaluation of reader performance on MDCT in characterization of cystic pancreatic lesions and prediction of cyst biologic aggressiveness. AJR Am J Roentgenol 2011;197(1):W53–61.

12. Macari M, Spieler B, Kim D, et al. Dual-source dual-energy MDCT of pancreatic adenocarcinoma: initial observations with data generated at 80 kVp and at simulated weighted-average 120 kVp. AJR Am J Roentgenol 2010;194:W27–32.

13. Frellesen C, Fessler F, Hardie AD, et al. Dual-energy CT of the pancreas: improved carcinoma-to-pancreas contrast with a noise-optimized monoenergetic reconstruction algorithm. Eur J Radiol 2015; 84(11):2052–8.

14. Klauss M, Stiller W, Pahn G, et al. Dual-energy perfusion-CT of pancreatic adenocarcinoma. Eur J Radiol 2013;82(2):208–14.

15. Marin D, Nelson RC, Barnhart H, et al. Detection of pancreatic tumors, image quality, and radiation dose during the pancreatic parenchymal phase: effect of a low-tube-voltage, high-tube-current CT technique – Preliminary results. Radiology 2010; 256(2):450–60.

16. Raju R, Thompson AG, Lee K, et al. Reduced iodine load with CT coronary angiography using dual-energy imaging: a prospective randomized trial compared with standard coronary CT angiography. J Cardiovasc Comput Tomogr 2014;8(4):282–8.

17. Matsumoto K, Jinzaki M, Tanami Y, et al. Virtual monochromatic spectral imaging with fast kilovoltage switching: improved image quality as compared with that obtained with conventional 120-kVp CT. Radiology 2011;259:257–62.

18. Matsubavashi H. Familial pancreatic cancer and hereditary syndromes: screening strategy for high-risk individuals. J Gastroenterol 2011;46(11): 1249–59.

19. O'Neill E, Hammond N, Miller F. MR Imaging of the pancreas. Radiol Clin North Am 2014;52: 757–77.

20. Patel BN, Gupta RT, Zani S, et al. How the radiologist can add value in the evaluation of the pre- and post-surgical pancreas. Abdom Imaging 2015;40: 2932–44.

21. Choi TW, Lee JM, Kim JH, et al. Comparison of multidetector CT and gadobutrol-enhanced MR imaging for evaluation of small, solid pancreatic lesions. Korean J Radiol 2016;17(4):509–21.

22. Lee HJ, Kim MJ, Choi JY, et al. Relative accuracy of CT and MRI in the differentiation of benign from malignant pancreatic cystic lesions. Clin Radiol 2011; 66:315–21.

23. Visser BC, Yeh BM, Qayyum A, et al. Characterization of cystic pancreatic masses: relative accuracy of CT and MRI. AJR Am J Roentgenol 2007;189: 648–56.

24. Anupindi SA, Bedoya MA, Lindell RB, et al. Whole-body MRI as a tool for cancer screening in children with genetic cancer-predisposing conditions. AJR Am J Roentgenol 2015;205:400–8.

25. DeWitt J, Deveraux B, Chriswell M, et al. Comparison of endoscopic ultrasonography and multidetector tomography for detecting and staging pancreatic cancer. Ann Intern Med 2004;141: 753–63.

26. Kim YC, Choi JY, Chung YE, et al. Comparison of MRI and endoscopic ultrasound in the characterization of pancreatic cystic lesions. AJR Am J Roentgenol 2010;195(4):947–52.

27. Sahani DV, Kambadakone A, Macari M, et al. Diagnosis and management of cystic pancreatic lesions. AJR Am J Roentgenol 2013;200(2):343–54.

28. Sakorafas GH, Smyrniotis V, Reid-Lombardo KM, et al. Primary pancreatic cystic neoplasms revisited

29. Tanaka M, Chari S, Adsay V, et al. International consensus guidelines for management of intraductal papillary mucinous neoplasms and mucinous cystic neoplasms of the pancreas. Pancreatology 2006;6: 17–32.

30. Megibow AJ, Baker ME, Morgan DE, et al. Management of incidental pancreatic cysts: a white paper of the ACR Incidental Findings Committee. J Am Coll Radiol 2017;14(7):911–23.

31. Tanaka M, Fernandez-del Castillo C, Adsay V, et al. International consensus guidelines 2012 for the management of IPMN and MCN of the pancreas. Pancreatology 2012;12(3):183–97.

32. Vullierme MP, Lagadec M. Predisposing factors for pancreatic adenocarcinoma: what is the role of imaging? Diagn Interv Imaging 2016;97: 1233–40.

33. Rebours V, Gaujoux S, d'Assignies G, et al. Obesity and fatty pancreatic infiltration are risk factors for PanIN. Clin Cancer Res 2015;21(15):3522–8.

34. Sakorafas GH, Smyrniotis V, Reid-Lombardo KM, et al. Primary pancreatic cystic neoplasms revisited: part II. Mucinous cystic neoplasms. Surg Oncol 2011;20:e93–101.

35. Sakorafas GH, Smyrniotis V, Reid-Lombardo KM, et al. Primary pancreatic cystic neoplasms revisited part I, serous cystic neoplasms. Surg Oncol 2011; 20:e84–92.

36. Lee SE, Jang JY, Hwang DW, et al. Clinical features and outcome of solid pseudopapillary neoplasm: differences between adults and children. Arch Surg 2008;143:1218.

37. Kim MJ, Choi DW, Choi SH, et al. Surgical treatment of solid pseudopapillary neoplasms of the pancreas and risk factors for malignancy. Br J Surg 2014;101: 1266–71.

38. Connor A, Gallinger S. Hereditary pancreatic cancer syndromes. Surg Oncol Clin N Am 2015;24: 733–64.

39. Giardello FM, Brensinger JD, Tersmette AC, et al. Very high risk of cancer in familial Peutz-Jeghers syndrome. Gastroenterology 2000;119:1447–53.

40. Grover S, Syngal S. Hereditary pancreatic cancer. Gastroenterology 2010;139(4):1076–80.

41. Templeton AW, Brentall TA. Screening and surgical outcomes of familial pancreatic cancer. Surg Clin North Am 2013;93(3):629–45.

42. Peterson GM. Familial pancreatic cancer. Semin Oncol 2016;43(5):548–53.

43. Lynch HT, Fusaro RM, Lynch JF, et al. Pancreatic cancer and the FAMMM syndrome. Fam Cancer 2008;7:103–12.

44. Kastrinos F, Mukherjee B, Tayob N, et al. Risk of pancreatic cancer in families with Lynch Syndrome. JAMA 2009;302:1790–5.

part III, intraductal papillary mucinous neoplasms. Surg Oncol 2011;20:e109–18.

45. Chang MC, Wong JM, Chang YT. Screening and early detection of pancreatic cancer in high risk population. World J Gastroenterol 2014;20(9): 2358–64.

46. Ulrich CD. Pancreatic cancer in hereditary pancreatitis: consensus guidelines for prevention, screening, and treatment. Pancreatology 2001;1: 416–22.

47. Bartsch DK, Gress TM, Langer P. Familial pancreatic cancer – current knowledge. Nat Rev Gastroenterol Hepatol 2012;9:445–53.

48. Brune KA, Lau B, Palmisano E, et al. Importance of age of onset in pancreatic cancer kindreds. J Natl Cancer Inst 2010;102:119–26.

49. Kim JH, Park SH, Yu ES, et al. Visually isoattenuating pancreatic adenocarcinoma at dynamic-enhanced CT: frequency, clinical and pathologic characteristics, and diagnosis at imaging examinations. Radiology 2010;257(1):87–96.

50. Ichikawa T, Sou H, Araki T, et al. Duct penetrating sign at MRCP: usefulness for differentiating inflammatory pancreatic mass from pancreatic carcinomas. Radiology 2010;221(1):107–16.

51. Anand N, Sampath K, Wu BU. Cyst features and risk of malignancy in intraductal papillary mucinous neoplasms of the pancreas: a meta-analysis. Clin Gastroenterol Hepatol 2013;11:913–21.

52. Kim KW, Park SH, Pyo J, et al. Imaging features to distinguish malignant and benign branch-duct type intraductal papillary mucinous neoplasms of the pancreas: a meta-analysis. Ann Surg 2014;259(1): 72–81.

53. Sadowski S, Triponez F. Management of pancreatic neuroendocrine tumors in patients with MEN 1. Gland Surg 2015;4(1):63–8.

54. Lonser RR, Glenn GM, Walther M, et al. von Hippel-Lindau disease. Lancet 2003;361(9374):2059–67.

55. Davenport MS, Caoili EM, Cohan RH, et al. Pancreatic manifestations of von Hippel-Lindau disease – effect of imaging on clinical management. J Comput Assist Tomogr 2010;34(4):517–22.

56. Wiedenmann B, Pavel M, Kos-Kudla B. From targets to treatments: a review of molecular targets in pancreatic neuroendocrine tumors. Neuroendocrinology 2011;94:177–90.

57. Koc G, Sugimoto S, Kuperman R, et al. Pancreatic tumors in children and young adults with tuberous sclerosis complex. Pediatr Radiol 2017;47:39–45.

58. Wang Y, Chen ZE, Yaghmai V, et al. Diffusion-weighted MR imaging in pancreatic endocrine tumors correlated with histopathologic characteristics. J Magn Reson Imaging 2011;33(5):1071–9.

59. D'Onofrio M, De Robertis R, Capelli P, et al. Uncommon presentations of common pancreatic neoplasms: a pictorial essay. Abdom Imaging 2015; 40(6):1629–44.

60. Kim JH, Eun HW, Kim YJ, et al. Staging accuracy of MR for pancreatic neuroendocrine tumor and imaging findings according to the tumor grade. Abdom Imaging 2013;38:1106–14.

61. Lotfalizadeh E, Ronot M, Wagner M, et al. Prediction of pancreatic neuroendocrine tumor grade with MR imaging features: added value of diffusion-weighted imaging. Eur Radiol 2017;27(4):1748–59.

Imaging and Screening of Kidney Cancer

Alberto Diaz de Leon, MD, Ivan Pedrosa, MD, PhD*

KEYWORDS

- Kidney cancer • MR imaging • Computed tomography imaging • Bosniak classification • Screening
- Active surveillance

KEY POINTS

- Renal cell carcinoma (RCC) represents a heterogeneous disease spectrum with broad clinical outcomes and various appearances on imaging.
- Computed tomography and magnetic resonance allow detailed pretreatment and posttreatment assessment of RCC.
- The current classification system of cystic-appearing renal masses attempts to provide uniform terminology and guidance for management.
- Increasing data support active surveillance in a select subgroup of patients and have provided further insight into the natural history of RCC.

INTRODUCTION

Renal cell carcinoma (RCC) shows a diverse and heterogeneous disease spectrum. Insight into the behavior of RCC has yielded a better understanding of the potential risk factors, natural history of disease, and imaging features. After resection, many patients do well and remain disease-free, but in some patients recurrent/metastatic disease occurs even decades after surgical resection of the primary tumor. Furthermore, patients with a resected RCC are more likely than the general population to develop additional renal tumors after resection. Moreover, tumors being followed with active surveillance may remain stable for several years, slowly grow, or rapidly enlarge. Radiologists must assume a vital role in the management of patients with RCC, because they can be involved in all facets of care, including the diagnosis, treatment, and surveillance of RCC. This article provides a brief review of the epidemiologic, clinical, and imaging features of RCC.

EPIDEMIOLOGY

Incidence

RCC accounts for approximately 90% of all renal malignancies and is the 13th most common malignancy worldwide.[1] The incidence of renal cancer is highest in developed countries, with rates generally higher in Europe and North America than in India, Africa, and China.[2] In the United States, the incidence of kidney cancer increased by an average of 1.1% from 2004 to 2013, and it was estimated that close to 63,000 new cases were diagnosed in 2016.[1] It is speculated that an increase in cross-sectional imaging has in part resulted in the increase in incidence, with most RCCs being found incidentally, and, as a result, these tumors are being diagnosed at an earlier stage and smaller size.[3–6]

The current treatment model is based on the hypothesis that early intervention should yield better outcomes in survival, because a smaller tumor size at diagnosis has been associated with an

Disclosure: The authors have nothing to disclose.
Department of Radiology, University of Texas Southwestern Medical Center, 2201 Inwood Road, 2nd Floor, Suite 202, Dallas, TX 75390-9085, USA
* Corresponding author.
E-mail address: Ivan.Pedrosa@utsouthwestern.edu

Radiol Clin N Am 55 (2017) 1235–1250
http://dx.doi.org/10.1016/j.rcl.2017.06.007

improvement in 5-year survival among recently diagnosed patients.[7] The 5-year survival rate for kidney cancer was reported to be as high as 74% from 2005 to 2011, increased from 57% between 1987 and 1989. However, interpreting the overall outcomes of patients with RCC has been challenging because population-based mortality data do not support the aforementioned hypothesis. Although the 5-year survival has improved, the overall mortalities have shown minimal (if any) change during the same time period (**Fig. 1**),[8] suggesting that the higher survival proportion may reflect overdiagnosis rather than a survival benefit.[9,10]

Risk Factors

Multiple factors have been implicated in an increased risk of RCC, such as nutrition and diet, but only a few established risk factors have been confirmed. Age is considered to be a risk factor, because the incidences of RCC in Europe and United States increase consistently with age and plateau near 70 to 75 years of age.[11] The estimated risk of RCC for men between the ages of 50 and 59 years is around 0.3% compared with 1.3% for individuals 70 years and older.[1] Age-controlled incidences of RCC also indicate a 2:1 predominance of men compared with women.[2,8]

Smoking is an established risk factor for RCC with a described dose-response relationship.[12] There are limited data to suggest that cessation may reduce the risk, but only among long-term quitters of 10 years or more.[13] Several case control and prospective studies have shown hypertension and obesity to be risk factors as well.[11,14]

The incidence of RCC in patients with acquired renal cystic disease (ARCD) has been reported to be 3 to 6 times higher than in the general population,[15,16] and this risk may not decrease after renal transplant.[17] RCC in the setting of ARCD tends to be diagnosed at a younger age and show favorable histologic features and prognosis.[18]

Several occupational and environmental risk factors have been suggested as well. The most extensively studied is trichloroethylene, a metal degreaser and chemical additive. There have been an number of studies reporting an increased risk of RCC with increased levels of exposure to this agent but a clear mechanism has not yet been elucidated.[19,20] A recent meta-analysis suggested that high cadmium exposure was associated with an increased risk for renal cancer as well.[21]

Genetic predisposition

Numerous familial/hereditary renal cancer syndromes have been described but are overall rare and account for less than 5% of all RCCs.[22]

Patients with hereditary cancer syndromes tend to present at an earlier age and are more likely to have multifocal disease compared with those with non-syndromic RCC. Although a complete discussion of the various syndromes is beyond the scope of this article, readers should be aware that each of these syndromes tends to be associated with specific histologic subtypes of RCC because of their underlying genetic alterations and that those neoplasms are associated with variable levels of aggressiveness. A few examples are provided in **Table 1**.

IMAGING OF RENAL CELL CARCINOMA

In the evaluation of renal masses, one should seek to accomplish 2 main goals: lesion detection and classification. An optimal imaging protocol facilitates the identification of contrast enhancement, the primary criterion for diagnosing RCC, and assesses the degree of vascularity, which may be used to suggest a specific subtype of RCC. In addition, the radiology report must provide accurate information about tumor staging and renal vascular anatomy to facilitate a potential surgical and/or ablation intervention.

Imaging Protocols

Computed tomography

Computed tomography (CT) imaging protocols used for the evaluation of renal masses have been described elsewhere.[23–25] A conventional CT protocol routinely includes precontrast and multiphasic postcontrast images. Volumetric data sets acquired by modern CT scanners can be reconstructed in multiple planes and be of variable slice thickness, preserving excellent image quality.

Precontrast images are used to obtain a baseline attenuation value in the lesion of interest and help identify the presence of calcifications, hemorrhage, and/or fat. Thin slices (ie, 2–3 mm) may facilitate the detection of fat and therefore may help in the characterization of renal masses.[26] For the detection of a renal mass and determination of contrast enhancement, postcontrast images should be obtained during the nephrographic phase (60–90 seconds after administration of intravenous (IV) contrast). During the corticomedullary phase (acquired 20–45 seconds after IV contrast injection), there is peak enhancement of the renal cortex, readily distinguishable from the relatively hypovascular medulla, and these images are helpful in determining the vascularity of the lesion, delineating vascular anatomy, and identifying hypervascular metastases elsewhere in the abdomen. However, peripheral hypervascular masses may be of similar attenuation to, and obscured by, the renal cortex, and small central

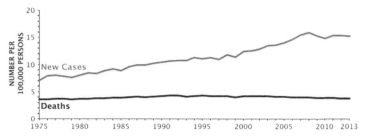

Fig. 1. Incidence in kidney cancer in the United States. A sustained increased in the incidence of kidney cancer has not translated into a decreased mortality. (*Data from* the Surveillance, Epidemiology, and End Results [SEER] database from the National Cancer Institute [NCI]. Available at: http://seer.cancer.gov/). Accessed January 25, 2017.

hypovascular lesions may be mistaken for the relatively hypoattenuating medulla.[25,27] Moreover, the added radiation dose of a routine acquisition during the corticomedullary phase may not be justified. Uniform renal parenchymal enhancement during the nephrographic phase better delineates otherwise subtle lesions that may have been overlooked during the corticomedullary phase and is useful in showing enhancement in hypovascular neoplasms.[25] Excretory phase images (3–5 minutes after IV contrast injection) can be obtained as well and may be helpful in identifying potential disease in the collecting system and ureter.

With the increasing use of dual-energy CT (DECT), the conventional multiphasic CT may soon be modified. Several studies support the use of virtual unenhanced data sets as a surrogate for the standard precontrast acquisition, which result in a decrease in radiation dose.[28–30] However, small differences in measured quantitative values between virtual and conventional unenhanced images have been reported,[29,30] and further studies are required before the routine implementation of virtual unenhanced images in clinical practice.

Magnetic resonance imaging

The standard sequences in a multiparametric MR (mpMR) imaging protocol have been described elsewhere.[31,32] The ideal mpMR imaging protocol includes conventional sequences, such as T2-weighted and chemical-shift imaging, combined with multiphasic contrast-enhanced images to provide a comprehensive evaluation of renal neoplasms. Appropriately performed, mpMR imaging may be able to provide information beyond what can be achieved with CT alone, but achieving a high-quality examination can be more challenging and depends on factors beyond sequence selection, including adequate patient cooperation.

T2-weighted spin-echo acquisitions can be performed using either multishot or single-shot techniques, with or without fat suppression. Although multishot sequences provide greater image contrast, signal-to-noise ratio (SNR), and spatial resolution, single-shot fast spin-echo/half-Fourier single-shot turbo spin-echo sequences are routinely used at the authors' institution when imaging the upper abdomen to help mitigate image degradation caused by respiratory motion.

Gradient-recalled echo techniques allow rapid imaging and adequate SNR and can be used to acquire two-dimensional T1-weighted in-phase (IP) and opposed-phase (OP) images for detection of intralesional fat.[33] Three-dimensional (3D) dual-echo Dixon-based acquisitions can also be used to obtain thinner, contiguous slices in a single

Table 1
Hereditary renal cell carcinoma syndromes

Syndrome	Gene	RCC Subtype
von Hippel-Lindau	*VHL*	Clear cell RCC
Birt-Hogg-Dube	*FLCN*	Chromophobe, oncocytoma, hybrid RCC with features of both chromophobe and oncocytoma, clear cell RCC
Hereditary papillary RCC	*MET*	Type 1 papillary RCC
Hereditary leiomyomatosis and RCC	*FH*	Type 2 papillary RCC
Succinate dehydrogenase–deficient renal cancer	*SDHB* *SDHD* *SDHC*	Clear cell RCC, oncocytic neoplasm, chromophobe RCC

Abbreviations: FH, fumarate hydratase; *FLCN*, folliculin; *MET*, MET proto-oncogene; *SDHB*, succinate dehydrogenase complex iron sulfur subunit B; *SDHC*, succinate dehydrogenase complex subunit C; *SDHD*, succinate dehydrogenase complex subunit D; *VHL*, von Hippel-Lindau tumor suppressor.

breath hold and can be reconstructed into water, fat, IP, and OP imaging data sets.[34]

For multiphasic postcontrast imaging, the authors prefer to use 3D fat-saturated spoiled gradient echo techniques to acquire T1-weighted images in the coronal plane. However, these can be acquired in the axial plane as well. These images are acquired during the corticomedullary phase, which is timed to the arrival of contrast to the kidneys using an MR fluoroscopic technique, in addition to early and late nephrographic phases. A Dixon-based fat-saturation technique provides more homogeneous fat suppression over a larger field of view.

The role of diffusion-weighted imaging (DWI) for the detection and characterization of renal masses continues to evolve. Some investigators have reported some value in the determination of the histologic diagnosis in renal masses[35,36] and the characterization of high-grade RCC.[37] However, a recent meta-analysis indicated only moderate diagnostic accuracy in the characterization of renal masses and determination of high-grade clear cell histology.[38] The lack of standardization of the DWI acquisition protocols across different MR imaging vendors and different medical centers is likely responsible, at least in part, for the less than optimal diagnostic performance. Breath-hold, single-shot, echo-planar imaging techniques allow rapid DWI acquisitions and help limit motion artifact. However, the number of signal averages and/or b-values may be limited by the duration of the breath-hold, resulting in poor SNR. Alternatively, free-breathing techniques may be incorporated to provide multiple signal averages, thereby improving SNR and contrast-to-noise ratio, but at the cost of longer acquisition times.

Characterization of Enhancement

The fundamental principle in diagnosing RCC relies on identifying the presence of enhancement within a renal lesion. MR imaging has a potential advantage compared with conventional CT because its sensitivity to detect small amounts of gadolinium is higher than that of CT for iodinated contrast. Furthermore, subtraction images, which are created by digitally subtracting the unenhanced image from the corresponding postcontrast image, allow the removal of any native T1 signal intensity from the postcontrast image, thereby displaying signal solely caused by enhancement. However, this technique is highly dependent on adequate and reproducible breath holds for accurate coregistration of images; if this is not fulfilled, misregistration may occur and thus determination of enhancement on these images is not reliable. Alternatively, if subtraction images are unavailable or of poor quality, determining the percentage change in signal intensity within the lesion is an additional method for determining enhancement; an increase greater than or equal to 15% in signal intensity on postcontrast images compared with precontrast images indicates enhancement on MR imaging examinations.[39]

Showing enhancement on CT can be complicated by multiple factors. First, the definition of enhancement varies. In the past, a change in 10 Hounsfield units (HU) was suggested as a threshold for determining enhancement.[40] Subsequent studies showed that the attenuation in cysts may artificially increase by more than 10 HU between unenhanced and postcontrast images because of beam-hardening effects caused by the marked enhancement of the adjacent renal parenchyma, and the apparent increase in attenuation may be more pronounced in small and completely intrarenal lesions.[41–43] As such, some investigators have suggested this threshold be increased to 15 to 20 HU,[42,44] but others still advocate using 10 HU.[41] Because identifying enhancement should be unequivocal due to the significant implications in the management of a renal lesion, some investigators suggest this threshold should be further increased to greater than 20 HU and a change between 10 and 20 HU considered as equivocal and potentially requiring further imaging with MR.[45]

DECT may help overcome these limitations of conventional CT. By using the image data acquired at 2 different energy levels, virtual monochromatic images simulating the attenuation of an ideal monochromatic beam may be reconstructed from the DECT data set.[46] There have been an increasing number of studies describing the utility of these virtual monochromatic data sets in mitigating the effect of beam hardening for small, intrarenal lesions.[47–49] In addition, DECT image data can be reconstructed to generate material density images. This technique can be used to produce the previously described virtual unenhanced, water-only image but can also be used to create an iodine-only image (**Fig. 2**).[50] This ability makes it possible to obtain a direct quantification of iodine concentration within a renal lesion, thereby allowing the identification and quantification of otherwise subtle enhancement in hypovascular or hyperattenuating renal lesions.[51–53]

Characterization of Cystic Renal Cell Carcinoma

Nomenclature

The definition of cystic RCC is highly variable and the term may include a variety of pathologic

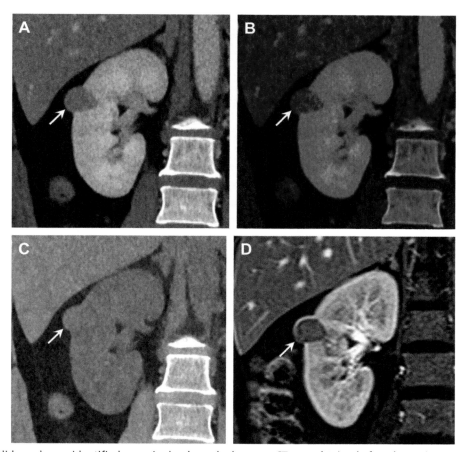

Fig. 2. Solid renal mass identified on a single-phase dual-energy CT scan obtained after the patient presented to the emergency room with abdominal pain. (*A*) Postcontrast coronal CT image of the upper abdomen, obtained during the portal venous phase, shows a partially exophytic mass (*white arrow*) arising from the upper-mid right kidney, which appears hypoattenuating relative to the renal parenchyma, but shows an attenuation near 80 HU. (*B*) Reconstructed iodine-only image clearly shows iodine accumulation within the lesion (1.8 mg/mL), consistent with a solid renal neoplasm (*white arrow*). (*C*) On the reconstructed virtual non-contrast image, the mass (*white arrow*) appears isoattenuating to hyperattenuating (near 40 HU). The attenuation difference between this reconstructed virtual non-contrast image and the postcontrast image (*A*) also confirms that the lesion corresponds with a solid, enhancing mass. (*D*) Postcontrast subtraction MR image from a subsequently performed MR scan confirms enhancement within the mass. The patient is scheduled to undergo a percutaneous biopsy and radiofrequency ablation in the near future.

entities, such as multilocular cystic RCC or one of the more common subtypes of RCC, including clear cell and papillary, with cystic components. This distinction is not solely an academic exercise; as discussed later, there are increasing data to support that cystic renal neoplasms show a more indolent pattern of behavior and favorable prognosis compared with solid renal tumors. This difference is best exemplified by multilocular cystic RCC, a specific subtype now sanctioned by the World Health Organization as a tumor of low malignant potential, more specifically multilocular cystic renal neoplasm of low malignant potential.[54] However, this neoplasm is composed entirely of cysts whose walls are lined by a single layer of clear cells and septa may contain groups of clear cells but no expansile growth. Specifically, a solid mass–forming component should be absent (**Fig. 3**).[54] Importantly, there is no reported evidence in the literature of metastatic disease caused by this tumor.

Up to 15% of all RCCs may contain a cystic component[55] but there is no uniform agreement as to what amount of cystic and/or solid component should be present to separate a solid mass with cystic change from a complex cystic mass with a solid component by imaging. Prior studies evaluating the prognosis of patients with cystic

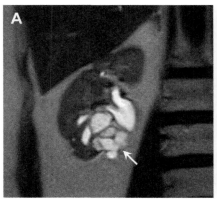
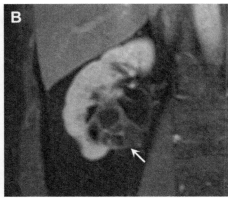

Fig. 3. Multilocular cystic neoplasm of low malignant potential. Coronal (*A*) T2-weighted and (*B*) T1-weighted postcontrast images of the right kidney show a complex cystic mass in the medial lower pole (*arrows*) containing several thickened, enhancing septations without a discrete nodular component. The mass was resected and confirmed to represent a multilocular cystic neoplasm of low malignant potential (International Society of Urological Pathology [ISUP] grade 1).

RCC have proposed a variable percentage of cystic components ranging from 75% to 90%.[56–58]

However, regardless of the threshold chosen, the more fundamental issue of identifying a region of true cystic change on preoperative imaging persists. What may be interpreted as a region of cystic change on imaging may correspond with a variety of lesion characteristics, including necrosis and hemorrhage, on histopathology. A recent retrospective study by Park and colleagues[59] evaluating the postoperative outcome of cystic renal neoplasms found a cystic proportion greater than or equal to 45% on the preoperative CT to be an independent prognostic factor for survival, which is a step in the right direction. Future studies are needed to define specific imaging phenotypes, including those with variable degrees of cystic component, and correlate them with outcome.

Imaging features

The Bosniak renal cyst classification system continues to be used when evaluating a cystic-appearing renal mass. Developed in 1986 by Morton Bosniak,[40] the system suggested a standardized nomenclature to classify and guide management of renal cystic lesions based on certain imaging features. The classification system describes 5 different categories of cystic lesions (I, II, IIF, III, and IV) with the increasing number corresponding with increase in complexity within the lesion and higher likelihood of malignancy. The categories are differentiated based on the presence and morphologic features of calcifications and septations, in addition to the degree of septal enhancement (ie, perceived vs measurable) and precontrast attenuation. However, the amount of calcification in a renal cystic lesion and/or change

in this amount over time was later shown to be not predictive of malignancy.

A Bosniak I cyst corresponds with a simple cyst. These cysts have a thin, smooth wall and fluid attenuation/signal without septa, enhancement, or calcification. Category II cysts are minimally complex cysts. These cysts can have a few and thin (<3 mm) septations with perceived, but not measurable, enhancement. Small, border-forming calcifications may be present. This category also includes small (≤3 cm) homogeneously hyperattenuating, nonenhancing lesions. Both category I and II cysts are considered benign and require no additional follow-up imaging.

Bosniak IIF includes mildly complex cysts, which require follow-up imaging. These cysts can have multiple thin or minimally thickened septa with perceived enhancement. Thick/nodular calcifications may also be present. The large (>3 cm), nonenhancing, hyperattenuating cysts are included in this category as well. Most Bosniak IIF cysts are benign,[60] but require follow-up imaging for confirmation. However, the interval and duration of follow-up imaging have not been clearly defined. In a recent meta-analysis up to 7% of these lesions were malignant.[61]

Bosniak III lesions include cysts with multiple and thick, enhancing septa and/or thick walls. The incidence of malignancy in resected Bosniak III lesions is overall higher than in Bosniak IIF cysts, but is highly variable, with rates reported between 30% and 100%.[62,63] In addition, category IV lesions include cystic lesions with enhancing soft tissue components, which may be adjacent to or separate from the wall or septa (**Fig. 4**). Lesions included in this category are considered malignant until proved otherwise. In the past, surgical

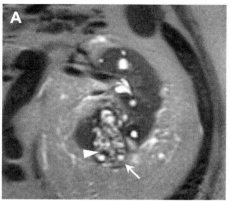
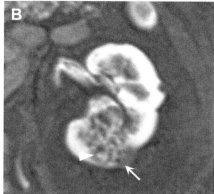

Fig. 4. Bosniak IV cyst in the left kidney. Coronal (*A*) T2-weighted (*B*) postcontrast images show a complex cystic lesion in the lower pole of the left kidney containing multiple thickened septations (*arrows*), in addition to several more discrete-appearing nodules within one of the septa (*arrowheads*), consistent with a Bosniak IV cyst. The lesion was resected and found to represent a clear cell RCC (ISUP grade 2). Note a few additional simple Bosniak I cysts in the left kidney.

resection has been the suggested management of category III and IV lesions, given their increased likelihood of malignancy.

Both clear cell RCC (ccRCC) and papillary RCC (pRCC) may present as a predominantly cystic mass. A complex, predominantly cystic mass with avidly enhancing, irregular, and nodular septa is said to be highly specific (94%) for low-grade ccRCC.[64] A characteristic appearance of pRCC is a cystic-appearing hemorrhagic mass with a hypo-enhancing mural nodule, which has been described to have a specificity of 94% as well (**Fig. 5**).

Characterization of Solid Renal Cell Carcinoma

The imaging characteristics of RCC are highly variable, but certain imaging features on CT and MR imaging may be used to favor a particular subtype. The degree of enhancement has been consistently shown as a means to differentiate certain subtypes of RCC. An advantage of MR imaging compared with CT is that tissue signal characteristics on different sequences can be used in conjunction with the degree of enhancement to assist in subtyping.

ccRCC is a hypervascular subtype, and this is reflected in its pattern of enhancement. On multiphasic imaging, the peak enhancement of ccRCC occurs during the corticomedullary phase, as much as or greater than the renal cortex.[65–68] pRCC is a hypovascular neoplasm and almost always hypoenhancing during the corticomedullary phase with its peak enhancement occurring during the nephrographic phase. Chromophobe RCC

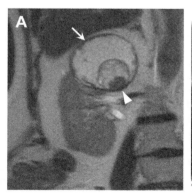
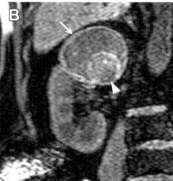
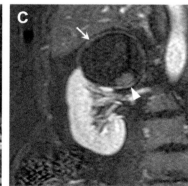

Fig. 5. Papillary renal cell carcinoma (pRCC). (*A*) Coronal T2-weighted image shows a complex cystic-appearing mass in the upper pole of the right kidney (*white arrow*) with thickened walls, septa, and a possible mural nodule along its inferior wall (*white arrowhead*). (*B*) Coronal precontrast fat-saturated gradient echo image shows areas of high signal intensity within the renal lesion (*asterisk*), suggestive of hemorrhagic contents. (*C*) Postcontrast subtraction image shows an irregular-appearing and hypo-enhancing mural nodule along its inferior wall (*white arrowhead*). The mass was subsequently resected and confirmed to represent a pRCC (with features of type 1 and type 2; ISUP grade 3).

(chrRCC) can show variable patterns of enhancement, but tends to be less vascular than ccRCC and show an intermediate degree of enhancement (50%–60% of that of the renal cortex) during the corticomedullary phase.[65,68]

On CT, several methods have been suggested to distinguish pRCC from ccRCC. Using multiphasic threshold levels of 55 HU during the corticomedullary phase, 65 HU during the nephrographic phase, and 55 HU in the excretory phase was reported to have an accuracy of 85%, sensitivity of 94%, a positive predictive value of 86%, and a negative predictive value of 81% to distinguish these two subtypes.[65] In a separate study, using a threshold of 100 HU on the corticomedullary phase to distinguish ccRCC and pRCC provided an accuracy of 95.7%, sensitivity of 98.3%, and specificity 92%.[69] Iodine quantification with DECT may also play a role in differentiating ccRCC from pRCC. Using a tumor iodine concentration threshold of 0.9 mg/mL yielded a sensitivity of 98.2%, specificity of 86.3%, positive predictive value of 95.8%, and a negative predictive value of 93.7%.[70]

On MR imaging, ccRCC can show variable signal intensity on T1-weighted and T2-weighted images, but commonly shows hyperintense signal on the latter, in addition to avid enhancement during the corticomedullary phase.[68] Intracytoplasmic deposition of lipids in ccRCC results in a characteristic appearance on chemical-shift imaging with areas containing intravoxel fat appearing hypointense on the OP images relative to the IP images.[71] pRCC most often shows a lower signal intensity relative to the renal cortex on T2-weighted images in the vascularized portions of the tumor. On T1-weighted images, pRCC commonly shows nonenhancing areas of hyperintense signal because of intralesional hemorrhage. chrRCC can show variable patterns of signal intensity and can appear hypointense to hyperintense relative to renal cortex on T2-weighted imaging. Papillary tumors frequently show marked restriction on DWI compared with ccRCCs.[36]

Several imaging features have been described that suggest a higher grade of tumor. The presence of a central area of nonenhancement, retroperitoneal collateral vessels, and venous invasion is associated with high-grade ccRCC.[64] Irregularity or interruption of the tumor pseudocapsule, a rim of normal renal parenchyma surrounding the tumor, suggests locally advanced disease and a high nuclear grade.[72] On DECT, a significant correlation between iodine concentration and Fuhrman tumor grade for both ccRCC and pRCC has been described.[70] Focal areas of marked restricted diffusion have been correlated with high-grade ccRCC.[37]

NATURAL HISTORY AND ACTIVE SURVEILLANCE

The greatest increase in incidentally detected renal masses has been in the small and localized tumors (≤4 cm), which now account for greater than 50% of all renal masses identified.[11] Approximately 20% to 30% of these small renal masses (SRMs) are benign and most show an indolent growth pattern,[73–75] which has resulted in a growing body of literature evaluating active surveillance for the management of SRMs and in which insight into the natural history of RCC is being derived. However, near 20% of SRMs show an aggressive, malignant behavior.[75,76] Patients more than 70 years of age have been found to be at an increased risk for high-stage and high-grade disease. Similarly, it is patients in this population in whom most SRMs are now being diagnosed and who are most likely to have comorbidities and increased surgical risk.[77,78] Therefore, there is a need to develop biomarkers that inform on the biology of SRM and predict their natural history.

Active surveillance is preferentially reserved for patients who are unable to undergo surgery because of competing risks from comorbidities or who are unwilling.[79] For those placed on active surveillance, the American Urological Association (AUA) and National Comprehensive Cancer Network (NCCN) guidelines recommend abdominal imaging with CT or MR imaging within 6 months from initiation of active surveillance and subsequent imaging (CT, MR imaging, or ultrasonography) performed annually thereafter for as long as the patient is on active surveillance.[80,81] During this time, the size of the lesion should be closely monitored, because growth kinetics are a commonly cited surrogate for metastatic potential and a potential indication for further intervention. Although the growth rates for SRMs are highly variable, several studies have reported a mean annual growth rate varying between 0.3 cm/y and 0.4 cm/y.[77,82,83] One systematic review of lesions on active surveillance that progressed to metastatic disease showed a significantly higher growth rate (0.8 cm/y) compared with those with favorable outcomes (0.3 cm/y).[84]

Apart from growth rate and size, imaging features to predict outcome are limited, but there is an increasing number of studies suggesting that cystic RCC may follow a more favorable course of disease. Multiple studies have reported an excellent prognosis in patients with cystic RCC after surgery, regardless of size, with an exceedingly rare incidence of metastasis.[57,58,85–87]

FOLLOW-UP AFTER THERAPY
Patterns of Recurrence

Local or systemic recurrence occurs in approximately 30% of patients who undergo surgical resection for localized RCC.[88] The most common sites of metastases are lung (45%), bone (30%), lymph node (22%), liver (20%), adrenal (9%), and brain (8%).[89] As with most malignancies, the greatest risk of recurrence is early in the posttreatment setting, with most recurrences occurring less than 3 years after surgery.[90,91] The timing of recurrence is related to the tumor stage, with reported median times to recurrence for T1, T2, and T3 tumors of 38, 32, and 17 months, respectively.[92] The risk is affected by several factors, including tumor grade and stage, presence of nodal metastases, and RCC subtypes. For tumor stages I to IV, the reported 5-year cancer-specific survival rates are 91%, 74%, 67%, and 32%, respectively.[93] Tumors with sarcomatoid differentiation, medullary carcinoma, and collecting duct carcinoma all show a higher risk for metastatic disease.[94] Late recurrences (ie, >5 years after surgery) occur in patients with smaller masses, lower stage, and lower nuclear grade than those with earlier recurrence/metastatic disease.[95]

For SRMs, partial and radical nephrectomies show similar risks for progression and renal cancer–related deaths, with the former's risks estimated to be 4.5% and 3%, respectively.[96] The overall failure rate for ablative therapies, including radiofrequency ablation and cryoablation, has been reported to range from 2% to 10%.[97] However, assessing the overall risk for local recurrence, development of metastatic disease, and death from T1a RCC after ablation is confounded by the different techniques available for ablation, lack of pretreatment biopsy confirmation of tumor, lack of uniform definition of a local recurrence, and difficulty in assessing recurrent/residual tumor on biopsy or radiographic imaging.

Surveillance Strategies After Therapy

Presently, there are no universally accepted guidelines for follow-up imaging after therapy, and there have been no prospective or randomized controlled trials to clarify what imaging surveillance protocol is the most efficacious. Most guidelines, including the AUA and NCCN guidelines, suggest surveillance strategies based on risk-adapted protocols, which stratify patients into groups based on TNM (tumor, node, metastasis) staging.

For T1a and T1b tumors with negative lymph nodes, several guidelines suggest less frequent follow-up imaging because of the low risk for recurrence. Typically, a chest radiograph may be obtained every 6 to 12 months for 3 years and then annually until year 5. Baseline abdominal imaging is recommended within 3 to 12 months following a partial or radical nephrectomy. Subsequent imaging varies depending on individual risk factors and type of surgery. For partial nephrectomy, if the initial post-surgical baseline imaging was negative, abdominal surveillance imaging may be performed at yearly intervals for 3 years. After radical nephrectomy, subsequent imaging after a negative baseline study is considered optional.[81] For T2 through T4 tumors, or any T stage with positive lymph nodes, AUA and NCCN suggest baseline chest and abdominal imaging within 3 to 6 months following surgery. Continued follow-up imaging is suggested every 3 to 6 months for at least 3 years, and then annually thereafter for up to 5 years.[80,81]

After ablative therapies, the AUA and NCCN recommend cross-sectional imaging at 3 and 6 months after therapy. If treatment success is documented by imaging, abdominal and chest radiographs are then recommended annually for 5 years with further imaging considered optional.

Imaging Appearance

Assessing for recurrence on imaging requires evaluation with at least dual-phase (arterial and portal venous) postcontrast imaging, as metastatic lesions tend to show enhancement characteristics similar to those of the primary tumor. One study reported 9% ccRCC metastases in the liver or pancreas were seen only on arterial phase imaging.[98] If ablative therapies were used for the primary lesion, precontrast imaging should be included to provide baseline attenuation values.

On CT imaging, evaluating the ablation zone requires careful review of precontrast and postcontrast phases. After a successful ablation, the zone of ablation should appear as a region of increased attenuation (>40 HU) on the unenhanced studies surrounded by a rim of fat attenuation.[99] On MR imaging, the ablation zone often shows heterogeneous hyperintense signal on T1-weighted and hypointense signal on T2-weighted images.[100] A thin, smooth rim of enhancement surrounding the ablation may be encountered and should be considered a benign finding. After radiofrequency ablation, a characteristic thin rim of soft tissue is present around the area of preserved fat that surrounds the ablation zone, which has been described as the halo sign, and can be confused with the appearance of an angiomyolipoma (**Fig. 6**).[101] An enlarging nodular or crescentic area of enhancement should be considered recurrent disease until proved otherwise.[99,100]

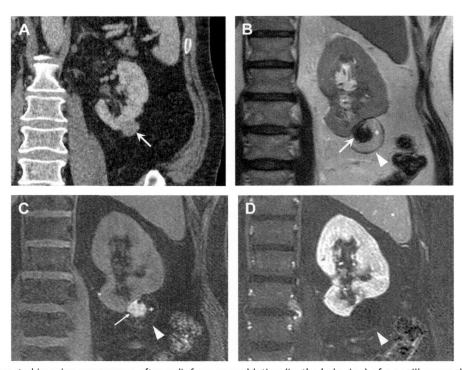

Fig. 6. Expected imaging appearance after radiofrequency ablation (ie, the halo sign) of a papillary renal cell carcinoma (pRCC). (*A*) Coronal postcontrast CT image acquired during the nephrographic phase shows a hypoenhancing mass (*white arrow*) compared with the precontrast image (not shown) arising from the lower pole of the kidney, proved to be a pRCC (type 1; ISUP grade 3) on a biopsy performed immediately before radiofrequency ablation. On the MR imaging performed 3 months after ablation, (*B*) coronal T2-weighted, (*C*) coronal precontrast T1-weighted, and (*D*) coronal postcontrast subtraction images show the treated tumor as a masslike, nonenhancing region of coagulative necrosis (hypointense on T2-weighted and hyperintense on T1-weighted images) surrounded by fat (*white asterisk*). Note the overlying thin, subtle rim of enhancement (*white arrowhead*) representing fibrous tissue and defining the region of the ablation zone.

RCC can metastasize to virtually any part of the human body, with case reports documenting recurrence in the subcutaneous tissues, oral cavity, and testicle.[102–104] However, the lungs are the most common site of metastatic disease in RCC.[105] The appearance of RCC metastases in the lung can manifest in a variety of manners, from a small and well-defined nodule to an irregularly shaped mass, and can enhance avidly.[106] It is important to recognize that patients with RCC may develop primary lung tumors given the known association of smoking to both neoplasms. This possibility should be considered in the presence of a single pulmonary nodule and in those patients in whom a single pulmonary nodule shows progression in the setting of stable disease/response elsewhere.[107] Furthermore, primary lung neoplasms tend to show a spiculated appearance compared with the more common smooth, rounded appearance of lung RCC metastases.

Bones metastases are common, affecting up to 32% of patients with metastatic disease.[108] Most often they present as a lytic lesion with a soft tissue component. Detection of lytic bone metastases is challenging given the frequent negative results with both CT and ^{99m}Tc-labeled bone scintigraphy.[109] Similarly, ^{18}F-labeled fluorodeoxyglucose PET has limited value because of inconsistent tumor uptake in RCC. ^{18}F-labeled sodium fluoride PET/CT is highly sensitive for osseous metastases, although it is not widely available or reimbursed.

Solid organ metastases in the abdomen and pelvis otherwise lack specific imaging characteristics and can have a variety of appearances, including a uniformly enhancing, hypervascular mass or a rim-enhancing and centrally necrotic lesion. Of note, the different RCC histologic subtypes show predilections for different organs,[110] including solid organs. For example, clear cell carcinoma metastases to the pancreas are common, whereas chrRCC has a predilection to metastasize to the liver.[110] Adrenal metastases are common in RCC and may become evident years after resection of the primary tumor.[95]

Antiangiogenic agents, such as tyrosine kinase inhibitors (TKIs), are being increasingly used in the treatment of metastatic RCC.[111] Tumor response with these agents may present with changes in perfusion with or without changes in size.[112] This response may be reflected by qualitative and semiquantitative decreases in enhancement on conventional postcontrast imaging, although more novel quantitative techniques to assess tissue perfusion have been described. On MR imaging, a decrease in tumor blood flow on arterial spin labeling, as soon as 1 month after therapy, and enhancement on dynamic contrast-enhanced MR imaging may predict a favorable outcome.[113,114] A recent study evaluating the use of DECT in patients on antiangiogenic therapy suggested that iodine maps may be more sensitive in the detection of an early response compared with traditional measurements of attenuation.[115] The use of automated segmentation algorithms to identify the amount of viable, enhancing tumor burden may facilitate the assessment of RCC response to TKIs.[116]

ROLE OF IMAGING IN SCREENING
General Population

There are no established guidelines for RCC screening in the general population. As with ovarian cancer, RCC is neither a common nor a rare disease, so screening the general population with CT or MR imaging is unlikely to show a positive impact on tumor-specific mortality, as highlighted by the increase in incidentally detected RCC having had a small effect on overall mortality. Moreover, an imaging screening protocol based on CT and/or MR imaging would be financially prohibitive, whereas ultrasonography is likely to not achieve enough sensitivity to serve in that role although addition of IV contrast may help. As nonsyndromic risk factors for RCC are further

elucidated, a targeted approach in screening may one day be established, but a large randomized controlled trial of renal cancer screening has yet to be performed.

Genetic Predisposition

The management of patients with an inherited predisposition to RCC requires a multidisciplinary approach and some form of routine imaging for lifelong surveillance of renal tumors. Annual screening with CT or MR imaging is recommended for most patients with a genetic predisposition, although the interval and age at which surveillance imaging begins vary.

For patients with hereditary leiomyomatosis and RCC (HLRCC) syndrome, screening begins at an early age, because tumors can be detected as early as 11 years of age and are often aggressive with distant metastases even when small.[117,118] As such, tumors identified in patients with HLRCC are resected with wide margins and not placed on active surveillance or ablated. The management for patients with succinate dehydrogenase–deficient kidney cancer is similar given its early age of onset (younger than 30 years of age) and association with aggressive renal tumors.[119]

In contradistinction, annual or biannual surveillance imaging in patients with Birt-Hogg-Dube syndrome is recommended, starting at the age of 20 years, and tumors are managed with active surveillance until 3 cm in size, similar to the management of individuals with von Hippel-Lindau syndrome.[120] In hereditary pRCC (HPRC) syndrome, tumors develop most often in the sixth and seventh decades of life, although early-onset families have been described (**Fig. 7**).[121] Tumors

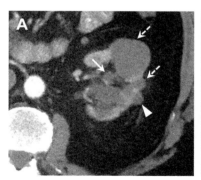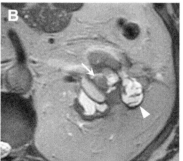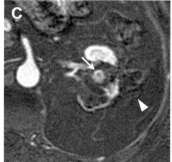

Fig. 7. Hereditary papillary renal cell carcinoma (HPRC) follow-up imaging. (*A*) Axial postcontrast CT image shows multiple hypoattenuating lesions exhibiting subtle hypoenhancement compared with the precontrast image (not shown). A total of 7 lesions were resected, 2 of which are shown on the image (*dashed arrows*) and represented pRCCs (type 1; ISUP grade 2). Two additional subcentimeter lesions (*solid arrow* and *arrowhead*) were described as too small to further characterize on this CT examination. Axial (*B*) T2-weighted and (*C*) postcontrast subtraction images obtained 6 months after the CT and surgical resection show interval enlargement of the more central lesion (*solid arrow*), which also shows unequivocal nodular enhancement on the subtraction postcontrast image. In addition, the more posterior cystic-appearing lesion seen on prior CT (*arrowhead*) has also enlarged and now shows multiple thickened septa.

in HPRC are more often slow growing and managed with active surveillance. To our knowledge, a screening protocol for HPRC has not been proposed.

SUMMARY

Further insight into RCC has provided an improved understanding of its complex epidemiologic, clinical, and imaging features. As knowledge of RCC continues to advance, screening protocols may one day be established in selected populations to help decrease the current mortality. Imaging biomarkers and further refinement of classification schema may help identify tumors with low likelihood of progressive disease that may benefit from active surveillance.

REFERENCES

1. Siegel RL, Miller KD, Jemal A. Cancer statistics, 2016. CA Cancer J Clin 2016;66(1):7–30.
2. Ferlay J, Shin HR, Bray F, et al. Estimates of worldwide burden of cancer in 2008: GLOBOCAN 2008. Int J Cancer 2010;127(12):2893–917.
3. Jayson M, Sanders H. Increased incidence of serendipitously discovered renal cell carcinoma. Urology 1998;51(2):203–5.
4. Tsui KH, Shvarts O, Smith RB, et al. Renal cell carcinoma: prognostic significance of incidentally detected tumors. J Urol 2000;163(2):426–30.
5. Smith SJ, Bosniak MA, Megibow AJ, et al. Renal cell carcinoma: earlier discovery and increased detection. Radiology 1989;170(3 Pt 1):699–703.
6. Hollingsworth JM, Miller DC, Daignault S, et al. Rising incidence of small renal masses: a need to reassess treatment effect. J Natl Cancer Inst 2006; 98(18):1331–4.
7. Nguyen MM, Gill IS, Ellison LM. The evolving presentation of renal carcinoma in the United States: trends from the surveillance, epidemiology, and end results program. J Urol 2006;176(6 Pt 1): 2397–400 [discussion: 2400].
8. Howlader N, Noone A, Krapcho M, et al. SEER cancer statistics review, 1975-2013. 2016. Available at: http://seer.cancer.gov/csr/1975_2013/. Accessed January 25, 2017.
9. Znaor A, Lortet-Tieulent J, Laversanne M, et al. International variations and trends in renal cell carcinoma incidence and mortality. Eur Urol 2015;67(3): 519–30.
10. Welch HG, Black WC. Overdiagnosis in cancer. J Natl Cancer Inst 2010;102(9):605–13.
11. Chow WH, Devesa SS. Contemporary epidemiology of renal cell cancer. Cancer J 2008;14(5): 288–301.
12. Hunt JD, van der Hel OL, McMillan GP, et al. Renal cell carcinoma in relation to cigarette smoking: meta-analysis of 24 studies. Int J Cancer 2005; 114(1):101–8.
13. Parker AS, Cerhan JR, Janney CA, et al. Smoking cessation and renal cell carcinoma. Ann Epidemiol 2003;13(4):245–51.
14. Chow WH, Gridley G, Fraumeni JF Jr, et al. Obesity, hypertension, and the risk of kidney cancer in men. N Engl J Med 2000;343(18):1305–11.
15. Port FK, Ragheb NE, Schwartz AG, et al. Neoplasms in dialysis patients: a population-based study. Am J Kidney Dis 1989;14(2):119–23.
16. Ishikawa I, Saito Y, Asaka M, et al. Twenty-year follow-up of acquired renal cystic disease. Clin Nephrol 2003;59(3):153–9.
17. Wong G, Chapman JR. Cancers after renal transplantation. Transplant Rev (Orlando) 2008;22(2): 141–9.
18. Neuzillet Y, Tillou X, Mathieu R, et al. Renal cell carcinoma (RCC) in patients with end-stage renal disease exhibits many favourable clinical, pathologic, and outcome features compared with RCC in the general population. Eur Urol 2011;60(2):366–73.
19. Chiu WA, Caldwell JC, Keshava N, et al. Key scientific issues in the health risk assessment of trichloroethylene. Environ Health Perspect 2006;114(9): 1445–9.
20. Scott CS, Chiu WA. Trichloroethylene cancer epidemiology: a consideration of select issues. Environ Health Perspect 2006;114(9):1471–8.
21. Song J, Luo H, Yin X, et al. Association between cadmium exposure and renal cancer risk: a meta-analysis of observational studies. Sci Rep 2015;5: 17976.
22. Lipworth L, Tarone RE, McLaughlin JK. The epidemiology of renal cell carcinoma. J Urol 2006;176(6 Pt 1):2353–8.
23. Ng CS, Wood CG, Silverman PM, et al. Renal cell carcinoma: diagnosis, staging, and surveillance. AJR Am J Roentgenol 2008;191(4):1220–32.
24. Szolar DH, Kammerhuber F, Altziebler S, et al. Multiphasic helical CT of the kidney: increased conspicuity for detection and characterization of small (< 3-cm) renal masses. Radiology 1997; 202(1):211–7.
25. Birnbaum BA, Jacobs JE, Ramchandani P. Multiphasic renal CT: comparison of renal mass enhancement during the corticomedullary and nephrographic phases. Radiology 1996;200(3): 753–8.
26. Kurosaki Y, Tanaka Y, Kuramoto K, et al. Improved CT fat detection in small kidney angiomyolipomas using thin sections and single voxel measurements. J Comput Assist Tomogr 1993;17(5):745–8.
27. Yuh BI, Cohan RH. Different phases of renal enhancement: role in detecting and characterizing

renal masses during helical CT. AJR Am J Roentgenol 1999;173(3):747–55.

28. Ascenti G, Mazziotti S, Mileto A, et al. Dual-source dual-energy CT evaluation of complex cystic renal masses. AJR Am J Roentgenol 2012;199(5):1026–34.

29. Ascenti G, Mileto A, Gaeta M, et al. Single-phase dual-energy CT urography in the evaluation of haematuria. Clin Radiol 2013;68(2):e87–94.

30. Graser A, Johnson TR, Hecht EM, et al. Dual-energy CT in patients suspected of having renal masses: can virtual nonenhanced images replace true nonenhanced images? Radiology 2009; 252(2):433–40.

31. Sun MR, Pedrosa I. Magnetic resonance imaging of renal masses. Semin Ultrasound CT MR 2009; 30(4):326–51.

32. Ramamurthy NK, Moosavi B, McInnes MD, et al. Multiparametric MRI of solid renal masses: pearls and pitfalls. Clin Radiol 2015;70(3):304–16.

33. Zhang J, Pedrosa I, Rofsky NM. MR techniques for renal imaging. Radiol Clin North Am 2003;41(5):877–907.

34. Rosenkrantz AB, Raj S, Babb JS, et al. Comparison of 3D two-point Dixon and standard 2D dual-echo breath-hold sequences for detection and quantification of fat content in renal angiomyolipoma. Eur J Radiol 2012;81(1):47–51.

35. Taouli B, Sandberg A, Stemmer A, et al. Diffusion-weighted imaging of the liver: comparison of navigator triggered and breathhold acquisitions. J Magn Reson Imaging 2009;30(3):561–8.

36. Wang H, Cheng L, Zhang X, et al. Renal cell carcinoma: diffusion-weighted MR imaging for subtype differentiation at 3.0 T. Radiology 2010;257(1):135–43.

37. Rosenkrantz AB, Niver BE, Fitzgerald EF, et al. Utility of the apparent diffusion coefficient for distinguishing clear cell renal cell carcinoma of low and high nuclear grade. AJR Am J Roentgenol 2010;195(5):W344–51.

38. Kang SK, Zhang A, Pandharipande PV, et al. DWI for renal mass characterization: systematic review and meta-analysis of diagnostic test performance. AJR Am J Roentgenol 2015;205(2):317–24.

39. Ho VB, Allen SF, Hood MN, et al. Renal masses: quantitative assessment of enhancement with dynamic MR imaging. Radiology 2002;224(3):695–700.

40. Bosniak MA. The current radiological approach to renal cysts. Radiology 1986;158(1):1–10.

41. Chung EP, Herts BR, Linnell G, et al. Analysis of changes in attenuation of proven renal cysts on different scanning phases of triphasic MDCT. AJR Am J Roentgenol 2004;182(2):405–10.

42. Maki DD, Birnbaum BA, Chakraborty DP, et al. Renal cyst pseudoenhancement: beam-hardening effects on CT numbers. Radiology 1999;213(2):468–72.

43. Bosniak MA. The small (less than or equal to 3.0 cm) renal parenchymal tumor: detection, diagnosis, and controversies. Radiology 1991;179(2):307–17.

44. Bae KT, Heiken JP, Siegel CL, et al. Renal cysts: is attenuation artifactually increased on contrast-enhanced CT images? Radiology 2000;216(3):792–6.

45. Israel GM, Bosniak MA. How I do it: evaluating renal masses. Radiology 2005;236(2):441–50.

46. Yu L, Christner JA, Leng S, et al. Virtual monochromatic imaging in dual-source dual-energy CT: radiation dose and image quality. Med Phys 2011; 38(12):6371–9.

47. Jung DC, Oh YT, Kim MD, et al. Usefulness of the virtual monochromatic image in dual-energy spectral CT for decreasing renal cyst pseudoenhancement: a phantom study. AJR Am J Roentgenol 2012;199(6):1316–9.

48. Mileto A, Nelson RC, Samei E, et al. Impact of dual-energy multi-detector row CT with virtual monochromatic imaging on renal cyst pseudoenhancement: in vitro and in vivo study. Radiology 2014;272(3):767–76.

49. Neville AM, Gupta RT, Miller CM, et al. Detection of renal lesion enhancement with dual-energy multi-detector CT. Radiology 2011;259(1):173–83.

50. Brown CL, Hartman RP, Dzyubak OP, et al. Dual-energy CT iodine overlay technique for characterization of renal masses as cyst or solid: a phantom feasibility study. Eur Radiol 2009;19(5):1289–95.

51. Graser A, Becker CR, Staehler M, et al. Single-phase dual-energy CT allows for characterization of renal masses as benign or malignant. Invest Radiol 2010;45(7):399–405.

52. Kaza RK, Caoili EM, Cohan RH, et al. Distinguishing enhancing from nonenhancing renal lesions with fast kilovoltage-switching dual-energy CT. AJR Am J Roentgenol 2011;197(6):1375–81.

53. Ascenti G, Mileto A, Krauss B, et al. Distinguishing enhancing from nonenhancing renal masses with dual-source dual-energy CT: iodine quantification versus standard enhancement measurements. Eur Radiol 2013;23(8):2288–95.

54. Moch H, Cubilla AL, Humphrey PA, et al. The 2016 WHO classification of tumours of the urinary system and male genital organs–part A: renal, penile, and testicular tumours. Eur Urol 2016;70(1):93–105.

55. Hartman DS, Davis CJ Jr, Johns T, et al. Cystic renal cell carcinoma. Urology 1986;28(2):145–53.

56. Corica FA, Iczkowski KA, Cheng L, et al. Cystic renal cell carcinoma is cured by resection: a study of 24 cases with long-term followup. J Urol 1999; 161(2):408–11.

57. Webster WS, Thompson RH, Cheville JC, et al. Surgical resection provides excellent outcomes for patients with cystic clear cell renal cell carcinoma. Urology 2007;70(5):900–4 [discussion: 904].

58. Jhaveri K, Gupta P, Elmi A, et al. Cystic renal cell carcinomas: do they grow, metastasize, or recur? AJR Am J Roentgenol 2013;201(2):W292–6.

59. Park JJ, Jeong BC, Kim CK, et al. Postoperative outcome of cystic renal cell carcinoma defined on preoperative imaging: a retrospective study. J Urol 2017;197(4):991–7.

60. Israel GM, Bosniak MA. Follow-up CT of moderately complex cystic lesions of the kidney (Bosniak category IIF). AJR Am J Roentgenol 2003;181(3):627–33.

61. Sevcenco S, Spick C, Helbich TH, et al. Malignancy rates and diagnostic performance of the Bosniak classification for the diagnosis of cystic renal lesions in computed tomography - a systematic review and meta-analysis. Eur Radiol 2017;27(6):2239–47.

62. Curry NS, Cochran ST, Bissada NK. Cystic renal masses: accurate Bosniak classification requires adequate renal CT. AJR Am J Roentgenol 2000;175(2):339–42.

63. Lang EK. Renal cyst puncture studies. Urol Clin North Am 1987;14(1):91–102.

64. Pedrosa I, Chou MT, Ngo L, et al. MR classification of renal masses with pathologic correlation. Eur Radiol 2008;18(2):365–75.

65. Young JR, Margolis D, Sauk S, et al. Clear cell renal cell carcinoma: discrimination from other renal cell carcinoma subtypes and oncocytoma at multiphasic multidetector CT. Radiology 2013;267(2):444–53.

66. Lee-Felker SA, Felker ER, Tan N, et al. Qualitative and quantitative MDCT features for differentiating clear cell renal cell carcinoma from other solid renal cortical masses. AJR Am J Roentgenol 2014;203(5):W516–24.

67. Zhang J, Lefkowitz RA, Ishill NM, et al. Solid renal cortical tumors: differentiation with CT. Radiology 2007;244(2):494–504.

68. Sun MR, Ngo L, Genega EM, et al. Renal cell carcinoma: dynamic contrast-enhanced MR imaging for differentiation of tumor subtypes–correlation with pathologic findings. Radiology 2009;250(3):793–802.

69. Ruppert-Kohlmayr AJ, Uggowitzer M, Meissnitzer T, et al. Differentiation of renal clear cell carcinoma and renal papillary carcinoma using quantitative CT enhancement parameters. AJR Am J Roentgenol 2004;183(5):1387–91.

70. Mileto A, Marin D, Alfaro-Cordoba M, et al. Iodine quantification to distinguish clear cell from papillary renal cell carcinoma at dual-energy multidetector CT: a multireader diagnostic performance study. Radiology 2014;273(3):813–20.

71. Pedrosa I, Sun MR, Spencer M, et al. MR imaging of renal masses: correlation with findings at surgery and pathologic analysis. Radiographics 2008;28(4):985–1003.

72. Roy C Sr, El Ghali S, Buy X, et al. Significance of the pseudocapsule on MRI of renal neoplasms and its potential application for local staging: a retrospective study. AJR Am J Roentgenol 2005;184(1):113–20.

73. Vasudevan A, Davies RJ, Shannon BA, et al. Incidental renal tumours: the frequency of benign lesions and the role of preoperative core biopsy. BJU Int 2006;97(5):946–9.

74. Kutikov A, Fossett LK, Ramchandani P, et al. Incidence of benign pathologic findings at partial nephrectomy for solitary renal mass presumed to be renal cell carcinoma on preoperative imaging. Urology 2006;68(4):737–40.

75. Remzi M, Ozsoy M, Klingler HC, et al. Are small renal tumors harmless? Analysis of histopathological features according to tumors 4 cm or less in diameter. J Urol 2006;176(3):896–9.

76. O'Malley RL, Godoy G, Phillips CK, et al. Is surveillance of small renal masses safe in the elderly? BJU Int 2010;105(8):1098–101.

77. Crispen PL, Viterbo R, Boorjian SA, et al. Natural history, growth kinetics, and outcomes of untreated clinically localized renal tumors under active surveillance. Cancer 2009;115(13):2844–52.

78. Laguna MP, Algaba F, Cadeddu J, et al. Current patterns of presentation and treatment of renal masses: a clinical research office of the Endourological Society prospective study. J Endourol 2014;28(7):861–70.

79. Campbell SC, Novick AC, Belldegrun A, et al. Guideline for management of the clinical T1 renal mass. J Urol 2009;182(4):1271–9.

80. Motzer RJ, Jonasch E, Agarwal N, et al. Kidney cancer, version 3.2015. J Natl Compr Canc Netw 2015;13(2):151–9.

81. Donat SM, Diaz M, Bishoff JT, et al. Follow-up for clinically localized renal neoplasms: AUA guideline. J Urol 2013;190(2):407–16.

82. Rosales JC, Haramis G, Moreno J, et al. Active surveillance for renal cortical neoplasms. J Urol 2010;183(5):1698–702.

83. Kouba E, Smith A, McRackan D, et al. Watchful waiting for solid renal masses: insight into the natural history and results of delayed intervention. J Urol 2007;177(2):466–70 [discussion: 470].

84. Smaldone MC, Kutikov A, Egleston BL, et al. Small renal masses progressing to metastases under active surveillance: a systematic review and pooled analysis. Cancer 2012;118(4):997–1006.

85. Winters BR, Gore JL, Holt SK, et al. Cystic renal cell carcinoma carries an excellent prognosis regardless of tumor size. Urol Oncol 2015;33(12):505. e9-13.

86. Han KR, Janzen NK, McWhorter VC, et al. Cystic renal cell carcinoma: biology and clinical behavior. Urol Oncol 2004;22(5):410–4.

87. Koga S, Nishikido M, Hayashi T, et al. Outcome of surgery in cystic renal cell carcinoma. Urology 2000;56(1):67–70.

88. Zisman A, Pantuck AJ, Wieder J, et al. Risk group assessment and clinical outcome algorithm to predict the natural history of patients with surgically resected renal cell carcinoma. J Clin Oncol 2002; 20(23):4559–66.

89. Bianchi M, Sun M, Jeldres C, et al. Distribution of metastatic sites in renal cell carcinoma: a population-based analysis. Ann Oncol 2012;23(4): 973–80.

90. Eggener SE, Yossepowitch O, Pettus JA, et al. Renal cell carcinoma recurrence after nephrectomy for localized disease: predicting survival from time of recurrence. J Clin Oncol 2006; 24(19):3101–6.

91. Klatte T, Lam JS, Shuch B, et al. Surveillance for renal cell carcinoma: why and how? When and how often? Urol Oncol 2008;26(5):550–4.

92. Levy DA, Slaton JW, Swanson DA, et al. Stage specific guidelines for surveillance after radical nephrectomy for local renal cell carcinoma. J Urol 1998;159(4):1163–7.

93. Lam JS, Shvarts O, Leppert JT, et al. Renal cell carcinoma 2005: new frontiers in staging, prognostication and targeted molecular therapy. J Urol 2005; 173(6):1853–62.

94. Janzen NK, Kim HL, Figlin RA, et al. Surveillance after radical or partial nephrectomy for localized renal cell carcinoma and management of recurrent disease. Urol Clin North Am 2003;30(4):843–52.

95. Kobayashi K, Saito T, Kitamura Y, et al. Clinicopathological features and outcomes in patients with late recurrence of renal cell carcinoma after radical surgery. Int J Urol 2016;23(2):132–7.

96. Van Poppel H, Da Pozzo L, Albrecht W, et al. A prospective, randomised EORTC intergroup phase 3 study comparing the oncologic outcome of elective nephron-sparing surgery and radical nephrectomy for low-stage renal cell carcinoma. Eur Urol 2011;59(4):543–52.

97. Matin SF, Ahrar K, Cadeddu JA, et al. Residual and recurrent disease following renal energy ablative therapy: a multi-institutional study. J Urol 2006; 176(5):1973–7.

98. Jain Y, Liew S, Taylor MB, et al. Is dual-phase abdominal CT necessary for the optimal detection of metastases from renal cell carcinoma? Clin Radiol 2011;66(11):1055–9.

99. Matsumoto ED, Watumull L, Johnson DB, et al. The radiographic evolution of radio frequency ablated renal tumors. J Urol 2004;172(1):45–8.

100. Svatek RS, Sims R, Anderson JK, et al. Magnetic resonance imaging characteristics of renal tumors after radiofrequency ablation. Urology 2006;67(3): 508–12.

101. Iannuccilli JD, Grand DJ, Dupuy DE, et al. Percutaneous ablation for small renal masses-imaging follow-up. Semin Intervent Radiol 2014;31(1):50–63.

102. Chan DY, Chua WJ. A rare subcutaneous manifestation of metastatic renal cell carcinoma. Case Rep Surg 2016;2016:6453975.

103. Guimaraes DM, Pontes FS, Miyahara LA, et al. Metastatic renal cell carcinoma to the oral cavity. J Craniofac Surg 2016;27(6):e533–4.

104. Dell'Atti L. Unusual ultrasound presentation of testicular metastasis from renal clear cell carcinoma. Rare Tumors 2016;8(3):6471.

105. Hafez KS, Novick AC, Campbell SC. Patterns of tumor recurrence and guidelines for followup after nephron sparing surgery for sporadic renal cell carcinoma. J Urol 1997;157(6):2067–70.

106. Saitoh H, Nakayama M, Nakamura K, et al. Distant metastasis of renal adenocarcinoma in nephrectomized cases. J Urol 1982;127(6):1092–5.

107. Bowman IA, Pedrosa I, Kapura P, et al. Renal cell carcinoma with pulmonary metastasis and metachronous non-small cell lung cancer. Clin Genitourin Cancer 2017;15(4):e675–80.

108. Woodward E, Jagdev S, McParland L, et al. Skeletal complications and survival in renal cancer patients with bone metastases. Bone 2011;48(1): 160–6.

109. Woolfenden JM, Pitt MJ, Durie BG, et al. Comparison of bone scintigraphy and radiography in multiple myeloma. Radiology 1980;134(3):723–8.

110. Hoffmann NE, Gillett MD, Cheville JC, et al. Differences in organ system of distant metastasis by renal cell carcinoma subtype. J Urol 2008;179(2): 474–7.

111. Aslam S, Eisen T. Vascular endothelial growth factor receptor tyrosine kinase inhibitors in metastatic renal cell cancer: latest results and clinical implications. Ther Adv Med Oncol 2013;5(6): 324–33.

112. Maksimovic O, Schraml C, Hartmann JT, et al. Evaluation of response in malignant tumors treated with the multitargeted tyrosine kinase inhibitor sorafenib: a multitechnique imaging assessment. AJR Am J Roentgenol 2010;194(1):5–14.

113. de Bazelaire C, Alsop DC, George D, et al. Magnetic resonance imaging-measured blood flow change after antiangiogenic therapy with PTK787/ZK 222584 correlates with clinical outcome in metastatic renal cell carcinoma. Clin Cancer Res 2008; 14(17):5548–54.

114. Flaherty KT, Rosen MA, Heitjan DF, et al. Pilot study of DCE-MRI to predict progression-free survival with sorafenib therapy in renal cell carcinoma. Cancer Biol Ther 2008;7(4):496–501.

115. Hellbach K, Sterzik A, Sommer W, et al. Dual energy CT allows for improved characterization of response to antiangiogenic treatment in patients with metastatic renal cell cancer. Eur Radiol 2017; 27(6):2532–7.

116. Smith AD, Zhang X, Bryan J, et al. Vascular tumor burden as a new quantitative CT biomarker for predicting metastatic RCC response to antiangiogenic therapy. Radiology 2016;281(2):484–98.

117. Alrashdi I, Levine S, Paterson J, et al. Hereditary leiomyomatosis and renal cell carcinoma: very early diagnosis of renal cancer in a paediatric patient. Fam Cancer 2010;9(2):239–43.

118. Grubb RL 3rd, Franks ME, Toro J, et al. Hereditary leiomyomatosis and renal cell cancer: a syndrome associated with an aggressive form of inherited renal cancer. J Urol 2007;177(6):2074–9 [discussion: 2079–80].

119. Ricketts CJ, Shuch B, Vocke CD, et al. Succinate dehydrogenase kidney cancer: an aggressive example of the Warburg effect in cancer. J Urol 2012;188(6):2063–71.

120. Menko FH, van Steensel MA, Giraud S, et al. Birt-Hogg-Dube syndrome: diagnosis and management. Lancet Oncol 2009;10(12):1199–206.

121. Schmidt L, Junker K, Weirich G, et al. Two North American families with hereditary papillary renal carcinoma and identical novel mutations in the MET proto-oncogene. Cancer Res 1998;58(8): 1719–22.

Imaging and Screening of Ovarian Cancer

Kathryn P. Lowry, MD[a],*, Susanna I. Lee, MD, PhD[b]

KEYWORDS

• Ovarian cancer • Cancer screening • Randomized trials • Transvaginal ultrasound

KEY POINTS

- Ovarian cancer screening has not been shown to decrease mortality in average-risk women and is not recommended by any North American professional society.
- Randomized trials of ovarian cancer screening have not been conducted in women at high risk for ovarian cancer. Women with BRCA mutation or a family history of ovarian cancer are considered at high risk.
- Some professional societies recommend consideration of screening women at high risk using annual transvaginal ultrasound and serum CA-125; however, there is no evidence of mortality benefit.
- Prophylactic bilateral salpingo-oophorectomy in high-risk women is the only intervention that has been proven to decrease ovarian cancer mortality.
- Currently, the role of imaging in ovarian cancer screening is for confirmation of a clinically suspected diagnosis; more importantly, imaging is used for definitive characterization of incidental benign adnexal lesions in order to decrease rates of surgical diagnosis.

INTRODUCTION

Epithelial ovarian cancer is a malignancy with low prevalence and high mortality: although only 1.3% of women will be diagnosed with ovarian cancer during their lifetime,[1] ovarian cancer is the leading cause of gynecologic malignancy in the United States with 14,080 deaths due to ovarian cancer projected for 2017.[2] The high mortality of ovarian cancer is attributed to the presence of distant metastases at the time of diagnosis. Although localized ovarian cancer has a good prognosis with 5-year survival estimates of 92%, more than half (60%) of ovarian cancers are metastatic at time of diagnosis,

which confers a much lower 5-year survival estimate of 29%.[2] This observation has fueled the effort to identify a diagnostic test that could be used to screen for ovarian cancer, in hopes of detecting disease at earlier stages when it is most treatable.

To date, ovarian cancer screening has not proven effective, due in part to its relatively low incidence rate, its pathophysiology, and the diagnostic test performance of currently available screening tools. The authors review what is known about the natural history of high-grade epithelial ovarian cancer, the results of the largest trials of ovarian cancer screening using transvaginal ultrasound (TVUS), as well as the current and future use of imaging in

Disclosures: K.P. Lowry has no conflicts of interest to disclose. S.I. Lee receives salary compensation as UptoDate editor from Wolters Kluwer.
[a] University of Washington School of Medicine, Seattle Cancer Care Alliance, 825 Eastlake Avenue East, G2-600, Seattle, WA 98109, USA; [b] Massachusetts General Hospital, Harvard Medical School, 55 Fruit Street, WAC 240, Boston, MA 02114, USA
* Corresponding author. 825 Eastlake Avenue East, G2-600, Seattle, WA 98109.
E-mail address: kplowry@uw.edu

ovarian cancer detection. They also summarize the current consensus recommendations for women at average and high risk for ovarian cancer.

PATHOPHYSIOLOGY OF OVARIAN CANCER

Although the natural history of the development and spread of ovarian cancer is not fully understood, it is clear that tumors classified as ovarian make up a heterogeneous group of diseases. More than 95% of ovarian cancers are epithelial in origin, with the remaining 5% comprising germ cell and sex cord-stromal tumors.[3] Of the epithelial tumors, serous tumors are most common, representing 40% of all epithelial tumors.[3] A 2-phenotype classification of serous carcinomas has been proposed that distinguishes between low- and high-grade serous tumors, which are thought to represent distinct diseases with markedly different biological behaviors.[3] Low-grade serous lesions may arise from precursor lesions and are associated with several mutations including B-raf proto-oncogene serine/threonine-protein kinase (BRAF) and v-Ki-ras2 Kirsten rat sarcoma viral oncogene homolog (KRAS).[3] Their rate of growth is more indolent, and thus, they are also more likely to be detected at early stage by screening (**Fig. 1**). In contrast, high-grade serous tumors are associated with tumor protein 53 mutations and progress rapidly, making early screen-detection difficult (**Fig. 2**).[3] Examination of specimens from prophylactic bilateral salpingo-oophorectomy (PBSO) in BRCA1/BRCA2 mutation carriers has suggested that high-grade serous tumors may actually arise from the fallopian tubes rather than the ovary.[4,5]

Models of the natural history and progression of ovarian cancer have been used to estimate the sojourn time of clinically occult ovarian cancer. Based on pooled data from studies of serous cancers discovered at PBSO, Brown and Palmer[6] estimated that ovarian cancers spend approximately 4 years as in situ, stage I and stage II tumors, during which time they are typically too small to visualize even on gross examination of the ovaries and fallopian tubes. At time of progression to stage III/IV, median diameter is approximately 3 cm. Based on these findings, the investigators estimate that a screening test would need to detect tumors less than 4 mm in diameter to achieve 80% sensitivity; to reduce cancer mortality by 50% would require detection of tumors 5 mm in size.[6] Moreover, the known discrepancy in the biologic behavior of low- and high-grade serous tumors may limit the effectiveness of current methods available for screening. Results from one Markov model of serous ovarian cancers incorporating this 2-phenotype model suggest

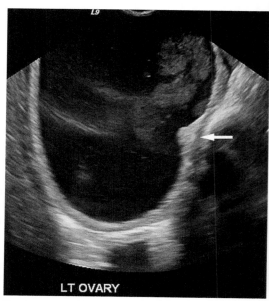

Fig. 1. Low-grade epithelial ovarian cancer. TVUS image of a 24-year-old woman presenting with symptoms of bloating and constipation shows a 12-cm complex left adnexal cyst with mural nodularity (*arrow*). Surgery and pathology showed grade 1 (of 3) mucinous cystadenocarcinoma confined to the left ovary. As the patient was stage IA at diagnosis, her likelihood of 5-year survival was approximately 94%.

that application of currently available screening technologies would only result in modest (6.4%–10.9%) reductions in ovarian cancer mortality. This potential limitation is further supported by the high rate of interval cancers seen in screening trials of women with BRCA mutations.[7]

RISK FACTORS FOR OVARIAN CANCER

Ovarian cancer risk increases with age: based on 2014 observed National Cancer Institute Surveillance, Epidemiology, and End Result data, ovarian cancer incidence rates increase from 6.1 per 100,000 women ages 20 to 49, to 22.8 per 100,000 women ages 50 to 64, to 36.6 per 100,000 women ages 65 to 74.[8] Large prospective observational studies have been conducted to identify other risk factors and protective factors for ovarian cancer. One study evaluating ovarian cancer risk in the US Nurses' Health Study and Nurses' Health Study II found increased risk of ovarian cancer (ROC) associated with higher age of natural menopause and estrogen use, and lower risk associated with parity, breastfeeding, history of tubal ligation, and hysterectomy.[9] Oral contraceptive pills (OCP) use has been consistently shown to be protective against ovarian cancer.[10,11] A meta-analysis of 45 epidemiologic studies

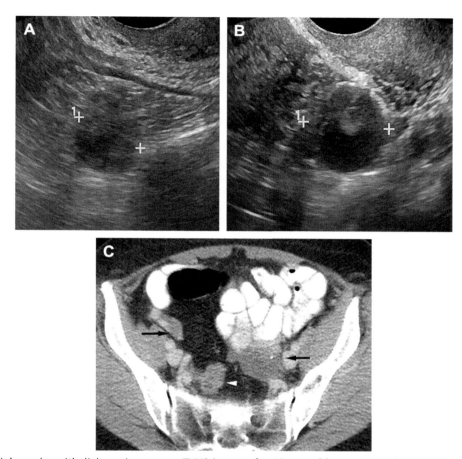

Fig. 2. High-grade epithelial ovarian cancer. TVUS image of a 48-year-old asymptomatic woman with fibroids demonstrates right (*A*) and left (*B*) ovaries (*caliper 1*) with minimally complex cysts thought to be physiologic. Both ovaries are normal in size measuring 1.8 cm on right and 2.1 cm on left. Pelvic image from CT with intravenous and oral contrast (*C*) performed 6 weeks later shows enhancing nodules in both ovaries (*arrows*) and in the peritoneum (*arrowhead*). Surgery and pathology showed grade 3 (of 3) serous cystadenocarcinoma involving ovaries, fallopian tubes, omentum, and abdominopelvic peritoneum. As the patient was stage IIIC at diagnosis, her likelihood of 5-year survival was approximately 40%.

estimated that 10 years of OCP use reduces ovarian cancer incidence before age 70 from 1.2 to 0.8 per 100 women, and for every 5000 women who use OCPs for 10 years, one ovarian cancer death is prevented.[10]

Approximately 10% to 15% of women with epithelial ovarian cancer carry a germline BRCA mutation.[11] Women with these mutations are at a markedly increased risk for ovarian cancer, with a lifetime risk of 40% in women with BRCA1 mutations and 18% for BRCA2 mutation carriers.[12] BRCA germline mutations are also associated with the development of high-grade serous carcinomas.[5]

OVARIAN CANCER BIOMARKERS

Serum cancer antigen 125 (CA-125) is the most studied biomarker for epithelial ovarian cancer.

Initial interest in CA-125 as a screening tool developed because of an observation in an early study that the marker is elevated in 80% of women with ovarian cancer but only 1% to 2% of the normal population.[13] However, subsequent studies demonstrated that although CA-125 is usually elevated in advanced disease, it is often normal in early-stage ovarian cancer.[14] Moreover, CA-125 is very nonspecific and can be elevated in several benign and malignant diseases (eg, ascites, endometriosis).[15] For these reasons, current use of CA-125 is largely restricted to monitoring for treatment response and disease recurrence in patients with known diagnosis of ovarian cancer.

More recent work has suggested that it is not the absolute level of CA-125 but the change in serum levels over time that may be useful in identifying clinically occult ovarian cancer. Menon and colleagues[16] published results from a randomized study of ovarian cancer screening using a ROC algorithm, which was initially developed from stored serum samples from the Stockholm Ovarian Cancer Screening study.[17] The algorithm estimates a woman's ROC by comparing her change in serum CA-125 levels over time with a change-point model in CA-125 estimated in age-matched ovarian cancer cases versus the flat CA-125 levels observed in controls. Women were randomly assigned to annual CA-125 screening with interpretation using the ROC algorithm; abnormal values prompted further evaluation with TVUS. Specificity of the ROC algorithm was 99.8%, and the positive predictive value (PPV) was 19%.[16]

Other serum biomarkers have been investigated as potential tools for ovarian cancer screening, but none to date have performed as well as CA-125. In an analysis of performance of a panel of 35 biomarkers in specimens from the Prostate, Lung, Colorectal, and Ovarian Cancer Screening Trial (PLCO), CA-125 was the best performing biomarker, followed by HE4, transthyretin, CA-15.3, and CA-72.4.[18]

In the past decade, biomarkers based on high-throughput technologies of genomics and proteomics have shown promise in early ovarian cancer detection. Assays of gene expression or hypermethylation and analyses of proteomic, microRNA, or metabolite expression profiles are all under various stages of development; but none are sufficiently mature for clinical use.[19] The known genetic heterogeneity of ovarian cancers represents one challenge in biomarker development yet to be addressed.[20] Current research strategies focus on improving both the sensitivity and the specificity of detection with assay panels comprising known and novel biomarkers of ovarian cancer.

TRIALS OF OVARIAN CANCER SCREENING IN WOMEN AT AVERAGE RISK

Ovarian cancer screening trials have predominantly evaluated the potential use of TVUS, with and without concurrent biomarker screening with serum CA-125 levels. Currently, there is no role for the use of other modalities such as computed tomography (CT) or magnetic resonance (MR) imaging to screen for ovarian cancer. Results from the largest randomized controlled trials of ovarian cancer screening in women at average risk are summarized below and in **Table 1**.

Shizuoka Cohort Study

In the Shizuoka Cohort study,[21] asymptomatic postmenopausal women in the Shizuoka district of Japan were randomized to either an intervention group receiving annual pelvic ultrasound (US) and serum CA-125 testing (n = 41,688) or a control group (n = 40,799). Women in the intervention arm were referred for gynecologic oncology evaluation for either an abnormal US finding (defined as ovarian size >4 cm with complex morphology) or an elevated CA-125 level. The primary study endpoint was detection of early-stage cancers. After a mean follow-up of 9.2 years, 27 cancers were detected in the screening arm and 32 cancers were detected in the control arm. There was no significant difference in the percentage of stage I cancers between the 2 groups (63% in the screening group vs 38% in the control group; P = .2285). Of note, 8 cancers were diagnosed in the intervention arm outside of the screening program presenting between the screening intervals. Mortality data from this trial are not yet available.

United States Prostate, Lung, Colorectal, and Ovarian Cancer Screening Trial

In the PLCO trial,[22] asymptomatic postmenopausal women were randomized to an intervention arm (n = 39,105) with annual screening with serum CA-125 for 6 years and annual TVUS for 4 years, versus a control arm (n = 39,111), who received usual care. US was considered abnormal based on any of the following findings: ovarian volume greater than 10 cm^3, cyst volume greater than 10 cm, presence of a solid area or papillary projection extending into the cavity of a cystic ovarian tumor, or any mixed solid and cystic component within a cystic ovarian tumor. CA-125 levels were considered abnormal if 35 U/mL or greater. The primary study endpoint was ovarian cancer mortality.

After a median follow-up of 12.4 years, 212 women in the intervention group were diagnosed with ovarian cancer compared with 176 women in the control group (incidence rates of 5.7 vs 4.7 cases per 100,000 person-years, respectively). Stage distribution of cancers was similar between the intervention and control arms, with most cancers in both arms being stage III/IV cancers (77% in the intervention arm and 78% in the control arm). Of cancers diagnosed in the intervention arm during the screening phase, 29% were interval cancers. There was no significant difference in ovarian cancer mortality between the 2 arms (3.1 deaths per 100,000 person-years in the intervention arm vs 2.6 per 100,000 person-years in the control arm).

United Kingdom Collaborative Trial of Ovarian Cancer Screening

In 2016, long-term results were reported for the United Kingdom Collaborative Trial of Ovarian

Table 1
Summary of largest ovarian cancer screening trials

Trial	Population	Design	Intervention	Primary Endpoint	Result
Shizuoka Cohort Study[21] (n = 82,487)	Asymptomatic postmenopausal women	Randomized controlled trial	Annual pelvic US and serum CA-125 levels	Detection of early (stage I) ovarian cancers	No significant difference in stage distribution between intervention and control group
PLCO[22] (n = 78,216)	Asymptomatic postmenopausal women	Randomized controlled trial	Annual serum CA-125 for 6 y and annual TVUS for 4 y	Ovarian cancer mortality	No significant difference in ovarian cancer mortality between the 2 arms
UKCTOCS[23] (n = 202,638)	Asymptomatic postmenopausal women	Randomized controlled trial	Annual serum CA-125 levels interpreted using a predefined algorithm, with follow-up TVUS as needed (multimodality) vs annual TVUS alone	Ovarian cancer mortality over a 14-y study period	No significant difference in ovarian cancer mortality at the end of the 14-y study period; a stage shift was seen in the multimodality arm
UK FOCSS[25] (n = 3563)	Women with first-degree relative with history of ovarian cancer	Prospective single-arm study	Annual serum CA-125 and TVUS	Test performance	Sensitivity: 81%–87.5% PPV: 25.5%

Cancer Screening (UKCTOCS),[23] the largest performed randomized controlled trial of ovarian cancer screening. In this study, asymptomatic postmenopausal women from 13 centers in National Health Service Trusts in the United Kingdom were assigned to 1 of 3 arms: multimodality screening using annual CA-125 with follow-up TVUS as indicated (n = 50,640), TVUS alone (50,639), or usual care (101,359). In the multimodality screening arm, CA-125 levels were interpreted using the ROC algorithm described above and in earlier work.[16] Screening US was considered abnormal based on the presence of complex ovarian morphology, simple cysts greater than 60 mL, or ascites. The primary endpoint was death due to ovarian cancer.

After a median follow-up of 11.1 years, a stage shift was observed in the multimodality screening group, with 40% of cancers diagnosed at stages I, II, or IIIA compared with 24% in the US group and 26% in the control group. However, there was no statistically significant difference in ovarian cancer mortality at the end of the 14-year study period. During the study period, 148 women died of ovarian cancer in the multimodality group (0.29%), compared with 154 (0.30%) in the US group and 347 (0.34%) in the control arm. In a post hoc analysis, the investigators noted a potential delayed survival benefit in the multimodality group compared with controls, with a 23% (95% confidence interval 1%–46%) decrease in ovarian cancer mortality in years 7 to 14 but no significant difference in mortality during years 0 to 7. Mortality in the US group was not significantly different from controls in either the early (years 0–7) or the late (years 7–14) study period.

OVARIAN CANCER SCREENING TRIALS IN HIGH-RISK POPULATIONS

To date, PBSO is the only intervention that has been proven effective and is estimated to reduce ovarian cancer mortality in high-risk women by 80% based on a recent meta-analysis.[24] Randomized trials of ovarian cancer screening in high-risk groups have not been conducted and are unlikely to be performed given the ethical concerns of assigning a high-risk group to a control arm that does not offer screening. Thus, data for screening in high-risk women are limited to prospective cohort study data.

The largest prospective trial of women at high risk for ovarian cancer is the United Kingdom Familial Ovarian Cancer Screening Study (FOCSS),[25] which enrolled 3563 women with an estimated lifetime ROC ≥10% based on family history or known genetic mutation. Women in the

study receive annual screening with a combination of serum CA-125 and TVUS. Results from first phase of the trial were reported in 2008, which showed that after a mean of 3.2 years of follow-up, 13 cancers were detected, of which 4 (30.8%) were stage I or II. The sensitivity of detection of ovarian/fallopian tube cancers was reported as 81.3% to 87.5%, depending on whether fallopian tube cancers detected at risk-reducing bilateral salpingo-oophorectomy were categorized as true negatives or false positives. PPV was 25.5%, which exceeds the 10% threshold that has been suggested as the minimum necessary for ovarian cancer screening to be acceptable. Of note, stage IIIc/IV cancers were more common in women who had not been screened within the prior year (85.7% vs 26.1% in those who had received screening within the preceding year). In light of this finding, the investigators highlight the importance of screening adherence and have reduced the screening interval to 4 months for the second phase of the trial, the results of which are not yet available.[25]

Other trials of ovarian cancer screening in high-risk women have shown less promise, largely because of high rates of interval cancers (ie, cancers presenting between screening events). For example, in one prospective study of 888 BRCA1 and BRCA2 mutation carriers undergoing annual screening with TVUS and serum CA-125, half of cancers detected (5/10) were interval cancers, which presented in women who had a normal screening examination within the preceding 3 to 10 months.[7] Most cancers (80%) were stage III or higher at diagnosis. In a recent subgroup analysis of women in the PLCO trial who reported a first-degree relative of ovarian cancer, no significant difference in ovarian cancer mortality was observed between the intervention and control arms.[26] There was suggestion of a stage shift and possible improved survival among women with ovarian cancer in women in the screening arm; however, as noted by the investigators, these findings are subject to epidemiologic biases.[26] Because of the lack of convincing evidence of a benefit of screening, most experts emphasize the benefit of PBSO for risk reduction over screening. More data are needed from prospective trials of ovarian cancer screening in high-risk populations to inform clinical decision making about imaging surveillance in women who choose not to undergo PBSO.

ADVERSE EFFECTS OF SCREENING

One of the barriers of implementing an ovarian cancer screening program at a population level is the potential harmful consequences of screening, particularly the number of surgeries performed in women without cancer. For example, in the PLCO screening arm, 3285 (8.5%) had a false positive test result. Of these, 1080 (33%) underwent surgical follow-up, and 163 women (15%) experienced at least one serious complication.[22] Screening complications were lower in the multimodality arm of the UKCTOCS,[23] which estimated rates of serious complications due to screening as 8.6 per 100,000 in the multimodality arm compared with 18.6 per 100,000 in the US-only group. False positive screens led to surgeries with normal adnexa or benign adnexal abnormality in 488 (1%) of women in the multimodality arm and 1634 (3.2%) of women in the US arm.[23] The overall effects of ovarian cancer screening on patient quality of life and societal health care expenditures have yet to be directly estimated in large trials.

CONSENSUS RECOMMENDATIONS

Because of the lack of evidence for a mortality benefit in multiple randomized controlled trials, ovarian cancer screening is not currently recommended for average-risk women by any North American professional society (**Table 2**). The US Preventive Services Task Force recommends against screening,[27] and this recommendation is endorsed by the Society of Gynecologic Oncology (SGO).[28] Similarly, the American College of Obstetricians and Gynecologists (ACOG),[29] the American Cancer Society,[30] and the Canadian Task Force on the Periodic Health Examination[31] also recommend against ovarian cancer screening women at average risk.

There is less consensus for screening recommendations for women at high ROC. The American Cancer Society notes that no screening test has proven effective or sufficiently accurate in the early detection of ovarian cancer but that for women at high risk, pelvic examination, TVUS evaluation, and serum CA-125 may be offered.[30] The SGO guidelines[28] recommend screening for BRCA mutation carriers or women with a first-degree relative with ovarian cancer using TVUS and CA-125 every 6 months beginning at ages 30 to 35 or 5 to 10 years earlier than the youngest age of diagnosis of ovarian cancer in the family. The National Comprehensive Cancer Network (NCCN) notes that the test performance of TVUS has not been shown sufficient to support a recommendation for ovarian cancer screening in women with BRCA mutations, but that screening with TVUS and/or serum CA-125 may be considered at the clinician's discretion starting at age 30 to 35. The NCCN also recommends strong consideration of PBSO in women with BRCA mutations once

---

Table 2
Recommendations from North American health care organizations regarding ovarian cancer screening

Organization	Recommendation
American Cancer Society[30]	Recommends against screening in average-risk women; screening may be offered to high-risk women, although it is not clear that there is a survival benefit
ACOG[29]	Recommends against screening in average-risk women; in high-risk women, recommends evaluation for known signs and symptoms of ovarian cancer, cites NCCN guidelines and acknowledges no evidence of survival benefit
Canadian Task Force on the Periodic Health Examination[31]	Recommends against screening
NCCN[32]	Notes that sensitivity and specificity of screening with TVUS has not been shown to be sufficient enough to warrant a positive recommendation, however, screening in BRCA mutation carriers can be considered starting at ages 30–35, at clinician's discretion
Society of Gynecologic Oncology[28]	Endorses US Preventive Services Task Force recommendation against screening in average-risk women; in high-risk women, recommends screening be considered with TVUS and CA-125 every 6 mo beginning at ages 30–35, or 5–10 y before the age of diagnosis of youngest family member; recommends women be counseled that screening has not been proven to decrease mortality and that PBSO should be considered
US Preventive Services Task Force[27]	Recommends against screening

childbearing is complete.[32] ACOG cites NCCN guidelines but states that there is no evidence that screening improves survival in high-risk populations.[29]

ADNEXAL IMAGING

Given the available data on screening, the future role of imaging in ovarian cancer screening is likely to be for further evaluation of women triaged based on abnormal biomarker results. This evaluation includes confirmation of suspected cancers and, perhaps more importantly, noninvasively characterizing benign adnexal lesions to prevent unnecessary salpingo-oophorectomy in women without cancer.

MR imaging has been shown to be the most accurate modality for diagnosis of adnexal lesions. Because it provides better tissue characterization and lesion localization than TVUS or CT, the contribution of MR imaging in adnexal mass evaluation is its specificity. A prospective trial demonstrated that both Doppler US and MR imaging were highly sensitive for identifying malignant lesions (100% with US and 96.6% with MR imaging), but the specificity of MR imaging was significantly greater (39.5% with US and 83.7% with MR imaging).[33] An important role of imaging in future ovarian cancer screening trials is to noninvasively characterize benign adnexal lesions and minimize the morbidity associated with screening.

SUMMARY

- Ovarian cancer screening with TVUS alone or in combination with serum CA-125 has not been shown to decrease mortality in average-risk postmenopausal women.
- No randomized trials of ovarian cancer screening have been conducted in women at high risk for ovarian cancer. Some professional societies recommend consideration of screening women at high risk (BRCA mutation or family history) using annual TVUS and serum CA-125. However, a mortality benefit with this approach is yet to be demonstrated in trials.
- PBSO is the only intervention that has been proven to decrease ovarian cancer–specific mortality in women at high risk.
- Should screening trials using serum or genetic biomarkers prove effective, imaging will likely play a role in future ovarian cancer screening to improve the specificity of the screening strategy by confirming a suspected positive diagnosis.

- Currently the most important role of imaging for women at risk for ovarian cancer is in noninvasive diagnosis of incidental benign adnexal lesions to minimize rates of surgery and the morbidity associated from screening.

REFERENCES

1. Howlader N, Noone AM, Krapcho M, et al, editors. SEER cancer statistics review, 1975-2014. Bethesda (MD): National Cancer Institute; 2017. Available at: https://seer.cancer.gov/csr/1975_2014/. Based on November 2016 SEER data submission, posted to the SEER Web site.
2. Siegel RL, Miller KD, Jemal A. Cancer Statistics, 2017. CA Cancer J Clin 2017;67(1):7–30.
3. Quirk JT, Natarajan N. Ovarian cancer incidence in the United States, 1992-1999. Gynecol Oncol 2005;97(2):519–23.
4. Crum CP, Drapkin R, Kindelberger D, et al. Lessons from BRCA: the tubal fimbria emerges as an origin for pelvic serous cancer. Clin Med Res 2007;5(1):35–44.
5. McCluggage WG. Morphological subtypes of ovarian carcinoma: a review with emphasis on new developments and pathogenesis. Pathology 2011;43(5):420–32.
6. Brown PO, Palmer C. The preclinical natural history of serous ovarian cancer: defining the target for early detection. PLoS Med 2009;6(7):e1000114.
7. Hermsen BB, Olivier RI, Verheijen RH, et al. No efficacy of annual gynaecological screening in BRCA1/2 mutation carriers; an observational follow-up study. Br J Cancer 2007;96(9):1335–42.
8. Fast Stats: an interactive tool for access to SEER cancer statistics. Surveillance Research Program, National Cancer Institute. Available at: https://seer.cancer.gov/faststats. Accessed April 15, 2017.
9. Gates MA, Rosner BA, Hecht JL, et al. Risk factors for epithelial ovarian cancer by histologic subtype. Am J Epidemiol 2010;171(1):45–53.
10. Collaborative Group on Epidemiological Studies of Ovarian Cancer, Beral V, Doll R, Hermon C, et al. Ovarian cancer and oral contraceptives: collaborative reanalysis of data from 45 epidemiological studies including 23,257 women with ovarian cancer and 87,303 controls. Lancet 2008;371(9609):303–14.
11. Moorman PG, Havrilesky LJ, Gierisch JM, et al. Oral contraceptives and risk of ovarian cancer and breast cancer among high-risk women: a systematic review and meta-analysis. J Clin Oncol 2013;31(33):4188–98.
12. Chen S, Parmigiani G. Meta-analysis of BRCA1 and BRCA2 penetrance. J Clin Oncol 2007;25(11):1329–33.

13. Bast RC Jr, Klug TL, St John E, et al. A radioimmunoassay using a monoclonal antibody to monitor the course of epithelial ovarian cancer. N Engl J Med 1983;309(15):883–7.

14. Woolas RP, Xu FJ, Jacobs IJ, et al. Elevation of multiple serum markers in patients with stage I ovarian cancer. J Natl Cancer Inst 1993;85(21):1748–51.

15. Clarke-Pearson DL. Clinical practice. Screening for ovarian cancer. N Engl J Med 2009;361(2):170–7.

16. Menon U, Skates SJ, Lewis S, et al. Prospective study using the risk of ovarian cancer algorithm to screen for ovarian cancer. J Clin Oncol 2005; 23(31):7919–26.

17. Skates SJ, Xu FJ, Yu YH, et al. Toward an optimal algorithm for ovarian cancer screening with longitudinal tumor markers. Cancer 1995;76(10 Suppl): 2004–10.

18. Yurkovetsky Z, Skates S, Lomakin A, et al. Development of a multimarker assay for early detection of ovarian cancer. J Clin Oncol 2010;28(13):2159–66.

19. Zhang B, Cai FF, Zhong XY. An overview of biomarkers for the ovarian cancer diagnosis. Eur J Obstet Gynecol Reprod Biol 2011;158(2):119–23.

20. Rojas V, Hirshfield KM, Ganesan S, et al. Molecular characterization of epithelial ovarian cancer: implications for diagnosis and treatment. Int J Mol Sci 2016;17(12) [pii:E2113].

21. Kobayashi H, Yamada Y, Sado T, et al. A randomized study of screening for ovarian cancer: a multicenter study in Japan. Int J Gynecol Cancer 2008;18(3): 414–20.

22. Buys SS, Partridge E, Black A, et al. Effect of screening on ovarian cancer mortality: the prostate, lung, colorectal and ovarian (PLCO) cancer screening randomized controlled trial. JAMA 2011; 305(22):2295–303.

23. Jacobs IJ, Menon U, Ryan A, et al. Ovarian cancer screening and mortality in the UK Collaborative Trial of Ovarian Cancer Screening (UKCTOCS): a randomised controlled trial. Lancet 2016;387(10022): 945–56.

24. Rebbeck TR, Kauff ND, Domchek SM. Meta-analysis of risk reduction estimates associated with risk-reducing salpingo-oophorectomy in BRCA1 or BRCA2 mutation carriers. J Natl Cancer Inst 2009; 101(2):80–7.

25. Rosenthal AN, Fraser L, Manchanda R, et al. Results of annual screening in phase I of the United Kingdom familial ovarian cancer screening study highlight the need for strict adherence to screening schedule. J Clin Oncol 2013;31(1):49–57.

26. Lai T, Kessel B, Ahn HJ, et al. Ovarian cancer screening in menopausal females with a family history of breast or ovarian cancer. J Gynecol Oncol 2016;27(4):e41.

27. Moyer VA, U.S. Preventive Services Task Force. Screening for ovarian cancer: U.S. preventive services task force reaffirmation recommendation statement. Ann Intern Med 2012;157(12):900–4.

28. Schorge JO, Modesitt SC, Coleman RL, et al. SGO White paper on ovarian cancer: etiology, screening and surveillance. Gynecol Oncol 2010;119(1):7–17.

29. American College of Obstetricians and Gynecologists Committee on Gynecologic Practice. Committee Opinion No. 477: the role of the obstetrician-gynecologist in the early detection of epithelial ovarian cancer. Obstet Gynecol 2011;117:742–6.

30. American Cancer Society. Ovarian cancer: early detection, diagnosis, and staging. Available at: https://www.cancer.org/content/dam/CRC/PDF/Public/ 8775.00.pdf. Accessed May 4, 2017.

31. Gladstone CQ. Screening for ovarian cancer. In: Goldbloom RB, editor. The Canadian task force on the periodic health examination. The Canadian guide to clinical preventive health care. Ottawa (Canada): Canada Communication Group; 1994. p. 870–81.

32. National Comprehensive Cancer Network. Genetic/ familial high-risk assessment: breast and ovarian. NCCN. Version 2.2017-December 7, 2016. Available at: https://www.nccn.org/professionals/physician_ gls/pdf/genetics_screening.pdf. Accessed May 4, 2017.

33. Sohaib SA, Mills TD, Sahdev A, et al. The role of magnetic resonance imaging and ultrasound in patients with adnexal masses. Clin Radiol 2005;60(3): 340–8.

Imaging and Screening of Thyroid Cancer

Qian Li, MD[a], Xueying Lin, MD[b], Yuhong Shao, MD[c], Feixiang Xiang, MD[d],
Anthony E. Samir, MD, MPH[a,*]

KEYWORDS

- Thyroid cancer • Ultrasonography • Screening • Overdiagnosis

KEY POINTS

- Ultrasound (US) is the first-line diagnostic tool for the diagnosis of thyroid diseases, especially for the differentiation of benign and malignant nodules.
- The relatively low aggressiveness of many thyroid cancers, however, coupled with the high sensitivity of sonography for focal thyroid lesions, can lead to cancer diagnosis and treatment with no effect on outcomes.
- The widespread use of US is recognized as the most important driver of thyroid cancer overdiagnosis.
- To avoid excessive diagnosis and overtreatment, US should not be used as a general community screening tool and should be reserved for patients at high risk of thyroid cancer and in the diagnostic management of incidentally discovered thyroid nodules.
- With integration of prescreening risk stratification and the rigorous application of consensus criteria for nodule biopsy, the value of the diagnostic US in thyroid disease evaluation is likely to be maximized.

INTRODUCTION

Thyroid cancer, with an estimated 64,300 new cases and 1980 deaths in 2016, is the most common endocrine malignancy in the United States.[1] According to the National Institutes of Health Surveillance, Epidemiology, and End Results database, in the past 20 years, thyroid cancer incidence has increased significantly in the United States. Canada, Australia, and Western Europe, and some Asian countries have seen a similar increase in incidence.[2,3] For example, thyroid cancer has become the most common cancer in South Korea, where the 2011 thyroid cancer diagnosis rate was 15 times higher than in 1993.[4]

Despite the rapid increase in diagnosis (>5% per year in both men and women), thyroid cancer death rates only increased slightly from 0.43 (per 100,000 population) in 2003 to 0.51 in 2012.[1] More than 40,000 people in South Korea were diagnosed with thyroid cancer in 2011, but only 400 died of thyroid cancer, a similar mortality to that seen in the prior decade.[4] Increased diagnosis without a corresponding change in mortality is suggestive of overdiagnosis. Several population-

Disclosure Statement: All authors listed have contributed sufficiently to the project to be included as authors. To the best of our knowledge, no conflict of interest, financial or other, exists.
[a] Department of Radiology, Massachusetts General Hospital, Harvard Medical School, White 270, 55 Fruit Street, Boston, MA 02114, USA; [b] Department of Ultrasound, Fujian Medical University Union Hospital, 29 Xinquan Road, Gulou District, Fuzhou, Fujian 350001, China; [c] Department of Ultrasound, Peking University First Hospital, 8 Xishiku Street, Xicheng District, Beijing 100034, China; [d] Department of Ultrasound, Union Hospital, Tongji Medical College, Huazhong University of Science and Technology, 1277 Jiefang Road, Jianghan District, Wuhan 430022, China
* Corresponding author. Abdominal Imaging and Intervention, Massachusetts General Hospital, Harvard Medical School, White 270, 55 Fruit Street, Boston, MA 02114.
E-mail address: ASAMIR@mgh.harvard.edu

Radiol Clin N Am 55 (2017) 1261–1271
http://dx.doi.org/10.1016/j.rcl.2017.06.002
0033-8389/17/© 2017 Elsevier Inc. All rights reserved.

based studies ascribe this to increasing utilization of sonography, fine-needle aspiration (FNA), and an increase in thyroid nodules found on nonthyroid imaging studies.[5,6] In some countries, thyroid ultrasound (US) is used as a screening tool as part of routine health maintenance.[4] This has led to an epidemic of overdiagnosed thyroid cancer,[7] in which a large number of clinically occult thyroid nodules, which are most papillary thyroid carcinomas (PTCs), are detected and aspirated.[8] Overdiagnosis leads to overtreatment: it is estimated in excess of 90% of thyroid cancer patients have their thyroid glands surgically removed,[4,9] even though the evidence that thyroidectomy alters outcomes in these patients is lacking. In addition to the surgical risks of overtreatment, overdiagnosis of low-risk cancers also leads to psychological morbidity and increases health care costs.[10] For these reasons, the role of thyroid US in thyroid cancer screening is limited.

NORMAL ANATOMY AND IMAGING TECHNIQUES OF THYROID CANCER
Normal Anatomy

The thyroid is a shield-shaped endocrine gland. It locates anteriorly in the neck, composed of left and right lobes, connected by a median isthmus. The weight of thyroid is approximately 25 g in adults, with lobar dimensions approximately 5 cm (length) × 3 cm (transverse) × 2 cm (anteroposterior). The isthmus varies from 0.6 cm to 1 cm sonographically. The thyroid hormones secreted by thyroid gland regulate the metabolic rate, protein synthesis, and other aspects, such as development.[11]

Ultrasound Imaging

US can image thyroid structures, internal/surrounding blood flow, and adjacent tissues. It has been widely applied for nodule detection, characterization, risk stratification, treatment monitoring, and post-thyroidectomy cancer surveillance. Compared with other imaging modalities, US has high spatial resolution, uses no ionizing radiation, and is low in cost. For these reasons, US is the first-line imaging tool for evaluation of the thyroid. Despite a lack of evidence for screening efficacy, and the significant harm potential associated with overdiagnosis, US is in common use in some countries as a screening tool for thyroid cancer.

IMAGING PROTOCOLS

Thyroid sonography is not recommended as a screening tool in asymptomatic patients. As a result, there is no published screening imaging or

screening work-up protocol. In the absence of evidence, several expert societies have issued recommendations regarding the interpretation of thyroid sonography. Two of the most commonly used systems have been published by the American Thyroid Association (ATA) and Society of Radiologists in Ultrasound (SRU). The ATA guidelines recommend FNA in specific circumstances, including (1) nodule greater than or equal to 1 cm in greatest dimension with a high suspicion sonographic pattern; (2) nodule greater than or equal to 1 cm in greatest dimension with an intermediate suspicion sonographic pattern; (3) nodule greater than or equal to 1.5 cm in greatest dimension with low suspicion sonographic pattern; and (4) nodules greater than or equal to 2 cm in greatest dimension with very low suspicion sonographic pattern (eg, spongiform). Observation without FNA is an option for nodules that do not meet these criteria.[12] The SRU guidelines are also widely used and are somewhat simpler than those published by the ATA. In the SRU criteria, FNA is recommended in: (1) a nodule ≥ 1.0 cm in largest diameter if microcalcifications are present, (2) a nodule ≥ 1.5 cm in largest diameter with any of the following signs: solid or almost entirely solid, or coarse calcifications within the nodule, (3) a nodule ≥ 2.0 cm in largest diameter and mixed solid and cystic, or almost entirely cystic with a solid mural component; or (4) the nodule has shown substantial growth since prior US examination.[13]

IMAGING FINDINGS/PATHOLOGY

On FNA, most thyroid nodules can be divided into benign (colloid) nodules, follicular lesions, and malignant nodules.[14] The role of thyroid sonography is to diagnose, localize, and risk-stratify nodules for potential biopsy. Risk stratification is accomplished through assessment of nodule size and sonographic features. Multiple sonographic characteristics have been proposed to identify malignant nodules (**Table 1**). A system that integrates these signs, the Thyroid Imaging Reporting and Data System (TIRADS) system, has been proposed, and the US patterns, definitions, and corresponding malignancy risks (TIRADS scores) are shown in **Table 1**.[15] The characteristic sonographic features of thyroid nodule malignancy have largely been derived from series of the most common thyroid malignancy, PTC. These sonographic findings are less common in other thyroid cancers, such as follicular variant of PTC and medullary and ATCs. The typical US features in these less common thyroid neoplasm are summarized (**Table 2**),[16] and some characteristic US features of malignant thyroid cancers are depicted (**Fig. 1**).

Table 1
Ten ultrasound patterns, their definitions, and corresponding Thyroid Imaging Reporting and Data System category

	Ultrasound Pattern	Definition	Thyroid Imaging Reporting and Data System Category
Benign and probably benign patterns			
1	Colloid type 1	Oval cyst with hyperechoic spot	2
2	Colloid type 2	Mixed oval spongiform isoechoic, vascularized nodule, nonexpansive, noncapsulated, with hyperechoic spots	2
3	Colloid type 3	Mixed hyperplastic expansive nodule, deforms the gland, with imprecise margins, absent capsule (or incomplete halo), with or without hyperechoic spots, solid isoechoic portion vascularized on color Doppler.	3
4	Hashimoto pseudonodule	Gland with US signs of Hashimoto thyroiditis (lobulated surface, decreased echogenicity	2
		Hypervascularized parenchyma with heterogeneous structure, and oval perithyroid lymph nodes). Benign condition (TIRADS 2)	3
		Hyperechoic pseudonodules: frequently multiple, partially surrounded by a halo, poorly vascularized, no calcifications, always benign	2
		Hypoechoic pseudonodules that for any reason (size, shape) appear different from the other hypoechoic thyroiditis focus dispersed within the parenchyma	3
Indeterminate/suspicious patterns			
5	De Quervain pattern	Hypoechoic unifocal lesion with ill-defined borders, without calcifications, vascularization variable (scarce in the initial phase due to edema, hypervascularized in the regeneration stage and avascular in the scarring stage; multifocal lesions in inflammatory clinical context are considered benign (TIRADS 2)	4A

(continued on next page)

Table 1
(continued)

	Ultrasound Pattern	Definition	Thyroid Imaging Reporting and Data System Category
6	Simple neoplastic pattern	Solid or mixed isoechoic nodules, always with a complete fine hypoechoic halo, vascularized (vessels on the periphery and intranodular branches)	4A
7	Suspicious neoplastic pattern	Solid or mixed, encapsulated, iso-, hypo-, or hyperechoic nodule with 1 or more of the following characteristics: thick capsule, irregular thickness of the capsule microcalcifications, or coarse calcifications • Hypervascularization — too homogeneous solid structure • Hypo- and hyperechoic areas within the same nodule (mosaic aspect)	4B
Malignant patterns			
8	Malignant type A	Solid hypoechoic nodule, well-circumscribed margins, irregular shape, or taller than wider.[17]	4B
		The presence of micro- and/or coarse calcifications and penetrating vessels increase suspicion.	4C
9	Malignant type B	Solid iso/hypoechoic nodule, ill-defined margins, no capsule, always with microcalcifications mainly on the periphery, hypervascularized on color Doppler variant: multiple microcalcifications (psammomas) dispersed in the parenchyma, without identifiable nodule	5
10	Malignant type C	Mixed or solid isoechoic nodule, nonencapsulated, vascularized with micro- or macrocalcifications (without hyperechoic spots)	4C

From Horvath E, Silva CF, Majlis S, et al. Prospective validation of the ultrasound based TIRADS (Thyroid Imaging Reporting And Data System) classification: results in surgically resected thyroid nodules. Eur Radiol 2016;27(6):2619–28.

DIAGNOSTIC CRITERIA

The TIRADS uses multiple sonographic features to risk-stratify thyroid nodules (**Table 3**).[15,18,19] This system has demonstrated good correlation with cytologic findings and good diagnostic performance for malignancy with sensitivity 88% and specificity of 49%.[16] TIRADS is limited, however, by complexity and the inherently subjective nature of the sonographic features evaluated.

Table 2
Ultrasound features in less common thyroid neoplasms

Thyroid Neoplasms	Sonographic Findings
The follicular variant of PTC	An oval shape, well-defined and regular margins, and an absence of microcalcifications, usually larger than the classic PTC
The tall cell variant of PTC	Deeply hypoechoic nodules with lobulated margins and microcalcifications. Extrathyroidal extension and lymph node metastases may also be evident at US examination.
The diffuse sclerosing variant of PTC	The gland may appear enlarged and diffusely hypoechoic, as in Hashimoto thyroiditis. Multiple fine and scattered hyperechoic microcalcifications may confer a starry night appearance to wide portions of the thyroid.
FTC	Hypoechogenicity is seen only in a minority (30%–35%) of FTCs, whereas a hypoechoic halo is reported in up to 87% of FTCs. Microcalcifications are rare in FTC; whereas macrocalcifications may be observed in 15%–20% of cases. Most FTCs are solid tumors, but a partially cystic component is more frequent (up to 18%) than in PTC (approximately 4%–6%). These characteristics are shared by both benign and malignant follicular lesions, but the presence of hypoechogenicity, the irregular thickness of the peripheral halo, and the large size are suggestive of an FTC
MTC	Solid content, oval-to-round shape, marked hypoechogenicity, and coarse calcifications were common features

Abbreviation: FTC, follicular and Hürthle cell tumor.
　Data from Gharib H, Papini E, Garber JR, et al. American Association of Clinical Endocrinologists, American College of Endocrinology, and Associazione Medici Endocrinologi Medical Guidelines for Clinical Practice for the Diagnosis and Management of Thyroid Nodules – 2016 Update. Endocrine Practice 2016;22(Suppl 1):1–60.

may be an effective tool in thyroid referral centers.[20] TIRADS may reduce the number of fine-needle aspiration biopsies (FNAB) but is designed as a diagnostic technique, other than to replace FNAB.[19,21]

Another simplified 3-class sonographic rating system for thyroid cancer risk is also commonly used (**Table 4**).[16] The diagnostic performance of these sonographic features for thyroid cancer is reduced by low sensitivity. In most thyroid nodules, sonographic signs are not clearly predictive of a malignant lesion, whereas the absence of suspicious characters is not diagnostic of benignity.[22] Although individual features have limited predictive power, the coexistence of 2 or more suspicious sonographic characters showed increase risk of thyroid cancer.[18,22,23]

Additionally, evaluation systems should not be applied in isolation and should always consider the available technical resources, clinical scenario, and patient preferences.

DIFFERENTIAL DIAGNOSIS

Thyroid nodules are found in approximately one-third of the adult population on US examination,

but less than 10% of these nodules are malignant.[22] US is commonly used to risk-stratify nodules based on the presence or absence of typical benign or malignant features. Usually, nodules with benign appearances are followed-up, and nodules with high-risk features undergo FNA.[16] Typical benign features on US include isoechoic spongiform appearance, defined as the presence of microcystic spaces occupying greater than 50% of the nodule, simple cysts with thin regular margins, predominantly cystic nodules that contain colloid (defined as a hyperechoic focus with a comet-tail sign), and regular eggshell calcification around the periphery of a nodule.[16] Sonographic features associated with malignancy are listed in **Table 1**.[15]

PEARLS, PITFALLS, AND VARIANTS
The Value of Ultrasound in Screening

It is estimated at least one-third of adults harbor small PTCs, and most of these remain occult throughout their lifetimes.[24] Routine screening of a population of individuals at low risk for thyroid cancer therefore seems unlikely to be cost-effective in the absence of technology to

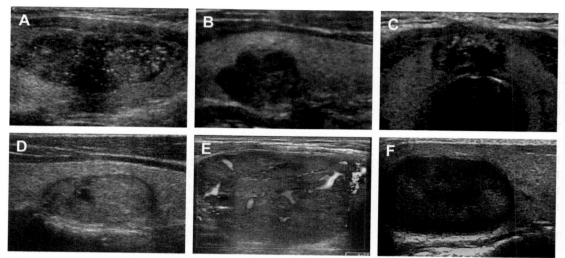

Fig. 1. US features of thyroid cancers. (A) PTC: solid, hypoechoic, heterogeneous nodules with ill-defined margins, microcalcifications; (B) PTC: solid hypoechoic, irregular nodules, without calcifications; (C) PTC: solid hypoechoic (relative to strap muscles anterior to the thyroid) nodule, with irregular calcifications and posterior shadowing; (D) the follicular variant of PTC: oval, well-defined, with a regular margin, no microcalcifications, usually larger than the classic PTC; (E) follicular and Hürthle cell tumors: solid, large size, hypoechogenicity, irregular peripheral halo, central vascularity, without microcalcifications; and (F) MTC: oval-to-round shape, solid, and markedly hypoechoic.

determine which of these malignancies poses a risk to long-term health outcomes. US is, therefore, primarily useful in higher-risk populations, in thyroid cancers with aggressive pathology, and in the diagnosis and management of incidentally discovered thyroid nodules.

Screening for patients with high risk of thyroid cancer

1. Radiation exposure—the thyroid gland is radiation sensitive, so a history of childhood irradiation, especially before the age of 15, is a risk factor for thyroid cancer development.[25] Potential sources of radiation exposure include medical use of radiation (eg, treatment of childhood malignancies and exposure to iodine 131 due to hypothyroidism), environmental exposure (eg, atomic weapons use in Nagasaki or Hiroshima, Japan), and nuclear power plant accidents.[26,27] The effects of radiation persist for several decades,[26] so regular screening is recommended in irradiated patients. The intensity of surveillance depends on risk factors, including radiation dose and age at exposure.[28,29]

2. Positive family history—the malignancy risk of a nodule increases if there is a history of thyroid cancer in a first-degree relative or a thyroid cancer syndrome family history, such as familial polyposis,[30] Carney complex, multiple endocrine neoplasia type 2, Werner syndrome, or Cowden syndrome.[31] A 10-fold increased thyroid cancer risk has been reported in patients whose first-degree relatives had thyroid cancer.[32] The standardized incidence ratio for papillary cancer was 3.2 with an involved parent, 6.2 with an involved sibling, and 11.2 for a woman with an involved sister.[33]

3. Age—age is a risk factor for thyroid malignancy, and US scanning is suggested for patients less than 14 or greater than 70 years of age who have palpable thyroid nodules, goiter, or cervical lymphadenopathy, due to high risk of the thyroid malignancy.[16]

4. Suspicious clinical signs—a history of rapid nodule growth or new-onset hoarseness and findings of fixation of the nodule to surrounding tissues, vocal cord paralysis, or presence of ipsilateral cervical lymphadenopathy should raise suspicion a nodule may be malignant. Palpable malignant nodules are typically larger than incidentally discovered nodules. This is important, because prognosis is associated with tumor size.[34,35] Small tumors usually have an excellent prognosis, with a low likelihood of recurrence.[24,36] In 1 study, the 20-year cancer-related mortality rates were 6%, 16%, and 50% for patients whose primary tumor diameters were 2 cm to 3.9 cm, 4 cm to 6.9 cm, or 7 cm or larger, respectively.[34] Extrathyroidal tumor invasion increases the risk of death 5-fold[37] and may cause substantial

Table 3
Thyroid Imaging Reporting and Data System categories

Categories	Ultrasound Findings	Cancer Risk (%)	Percent of Cancer on Surgery	Recommendations
TIRADS 1	Normal examination	0	0% (0/116)	Follow-up
TIRADS 2	Benign	0	1.79% (1/56)	Follow-up/FNAB
TIRADS 3	Probably benign	<5	76.13% (185/243)	FNAB
TIRADS 4	Suspicious	5–95	5.88% (1/17)	FNAB
TIRADS 4A	Low suspicion	5–10	62.82% (49/78)	FNAB
TIRADS 4B	Intermediate suspicion	11–65	5.88% (1/17)	FNAB
TIRADS 4C	High suspicion	66–95	91.22% (135/148)	FNAB
TIRADS 5	Suggestive of malignancy	>95	98.85% (86/87)	FNAB
TIRADS 6	FNAB-confirmed malignancy	100	—	—

From Horvath E, Silva CF, Majlis S, et al. Prospective validation of the ultrasound based TIRADS (Thyroid Imaging Reporting And Data System) classification: results in surgically resected thyroid nodules. Eur Radiol 2016;27(6):2619–28.

morbidity if there is involvement of the trachea, esophagus, recurrent laryngeal nerves, or spine. Palpable lymphadenopathy should suggest the possibility of a malignant lesion.

Table 4
Thyroid ultrasound features and risk of malignancy

Risk of Malignancy	Ultrasound Features
Low risk	Thyroid cyst
	Mostly cystic nodule with reverberation artifacts
	Isoechoic spongiform nodule
Intermediate risk	Isoechoic nodule with central vascularity
	Isoechoic nodule with macrocalcifications
	Isoechoic nodule with indeterminate hyperechoic spots
	Isoechoic nodule with elevated stiffness on elastography
High-risk	Marked hypoechogenicity
	Microcalcifications
	Irregular (speculated) margins
	More tall than wide
	Extracapsular growth
	Suspicious regional lymph node

Data from Gharib H, Papini E, Garber JR, et al. American Association of Clinical Endocrinologists, American College of Endocrinology, and Associazione Medici Endocrinologi Medical Guidelines for Clinical Practice for the Diagnosis and Management of Thyroid Nodules – 2016 Update. Endocrine Practice 2016;22(Suppl 1):1–60.

5. Distant metastases of thyroid cancers—2% to 10% of patients with thyroid cancer have metastases beyond the neck at the time of diagnosis, of which two-thirds are pulmonary and one-fourth skeletal. Rarer sites include brain, kidneys, liver, and adrenal glands. If thyroid cancer metastases are found, neck sonography is indicated.[38,39]

6. Other potential risk factors—other possible (but not proved) risk factors have been reported. Their relative importance seems small but incompletely defined.
   - Occupational and environmental exposures[40]
   - Hepatitis C virus chronic hepatitis[41]
   - Increased parity and late age at first pregnancy[42]
   - Graves disease in patients of 45 years of age or older: these patients are more likely to harbor locally advanced thyroid cancers than younger patients[43]

Thyroid cancers with aggressive pathology
Differentiated thyroid cancer (papillary and follicular cancers) has a good prognosis, especially if no regional metastases are found.[24] Medullary thyroid cancer (MTC), thyroid lymphoma, and anaplastic thyroid cancer (ATC) may show rapid progression and poor treatment outcomes.[44,45]

1. MTC: calcitonin is a specific diagnostic and prognostic marker for MTC and can be detected in both tumor specimens and serum.[45] Most MTCs are sporadic, but some are inherited from mutations of the RET proto-oncogene, which constitutes familial presentations.[31] So the calcitonin and familial history

may be the indicators of the US thyroid scanning.[46]

2. Thyroid lymphoma: Hashimoto thyroiditis has been reported its association with thyroid lymphoma, in which the risk of lymphoma is 60 times higher than in patients without thyroiditis.[47] US may be helpful in patients with Hashimoto thyroiditis to follow-up the potential lymphoma.

3. ATC: the value of sonography for ATC screening is unclear. Although approximately 20% of ATC patients have a history of differentiated thyroid cancer, and 20% to 30% have a coexisting differentiated cancer,[48,49] it is not clear that screening sonography reduces the incidence of ATC.

Management of incidentally discovered thyroid nodules

The incidental thyroid nodule is defined as a nodule identified by an imaging study but not previously detected.[50] Most are small and detected during other procedures for nonthyroid indications, such as carotid US, head-neck CT, or neck MR imaging. In a review of 97,908 imaging studies, it was reported that the prevalence of the thyroid incidentalomas was approximately 0.4%.[51] It has been reported that most incidental thyroid nodules are benign, and those patients diagnosed as malignant often exhibit indolent behavior. Therefore, incidentally discovered thyroid nodules contribute to the increasing incidence of thyroid cancer, and are likely to be an outsize contributor to needless overtreatment.

A system to guide evaluation of thyroid incidental nodules on CT, MR imaging, or fludeoxyglucose F 18–PET has been proposed.[52] In this system, the following nodules are recommended for further evaluation: (1) nodules with high-risk imaging features (suspicious lymph nodes, local invasion, and PET-avid nodule); (2) nodules greater than or equal to 1 cm in patients age less than 35 years; and (3) nodules greater than or equal to 1.5 cm in patients age greater than or equal to 35 years.[53]

Pitfalls of Ultrasound in Thyroid Cancer Screening

Current practice

At present, ultrasonography is considered useful in the following situations:

- To detect thyroid nodules
- To risk-stratify nodules for FNA
- To assist in FNA of thyroid nodules and cervical lymph nodes
- To monitor thyroid nodules

- To assist in thyroid cancer surgery planning
- To assist in thyroid cancer recurrence surveillance
- To screen high-risk groups for thyroid nodules (eg, childhood radiation exposure)

Because US has shown reasonably good diagnostic performance for nodule detection and risk stratification, with reported malignancy sensitivity of 80% to 86% and specificity of 84.6% to 95%,[23,50] current thyroid guideline recommendations still call for US in all patients with clinically suspected thyroid nodules.[12]

In some countries, US is used as a screening tool for thyroid cancer[3] and has become a key factor in driving thyroid malignancy diagnosis in asymptomatic patients.[12] In the past 3 decades, the prevalence of thyroid cancer has increased dramatically in many developed countries.[54] In the United States, the increasing incidence, indicated by the annual percent change, was 2.4% from 1980 to 1997% and 6.6% from 1997 to 2009 (including both genders).[54] The largest increase has been observed in South Korea: the incidence among people between 15 years and 79 years of age (standardized to the world population) increased from 12.2 cases per 100,000 persons in 1993 to 1997 to 59.9 cases per 100,000 persons in 2003 to 2007.[55]

Despite increasing diagnosis, thyroid cancer–related mortality rates have not changed substantially.[53] The literature strongly suggests US screening was the most important driver of overdiagnosis of thyroid cancer,[56,57] with increased diagnosis of subclinical and rarely lethal PTC,[54,56,58] especially microcarcinomas (<1 cm).[3]

The influence of overdiagnosis on clinical practice

Overdiagnosis exposes patients to harms of treatment, without expected benefit. A majority of patients who receive the diagnosis of thyroid cancer underwent thyroidectomy.[55] This procedure, although well-tolerated by most patients, causes voice problems or low calcium levels in approximately 1% to 10%. Additionally, postsurgery thyroid hormone replacement therapy has to be applied for the rest of the patients' lives.[56] A high percentage also receive other potentially harmful treatments, such as neck lymph-node dissection and radiotherapy.[55] Moreover, patients have to live with a diagnosis of cancer for the rest of their lives, which can create psychological morbidity.[59] Overdiagnosis of thyroid cancer may be costly over a patient's lifetime, depending on the complexity of intervention and follow-up.[54]

Methods of reducing the harms of overdiagnosis

The recognition that many well-differentiated thyroid nodules are indolent has led to a variety of approaches to reduce treatment-related harm. Some indolent thyroid tumors previously classified as noninvasive encapsulated papillary thyroid carcinoma (EFVPTC) were recently reclassified as noninvasive follicular thyroid neoplasm with papillary-like nuclear features. This reclassification to benignity will affect more than 45,000 patients worldwide each year and significantly reduce patients' psychological burden, medical expenses, and clinical consequences associated with a cancer diagnosis.[59] The updated 2015 ATA Management Guidelines for Patients with Thyroid Nodules and Differentiated Thyroid Cancer similarly attempts to reduce the number of microcarcinomas diagnosed. For example, cytologic examination is not recommended for nodules less than 1.0 cm in the absence of additional risk factors.[12]

SUGGESTIONS FOR REFERRING PHYSICIANS

Referring physicians should understand the value of US for thyroid nodule detection and risk stratification but should also appreciate the sonography has limitations and that many lesions diagnosed as cancer are indolent.

1. US screening of the thyroid in asymptomatic patients should not be used in patients at low risk of aggressive thyroid cancer. It is only potentially indicated in patients at high risk of developing thyroid cancers, in thyroid cancer with aggressive pathology, and for the management of incidentally discovered thyroid nodules.
2. Thyroid nodules should be referred for FNA according to consensus guidelines, of which the ATA[12] and SRU guidelines[13] are useful examples. When making management recommendations, radiologists should report which classification system was used.
3. An active surveillance approach can be considered in selected patients under appropriate specialist care. Recommended criteria include the absence of clinical lymph node metastases, absence of US signs of extrathyroid extension, and location of the nodule distant from the recurrent laryngeal nerve or trachea.[3]

SUMMARY

US is the first-line imaging tool to evaluate thyroid disease. Evidence-based sonographic practice requires a clear understanding of the potential harms of overdiagnosis and overtreatment. With careful clinical risk stratification prior to sonography and the rigorous application of diagnostic criteria and consensus interpretative guidelines, the value of diagnostic US for thyroid disease evaluation can be maximized and the harms of overdiagnosis minimized.

ACKNOWLEDGMENTS

The authors thank Jian Wu and Min Wu for article editing.

REFERENCES

1. Siegel RL, Miller KD, Jemal A. Cancer statistics, 2016. CA Cancer J Clin 2016;66(1):7–30.
2. Ibitoye R, Wilkins A. Thyroid papillary carcinoma after alemtuzumab therapy for MS. J Neurol 2014; 261(9):1828–9.
3. Leboulleux S, Tuttle RM, Pacini F, et al. Papillary thyroid microcarcinoma: time to shift from surgery to active surveillance? Lancet Diabetes Endocrinol 2016;4(11):933–42.
4. Ahn HS, Kim HJ, Welch HG. Korea's thyroid-cancer 'Epidemic' — screening and overdiagnosis. N Engl J Med 2014;371(19):1765–7.
5. Medici M, Liu X, Kwong N, et al. Long- versus short-interval follow-up of cytologically benign thyroid nodules: a prospective cohort study. BMC Med 2016;14(1):1420.
6. Zhang Y, Huang H, Sandler J, et al. Response to the commentary letter entitled "Diagnostic radiography and thyroid cancer – causation or simply an association?" to our article entitled 'Diagnostic radiography exposure increases the risk for thyroid microcarcinoma. Eur J Cancer Prev 2016;25(6):572–3.
7. Brito JP, Kim HJ, Han SJ, et al. Geographic distribution and evolution of thyroid cancer epidemic in South Korea. Thyroid 2016;26(6):864–5.
8. Gao S-Y, Zhang X-Y, Wei W, et al. Identification of benign and malignant thyroid nodules by in vivo iodine concentration measurement using single-source dual energy CT. Medicine (Baltimore) 2016; 95(39):e4816.
9. Cho BY, Choi HS, Park YJ, et al. Changes in the clinicopathological characteristics and outcomes of thyroid cancer in Korea over the past four decades. Thyroid 2013;23(7):797–804.
10. Davies L, Ouellette M, Hunter M, et al. The increasing incidence of small thyroid cancers: where are the cases coming from? Laryngoscope 2010;120(12):2446–51.
11. Loevner LAL, Kaplan SLS, Cunnane MEM, et al. Cross-sectional imaging of the thyroid gland. Neuroimaging Clin N Am 2008;18(3):445–61, vii.
12. Haugen BR, Alexander EK, Bible KC, et al. 2015 American Thyroid Association Management Guidelines for Adult Patients with Thyroid Nodules and

Differentiated Thyroid Cancer: The American Thyroid Association Guidelines Task Force on Thyroid Nodules and Differentiated Thyroid Cancer. Thyroid 2016;26(1):1–133.

13. Frates MCM, Benson CBC, Charboneau JWJ, et al. Management of thyroid nodules detected at US: Society of Radiologists in Ultrasound consensus conference statement. Radiology 2005;237:794–800.

14. Nam-Goong IS, Kim HY, Gong G, et al. Ultrasonography-guided fine-needle aspiration of thyroid incidentaloma: correlation with pathological findings. Clin Endocrinol (Oxf) 2004;60(1):21–8.

15. Horvath E, Silva CF, Majlis S, et al. Prospective validation of the ultrasound based TIRADS (Thyroid Imaging Reporting And Data System) classification: results in surgically resected thyroid nodules. Eur Radiol 2016;27:2619–28.

16. Gharib H, Papini E, Garber JR, et al. American Association of Clinical Endocrinologists, American College of Endocrinology, and Associazione Medici Endocrinologi Medical Guidelines for Clinical Practice for the Diagnosis and Management of Thyroid Nodules – 2016 Update. Endocr Pract 2016;22(5): 622–39.

17. Tessler FN, Middleton WD, Grant EG, et al. ACR thyroid imaging, reporting and data system (TI-RADS): white paper of the ACR TI-RADS committee. J Am Coll Radiol 2017;14(5):587–95.

18. Horvath E, Majlis S, Rossi R, et al. An ultrasonogram reporting system for thyroid nodules stratifying cancer risk for clinical management. J Clin Endocrinol Metab 2009;94(5):1748–51.

19. Grant EG, Tessler FN, Hoang JK, et al. Thyroid ultrasound reporting lexicon: white paper of the ACR Thyroid Imaging, Reporting and Data System (TI-RADS) Committee. J Am Coll Radiol 2015;12(12): 1272–9.

20. Russ G, Bigorgne C, Royer B, et al. Le système TI-RADS en échographie thyroïdienne. J Radiol 2011; 92(7–8):701–13.

21. Friedrich-Rust M, Meyer G, Dauth N, et al. Interobserver agreement of Thyroid Imaging Reporting and Data System (TIRADS) and strain elastography for the assessment of thyroid nodules. PLoS One 2013;8(10):e77927. Hendrikse J, ed.

22. Papini E, Guglielmi R, Bianchini A, et al. Risk of malignancy in nonpalpable thyroid nodules: predictive value of ultrasound and Color-Doppler features. J Clin Endocrinol Metab 2002;87(5):1941–6.

23. Moon W-J, Jung SL, Lee JH, et al. Benign and malignant thyroid nodules: us differentiation—multicenter retrospective study. Radiology 2008;247(3): 762–70.

24. Harach HR, Franssila KO, Wasenius VM. Occult papillary carcinoma of the thyroid. A "normal" finding in finland. A systematic autopsy study. Cancer 1985;56(3):531–8.

25. Vaccarella S, Franceschi S, Bray F, et al. Worldwide thyroid-cancer epidemic? the increasing impact of overdiagnosis. N Engl J Med 2016; 375(7):614–7.

26. Furukawa K, Preston D, Funamoto S, et al. Long-term trend of thyroid cancer risk among Japanese atomic-bomb survivors: 60 years after exposure. Int J Cancer 2013;132(5):1222–6.

27. Suzuki S. Childhood and adolescent thyroid cancer in Fukushima after the Fukushima Daiichi nuclear power plant accident: 5 years on. Clin Oncol (R Coll Radiol) 2016;28(4):263–71.

28. Zablotska LB, Ron E, Rozhko AV, et al. Thyroid cancer risk in Belarus among children and adolescents exposed to radioiodine after the Chornobyl accident. Br J Cancer 2011;104(1):181–7.

29. Taylor AJ, Croft AP, Palace AM, et al. Risk of thyroid cancer in survivors of childhood cancer: results from the British Childhood Cancer Survivor Study. Int J Cancer 2009;125(10):2400–5.

30. Herraiz M, Barbesino G, Faquin W, et al. Prevalence of thyroid cancer in familial adenomatous polyposis syndrome and the role of screening ultrasound examinations. Clin Gastroenterol Hepatol 2007;5(3):367–73.

31. Sadowski SM, He M, Gesuwan K, et al. Prospective screening in familial nonmedullary thyroid cancer. Surgery 2013;154(6):1194–8.

32. Pal T, Vogl FD, Chappuis PO, et al. Increased risk for nonmedullary thyroid cancer in the first degree relatives of prevalent cases of nonmedullary thyroid cancer: a hospital-based study. J Clin Endocrinol Metab 2001;86(11):5307–12.

33. Chen AY, Jemal A, Ward EM. Increasing incidence of differentiated thyroid cancer in the United States, 1988-2005. Cancer 2009;115(16):3801–7.

34. Ganly I, Wang L, Tuttle RM, et al. Invasion rather than nuclear features correlates with outcome in encapsulated follicular tumors: further evidence for the reclassification of the encapsulated papillary thyroid carcinoma follicular variant. Hum Pathol 2015;46(5):657–64.

35. Rivera M, Ricarte-Filho J, Knauf J, et al. Molecular genotyping of papillary thyroid carcinoma follicular variant according to its histological subtypes (encapsulated vs infiltrative) reveals distinct BRAF and RAS mutation patterns. Mod Pathol 2010; 23(9):1191–200.

36. Daniels G. What if many follicular variant papillary thyroid carcinomas are not malignant? A review of follicular variant papillary thyroid carcinoma and a proposal for a new classification. Endocr Pract 2011;17(5):768–87.

37. Ito Y, Kobayashi K, Tomoda C, et al. Ill-defined edge on ultrasonographic examination can be a marker of aggressive characteristic of papillary thyroid microcarcinoma. World J Surg 2005;29(8):1007–11 [discussion: 1011–2].

38. Ghossein R, Livolsi VA. Papillary thyroid carcinoma tall cell variant. Thyroid 2008;18(11):1179–81.

39. Johnson TL, Lloyd RV, Thompson NW, et al. Prognostic implications of the tall cell variant of papillary thyroid carcinoma. Am J Surg Pathol 1988;12(1):22–7.

40. Schneider AB, Sarne DH. Long-term risks for thyroid cancer and other neoplasms after exposure to radiation. Nat Clin Pract Endocrinol Metab 2005;1(2):82–91.

41. Hemminki K, Eng C, Chen B. Familial risks for non-medullary thyroid cancer. J Clin Endocrinol Metab 2005;90(10):5747–53.

42. Nagataki S, Nyström E. Epidemiology and primary prevention of thyroid cancer. Thyroid 2002;12(10): 889–96.

43. Kim WB, Han S-M, Kim TY, et al. Ultrasonographic screening for detection of thyroid cancer in patients with Graves' disease. Clin Endocrinol (Oxf) 2004; 60(6):719–25.

44. Machens A, Dralle H. Biological relevance of medullary thyroid microcarcinoma. J Clin Endocrinol Metab 2012;97(5):1547–53.

45. Kazaure HS, Roman SA, Sosa JA. Medullary thyroid microcarcinoma. Cancer 2011;118(3):620–7.

46. Sippel RS, Caron NR, Clark OH. An evidence-based approach to familial nonmedullary thyroid cancer: screening, clinical management, and follow-up. World J Surg 2007;31(5):924–33.

47. Pedersen RK, Pedersen NT. Primary non-Hodgkin's lymphoma of the thyroid gland: a population based study. Histopathology 1996;28(1):25–32.

48. McIver B, Hay ID, Giuffrida DF, et al. Anaplastic thyroid carcinoma: a 50-year experience at a single institution. Surgery 2001;130(6):1028–34.

49. Tan RK, Finley RK, Driscoll D, et al. Anaplastic carcinoma of the thyroid: a 24-year experience. Head Neck 1995;17(1):41–8.

50. Lee YH, Kim DW, In HS, et al. Differentiation between benign and malignant solid thyroid nodules using an US classification system. Korean J Radiol 2011;12(5):559–67.

51. Uppal A, White MG, Nagar S, et al. Benign and malignant thyroid incidentalomas are rare in routine clinical practice: a review of 97,908 imaging studies. Cancer Epidemiol Biomarkers Prev 2015;24(9): 1327–31.

52. Cooper DSD, Doherty GMG, Haugen BRB, et al. Revised American Thyroid Association management guidelines for patients with thyroid nodules and differentiated thyroid cancer. Thyroid 2009;19(11): 1167–214.

53. La Vecchia C, Malvezzi M, Bosetti C, et al. Thyroid cancer mortality and incidence: a global overview. Int J Cancer 2014;136(9):2187–95.

54. Pellegriti G, Frasca F, Regalbuto C, et al. Worldwide increasing incidence of thyroid cancer: update on epidemiology and risk factors. J Cancer Epidemiol 2013;2013(1):1–10.

55. Regenstein M, Nocella K, Jewers MM, et al. The cost of residency training in teaching health centers. N Engl J Med 2016;375(7):612–4.

56. Ahn HS, Kim HJ, Kim KH, et al. Thyroid cancer screening in South Korea increases detection of papillary cancers with no impact on other subtypes or thyroid cancer mortality. Thyroid 2016;26(11): 1535–40.

57. Mitman G. Ebola in a stew of fear. N Engl J Med 2014;371(19):1763–5.

58. Davies L. Overdiagnosis of thyroid cancer. BMJ 2016;355:i6312.

59. Nikiforov YE, Seethala RR, Tallini G, et al. Nomenclature revision for encapsulated follicular variant of papillary thyroid carcinoma: a paradigm shift to reduce overtreatment of indolent tumors. JAMA Oncol 2016;2:1023–9.

Imaging and Screening of Cancer of the Small Bowel

Jin Sil Kim, MD[a], Seong Ho Park, MD, PhD[a],*, Stephanie Hansel, MD, MS[b], Joel G. Fletcher, MD[c]

KEYWORDS

- Small bowel • Cancer • Screening • Surveillance • CT • MR

KEY POINTS

- Although population-based screening of asymptomatic patients for small bowel cancers is ineffective, targeted screening/surveillance strategies can be used in specific at-risk and symptomatic patient groups.
- Computed tomography (CT) and magnetic resonance (MR) enterography are currently the dominant radiologic techniques to detect small bowel cancers and are used in conjunction with push enteroscopy, capsule endoscopy, and balloon-assisted endoscopy.
- Radiologic screening/surveillance of small bowel adenocarcinoma can be applied to at-risk hereditary conditions as supplementary tools to endoscopy (upper, lower, push, capsule), tailored to the individual patient, and is relatively well established for Peutz-Jeghers syndrome.
- CT and MR enterography are often performed in patients with celiac disease after a gluten-free diet fails to evaluate for refractory celiac and to exclude enteropathy-associated T-cell lymphoma.
- Suspicion of small bowel bleeding in patients at increased risk for small bowel gastrointestinal stromal tumors (GISTs), such as familial GIST and neurofibromatosis type 1, should prompt referral to CT or MR enterography.

INTRODUCTION

Small bowel cancers are very rare despite the length and large mucosal surface of the small bowel and account for 3% to 6% of all gastrointestinal (GI) tract malignancies.[1] Adenocarcinoma, neuroendocrine neoplasms, lymphoma, and GI stromal tumors (GISTs) are the most prevalent primary small bowel cancers, with adenocarcinoma and neuroendocrine neoplasms accounting for nearly two-thirds of small bowel cancers.[1–7] According to the most recent US statistics, small bowel cancer is 24th in terms of incidence with an estimated 10,000 new patients a year.[7] Small bowel cancers are known to have bad prognosis and most patients already have advanced stages of disease at the time of initial diagnosis.[4,8,9] Delayed diagnosis of small bowel cancers is a real concern and is one of the main reasons for the lack of meaningful improvements in the oncologic outcomes of patients with small bowel cancer despite the overall advances in medicine.[4,8,9] Delayed diagnoses of small bowel cancer are associated with various factors,

Disclosure Statement: Nothing to disclose.

[a] Department of Radiology and Research Institute of Radiology, University of Ulsan College of Medicine, Asan Medical Center, 88, Olympic-ro 43-gil, Songpa-gu, Seoul 05505, South Korea; [b] Department of Gastroenterology and Hepatology, Mayo Clinic, 200 First Street, Southwest, Rochester, MN 55905, USA; [c] Department of Radiology, Mayo Clinic, 200 First Street, Southwest, Rochester, MN 55905, USA
* Corresponding author.
E-mail address: parksh.radiology@gmail.com

including the low incidence of the disease, difficult endoscopic access, lack of mucosal mass or abnormality, subtle radiologic features, and low index of clinical suspicion. As small bowel cancers are rare and their causes are largely unknown, routine population-based screening of asymptomatic patients to find precursor lesions or early cancers is ineffective and does not exist. However, targeted screening/surveillance strategies are used in specific at-risk and symptomatic patient populations using a wide variety of radiologic and endoscopic modalities. This article reviews issues regarding early diagnosis of small bowel cancers, with focus on state-of-the-art cross-sectional imaging techniques and their role in diagnosis and staging in the era of capsule endoscopy and balloon-assisted endoscopy, the primary endoscopic methods of small bowel visualization.

POTENTIAL IMAGING TESTS FOR SMALL BOWEL CANCERS

Barium fluoroscopy, including small bowel follow-through and barium enteroclysis, and cross-sectional imaging techniques, including computed tomography (CT) and magnetic resonance (MR) enterography (single or multiphase) and CT and MR enteroclysis, can be used to radiologically diagnose small bowel neoplasms; their performance and acquisition has been extensively described. Of these, CT and MR enterography are currently the dominant techniques. Barium fluoroscopy has a limited role in small bowel surveillance. Compared with barium fluoroscopy, CT and MR also have an advantage of multi-planar imaging with lack of superimposition and ability to evaluate the mesentery. Enteroclysis may cause substantial patient discomfort as it requires small bowel intubation, although it permits improved fluid distention of the bowel compared with per-oral administration of luminal contrast. Scan techniques for CT and MR enterography are well established and described elsewhere.[10–14] Regarding CT enterography, unlike the examination for inflammatory bowel diseases for which a single enteric-phase imaging to limit radiation exposure after an oral administration of neutral enteric contrast is the general standard,[13] CT enterography for small bowel cancers must be adjusted more to the specific individual indications, for example, multiphase (arterial, enteric, portal, or delayed phases) scans for a better characterization of the tumors or in case of suspected small bowel bleeding[10,11]; an omission of enteric contrast in case of overt bleeding for a speedy diagnosis[12]; and use of positive contrast in lieu of neutral contrast, when polyps and mucosal masses are the imaging target, to display filling defects similar to small bowel follow-through. MR enterography scan techniques are more homogeneous across different indications as they consist of similarly comprehensive sets of all potentially useful sequences,[14] which is because, unlike CT, multiple image acquisitions are not worrisome because MR does not incur radiation exposure.

A recent prospective study investigated the accuracy of MR enterography for detecting various small bowel neoplasms and reported fairly high per-patient sensitivity and specificity of 96%,[15] which were comparable with the published results obtained with MR enteroclysis[16,17] and CT enteroclysis[18] in the same clinical setting. There is a paucity of data regarding the direct comparison between CT enterography and MR enterography for the diagnosis of small bowel neoplasms. According to a recent prospective study comparing CT enterography and MR enterography for the detection of small bowel neoplasms, MR enterography demonstrated a higher accuracy compared with CT enterography.[19]

Push enteroscopy or extended upper endoscopy examines the entire duodenum and very proximal jejunum (depth of 80–120 cm).[20] This procedure is limited mainly by the extent of the examination; it is tolerated well by patients and can be performed with a pediatric colonoscope. Capsule endoscopy has been shown to be superior in detecting small bowel lesions in human and animal studies.[21,22] However, if a lesion is known to be in the reach of push enteroscopy, it can be used to obtain tissue.

Capsule endoscopy is a safe and minimally invasive modality for visualizing the entire small bowel. It is typically well tolerated by patients. The limitations of the procedure include diagnostic procedure (no therapeutic ability), potential of missing a lesion, decreased visualization if fluid or bubbles are retained in the lumen, false-positive findings, and capsule retention if stricture or significant inflammation present. Capsule endoscopy is well established as a procedure to assess for the cause of small bowel bleeding and is considered a first-line procedure for suspected small bowel bleeding.[23] There are mixed results for capsule endoscopy in the detection of small bowel tumors. In small retrospective and prospective single-center studies, CT enterography was shown to be superior to capsule endoscopy in the detection of small bowel tumors.[10,24] However, a large multicenter study of more than 1300 patients revealed capsule endoscopy effectively detected small bowel tumors not detected by other imaging studies.[25] Capsule endoscopy can play a complementary role to enterography in the detection of small bowel tumors and is likely better than cross-sectional enterography in identifying many non-neoplastic causes of small bowel bleeding.

Balloon-assisted endoscopy includes both single-balloon enteroscopy and double-balloon enteroscopy; both procedures can be performed in anterograde (oral route) or retrograde (anal route). With the single-balloon enteroscopy antegrade route, the small bowel can be visualized from the duodenum to the proximal jejunum; but with the double-balloon enteroscopy antegrade route, the proximal ileum may be reached. Total enteroscopy is possible but is not frequently achieved in the United States. Balloon-assisted endoscopy has both diagnostic and therapeutic capability; however, both procedures are invasive, time consuming, and require specialized training by a gastroenterologist. Balloon-assisted endoscopy is best used when a capsule endoscopy or imaging study has identified a small bowel tumor and tissue diagnosis (biopsy) is needed or if the tumor can be removed during the procedure so small bowel surgery is avoided.

Somatostatin receptor imaging with gallium 68 1,4,7,10-tetraazacyclododecane-1,4,7,10-tetraacetic acid PET/CT is an emerging molecular imaging technique to diagnose neuroendocrine tumors.[26,27] It has shown high accuracy for diagnosing neuroendocrine tumors in various locations,[27] but its role specifically for screening/surveillance of small bowel neuroendocrine tumors is yet unknown.

A proper selection of tests for a particular patient among the aforementioned various examinations should be tailored by patient preference and prior experience, local expertise and resources, surgical anatomy, and type of lesions suspected. Diagnostic algorithms and principles regarding appropriate use of these tests for screening/surveillance of small bowel tumors have been proposed for some clinical condition; but unified diagnostic algorithms are largely absent, largely owing to the need for a diagnostic approach tailored to patients with altered surgical anatomy, concurrent diseases, contraindications to screening, and different types of small bowel neoplasia. The several existing diagnostic algorithms are explained further later in the respective corresponding subtopics.

TARGETED SCREENING FOR SMALL BOWEL ADENOCARCINOMA
General Characteristics

Small bowel adenocarcinoma occurs slightly more frequently in men than in women, and the average age of diagnosis is about 60 years.[6,8] Most small bowel adenocarcinomas develop in the duodenum, most frequently in the second portion; the rest occur in the jejunum and ileum.[2,5,6,8,28] In patients with Crohn disease, most small bowel adenocarcinomas occur in the ileum because the ileum is the small bowel section that is most commonly involved by Crohn disease.[29–31]

Risk Factors

Some risk factors for small bowel adenocarcinoma are known,[4–6,32] but only approximately 20% of small bowel adenocarcinomas occur in the context of predisposing conditions.[5] Most patients do not have remarkable risk factors, and the causes of small bowel cancers are unknown in most patients.[5,8] The fact that most patients do not have apparent risk factors in addition to the rarity of the disease makes a true screening/surveillance for small bowel adenocarcinoma difficult. Several hereditary conditions, including familial adenomatous polyposis, hereditary nonpolyposis colorectal cancer (also known as Lynch syndrome), Peutz-Jeghers syndrome, MUTYH-associated polyposis, and cystic fibrosis, are well known to be associated with increased risk for small bowel adenocarcinoma. These patients often undergo combined and repeated radiologic and endoscopic screening/surveillance for small bowel adenocarcinoma. Other diseases, such as celiac disease, Crohn disease, and colon cancer, and smoking and alcohol confer an increased risk for small bowel adenocarcinoma; but because the absolute risk is very small, small bowel surveillance is not performed.

Surveillance in Hereditary Conditions at Risk for Adenocarcinoma

Even for the hereditary conditions that increase the risk of small bowel adenocarcinoma, the specifics of the screening/surveillance methods and timing are not firmly established, especially regarding the use of radiologic tests. A recent clinical guideline by the American College of Gastroenterology provides a comprehensive summary on the surveillance for these patients.[33] Although the guideline focuses on the use endoscopy, the principles may be similarly applied to CT and MR enterography. The specific details are beyond the scope of this article, and readers should refer to the guideline[33] for further information.

One disease in which the use of radiological examinations for screening/surveillance of small bowel adenocarcinoma is relatively well-established is Peutz-Jeghers syndrome. Peutz-Jeghers syndrome is an autosomal dominant condition characterized by the development of multiple hamartomatous polyps throughout the GI tract in conjunction with unique mucocutaneous pigmentation. Patients with Peutz-Jeghers syndrome are at high risk for intestinal as well as extraintestinal cancers, most notably gastric, small bowel, colorectal, pancreatic, breast, and uterus and ovary cancers.[34] Small bowel surveillance in Peutz-Jeghers syndrome has 2 purposes: (1) an early detection of small bowel cancer and (2) a detection of sizable polyps, which are prone to cause complications, such as intussusception/obstruction and bleeding, or may harbor a developing cancer. The former is a more important issue in older patients—the mean age at diagnosis for small bowel cancer in Peutz-Jeghers syndrome has been reported to be 37 years,[34] whereas the latter is more relevant to younger patients. There is no universal consensus regarding the frequency of small bowel screening/surveillance and the age of commencement in Peutz-Jeghers syndrome,[35] but several recommendations exist. A multinational European guideline recommends that small bowel screening/surveillance should be performed every 3 years if small bowel polyps are found at the initial examination, from 8 years of age or earlier if patients are symptomatic.[36] Another recommendation by Dutch investigators proposes small bowel screening/surveillance from 10 years of age with 2- to 3-year intervals.[34] This early onset small bowel screening/surveillance in Peutz-Jeghers syndrome focuses more on preventing complications from polyps, especially bowel obstruction and subsequent bowel surgery,[37] rather than early detection of adenocarcinomas.

Both barium follow-through (Fig. 1)[38] and MR enterography (Fig. 2)[39,40] have been shown to be accurate for detecting large (>1.0−1.5 cm) polyps in patients with Peutz-Jeghers syndrome even though they are inferior to capsule endoscopy for detecting smaller polyps. There are not yet remarkable data specific to CT (Fig. 3) or CT enterography, although these are expected to perform similarly to their MR counterparts given the technical similarities between CT and MR. Because polyps and mucosal masses are the imaging target, CT imaging can be performed with positive contrast to display filling defects similar to small bowel follow-through, which permits radiation dose reduction (ie, similar to CT colonography; Fig. 4). As the small bowel screening/surveillance

in Peutz-Jeghers syndrome starts at a fairly young age and is periodically repeated, MR enterography is currently a favored modality at most institutions.[36] Unlike endoscopy or barium follow-through, MR and CT enterography provide an opportunity to examine other abdominopelvic organs, such as the pancreas (Fig. 5), which also has an increased risk of developing cancer in patients with Peutz-Jeghers syndrome. Therefore, cross-sectional imaging could potentially be more beneficial. The imaging findings of adenocarcinomas arising from Peutz-Jeghers syndrome are not unique. Although no specific data on the relationship between polyp size and risk of adenocarcinoma in Peutz-Jeghers syndrome are present,[39] it is conventionally assumed that large polyps may have a greater risk of malignancy. Therefore, endoscopic or surgical removal is generally recommended for asymptomatic lesions greater than 1.0 to 1.5 cm both concerning their propensity for complications as well as the risk of cancer.[34,41]

Imaging Findings of Small Bowel Adenocarcinomas

Small bowel adenocarcinomas can have various morphologies. The most typical appearance of small bowel adenocarcinoma is an annular, constricting mass (apple-core lesion) (Figs. 6 and 7) that causes luminal narrowing that is often associated with upstream bowel dilatation. Even a small encircling adenocarcinoma can cause small bowel obstruction due to prominent intratumoral desmoplasia, and a small obstructing cancer should not

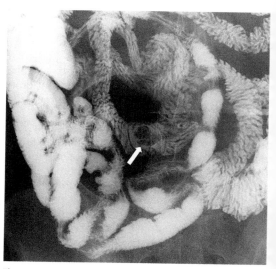

Fig. 1. A 2-cm hamartomatous polyp (*arrow*) in the jejunum seen on small bowel follow-through in a 26-year-old man with Peutz-Jeghers syndrome.

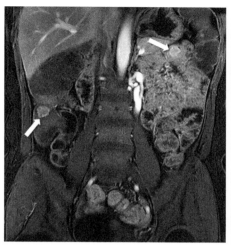
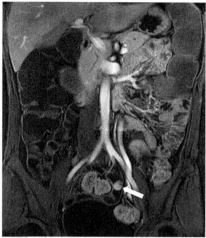

Fig. 2. Multiple hamartomatous polyps up to 2 cm in the jejunum (*upper arrow* in the left), ileum (*arrow* in the right), and ascending colon (*lower arrow* in the left), which are clearly seen on MR enterography (contrast-enhanced T1-weighted image) in a 50-year-old woman with Peutz-Jeghers syndrome.

be neglected. Less frequent morphologies include a rounded or lobulated polypoid mass (**Fig. 8**) or a noncircumferential ulcerative fungating mass (**Fig. 9**). Small bowel adenocarcinomas may reveal only subtle abnormalities at an imaging examination (**Figs. 10** and **11**), making their detection on imaging very challenging. Small bowel adenocarcinomas generally have an abrupt transition to the adjacent normal bowel wall, creating a shoulderlike or overhanging appearance of the tumor edges, which can be seen on both barium follow-through images (see **Fig. 6**)[42,43] and CT/MR images (see **Figs. 7** and **9**) and distinguishes cancers from inflammatory diseases. Compared with barium follow-through, CT and MR have an ability to directly evaluate the tumor extension through the small bowel wall into the adjacent mesentery. After intravenous administration of the contrast agent, the invading tumor appears as a lesion that is replacing the normal stratification of the thickened bowel wall (**Fig. 12**). Adenocarcinomas usually show moderate heterogeneous enhancement (see **Figs. 7, 9,** and **12**),[44] which has been described as progressive and delayed until the venous phase.[45] CT and MR can also show tumor metastasis to the liver, peritoneal space, lymph nodes, and other abdominopelvic organs in addition to revealing the

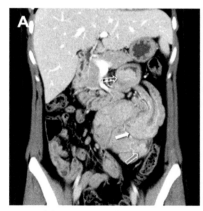
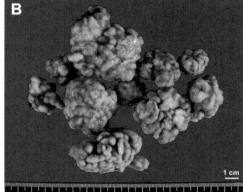

Fig. 3. A 20-year-old woman with Peutz-Jeghers syndrome presented with jejunal intussusception. (*A*) A 5-cm polyp (*solid white arrow*) associated with intussusception and 2 other slightly smaller polyps (*open arrows*) are noted in the jejunum on coronal contrast-enhanced CT. (*B*) Gross specimen image of surgically resected small bowel polyps.

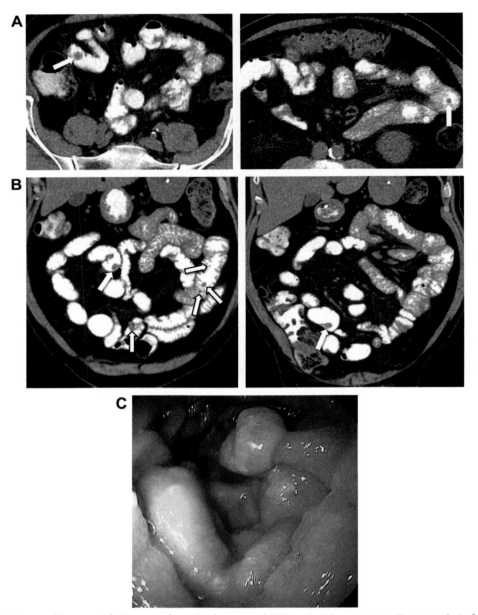

Fig. 4. A 69-year-old man with Peutz-Jeghers syndrome underwent positive-contrast CT enteroclysis for small bowel surveillance. (*A*) Axial low-dose images taken during filling of the small bowel demonstrate ileal and jejunal polyps (*arrows*). (*B*) Coronal images after complete small bowel distention demonstrate additional polyps (*arrows*). (*C*) Subsequent antegrade enteroscopy demonstrated multiple jejunal polyps, which were resected.

transmural extension, which is frequently noted in patients with small bowel adenocarcinomas.[8,9,46]

EXAMINATIONS OF PATIENTS WITH REFRACTORY CELIAC DISEASE
General Characteristics

Celiac disease is a chronic immune-mediated inflammatory enteropathy that affects nearly 1% of the US population and is treated with a gluten-free diet.[47] Patients with potential celiac disease are generally identified after positive serologic testing with tissue transglutaminase antibody.[48,49] Subsequently, definitive diagnosis is made after endoscopy and biopsy, with typical histologic findings of intraepithelial lymphocytes, villous atrophy, and crypt hyperplasia.[50,51] Approximately 10% to 30% of patients with celiac disease will not

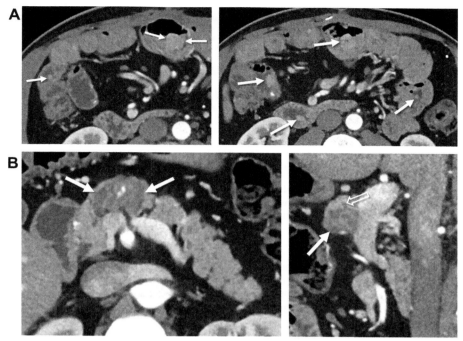

Fig. 5. A 47-year-old man with Peutz-Jeghers underwent contrast-enhanced CT enterography. (*A*) Multiple small bowel polyps of varying sizes were demonstrated (*arrows*). (*B*) Lobulated 3.7-cm cystic mass was found in the neck and body of the pancreas (*solid white arrows*) with enhancing septations and calcifications, with connection to the main pancreatic duct via a side branch duct (*open arrow*). Endoscopic ultrasound biopsy demonstrated adenocarcinoma with mucinous features.

respond immediately to a gluten-free diet for various reasons (called nonresponsive celiac disease), but approximately 1% to 2% of patients with celiac disease will develop refractory celiac disease.[52] Refractory celiac disease is divided into types 1 and 2, with type 2 characterized by clonal T-cell receptor gene rearrangement. Type 2 refractory celiac disease is associated with a poor prognosis and an approximately 50% 5-year survival rate owing to the development of enteropathy-associated T-cell lymphoma and, to a lesser extent, small bowel adenocarcinoma.

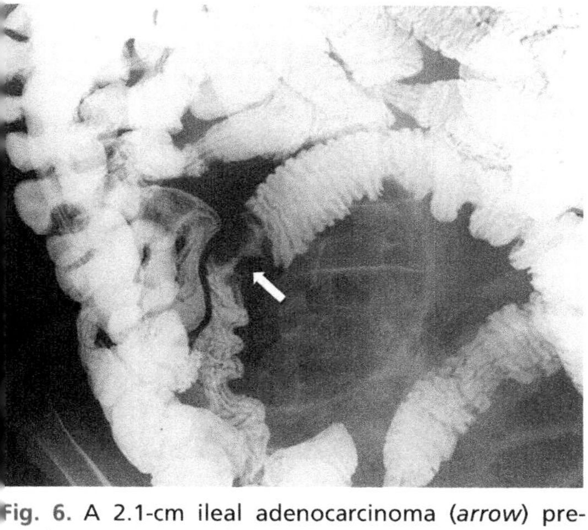

Imaging of Patients with Nonresponsive Celiac Disease

Upper endoscopy with biopsy is performed in patients with celiac after a gluten-free diet fails to alter patients' symptoms to evaluate for refractory celiac disease.[53] Cross-sectional enterography is often performed in practice in conjunction with endoscopy to evaluate for imaging findings of refractory celiac disease or to exclude a rare occurrence of enteropathy-associated T-cell lymphoma. Al-Bawardy and colleagues[54] recently performed a case-control study evaluating CT enterography findings in patients with refractory celiac disease and controls with healed celiac disease. They found that the presence of any of the typical fold pattern abnormalities seen in celiac disease was significantly more common in

Fig. 6. A 2.1-cm ileal adenocarcinoma (*arrow*) presenting as an apple-core lesion on small bowel follow-through in a 59-year-old man.

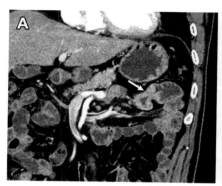
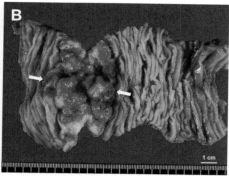

Fig. 7. A 47-year-old man with a jejunal adenocarcinoma presenting as an apple-core lesion. (*A*) A 4.3-cm luminal-encircling mass (*arrow*) is noted in the jejunum on coronal CT enterography. (*B*) Gross specimen image of the resected small intestine showing the luminal encircling tumor (*arrows*).

refractory versus healed celiac disease and that patients with type 2 disease were much more likely to have imaging features of ulcerative jejunitis (fold thickening and hyperenhancement; **Fig. 13**). Findings of a small bowel mass, focal and segmental mural thickening, and mesenteric fat infiltration should raise the concern for a small bowel malignancy in these patients.

Imaging Findings of Enteropathy-Associated T-Cell Lymphoma

The authors have observed enteropathy-associated T-cell lymphomas of the small bowel to have all of the morphologies described with other small bowel lymphomas.[55,56] Small bowel lymphomas are typically larger than adenocarcinomas and demonstrate only mild to moderate enhancement. Morphologically, small bowel lymphomas most often present with segmental bowel wall thickening, which can occur as a single lesion or involving multiple nearby small bowel loops (**Fig. 14**). Segmental small bowel wall thickening with aneurysmal ulceration invariably represents lymphoma. Less frequently, mesenteric adenopathy (sometimes without a clear small bowel mass), diffuse mesenteric fat infiltration, and ascites can be seen.

EXAMINATIONS OF SYMPTOMATIC PATIENTS AT RISK FOR GASTROINTESTINAL STROMAL TUMORS
General Characteristics

A variety of conditions increase the risk of small bowel GISTs. Familial GIST is autosomal dominant and often leads to the development of a single or multiple GISTs in middle age.[57,58] Additionally,

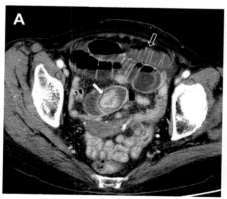
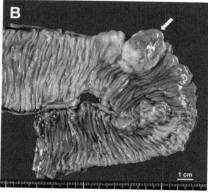

Fig. 8. An 84-year-old woman with a polypoid ileal adenocarcinoma. (*A*) A 3-cm lobulated polypoid mass (*solid white arrow*) is noted in the pelvic ileal loop on contrast-enhanced CT. Proximal small bowel is dilated (*open arrow*) due to intussusception (not shown) caused by the mass. (*B*) Gross specimen image of the resected small intestine showing the polypoid tumor (*arrow*).

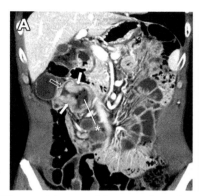
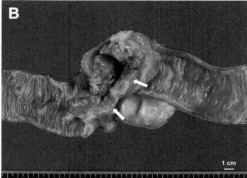

Fig. 9. A 64-year-old man with a noncircumferential ulcerative fungating ileal adenocarcinoma. (A) Coronal contrast-enhanced CT shows a large ulcerative fungating mass (solid white arrows) with a large deep central ulcer (asterisk) in the ileum. Normal appearance of the opposite wall (open arrow) is seen. (B) Gross specimen of the resected small intestine shows a 10 × 4-cm ulcerative fungating tumor (arrows).

about 5% of patients with neurofibromatosis type 1 (NF-1) will present with a small bowel GIST; GISTs can be seen in young females as part of the Carney triad (gastric or small bowel GIST, pulmonary chondroma, and extra-adrenal pheochromocytoma) or in males or females as part of the Carney-Stratakis syndrome (GIST and paraganglioma) (Figs. 15–17).[59] The occurrence of small bowel GIST is associated with the presence of other cancers both before and after GIST diagnosis,[60] including cancers of the GI and genitourinary tract. Cancers that occur with increased frequency before and after GIST diagnosis include other sarcomas, neuroendocrine neoplasms, and lymphomas. With the exception of familial GIST, the absolute incidence of GIST in any of these populations remains very low and routine

screening is not performed. Suspicion of small bowel bleeding should prompt referral to CT or MR enterography, particularly in patients with familial GIST and NF-1. Imaging surveillance is performed after GIST resection. Most GISTs occur sporadically in older individuals and are often detected with imaging for suspected small bowel bleeding or nonspecific abdominal complaints.

Imaging of Small Bowel Gastrointestinal Stromal Tumors

The imaging appearance of small bowel GISTs has been well-described.[61] GISTs appear as rounded small bowel masses, usually with an exo-enteric component and often an intraluminal component. They may contain ulcerations and generally enhance avidly. They are usually singular when

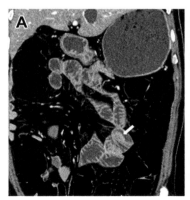
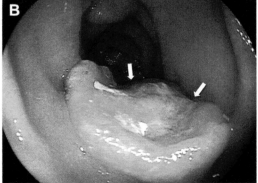

Fig. 10. A 75-year-old man with a small adenocarcinoma in the jejunum. (A) Coronal CT enterography shows a 1.7-cm plaquelike elevated lesion (arrow) in the jejunum. (B) Balloon-assisted endoscopy shows a corresponding small elevated lesion (arrows) with a shallow central ulcer in the jejunum. The lesion was confirmed to be an adenocarcinoma with an extension to the proper muscle layer by a surgery.

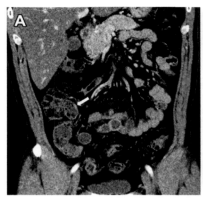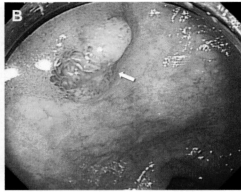

Fig. 11. A 48-year-old man with a tiny adenocarcinoma in the terminal ileum incidentally detected during colonoscopy. (A) Coronal contrast-enhanced CT shows a 1-cm subtle wall thickening with slightly increased enhancement (arrow) in the terminal ileum. This lesion could not be prospectively recognized. (B) Ileocolonoscopic view of the corresponding lesion (arrow). The lesion was confirmed to be an adenocarcinoma with an extension to the muscularis mucosa by a surgery.

sporadic but can be multifocal in familial GIST and NF-1. Vasconcelos and colleagues[62] recently reported on the Mayo Clinic experience with more than 100 small bowel GISTs and reported a dramatic increase in the diagnosis of nonmalignant small bowel GISTs after the use of multiphase CT enterography in patients with suspected small bowel bleeding (Fig. 18). Ulceration, internal air or enteric contrast, internal necrosis, and invasive borders were imaging findings associated with high-grade and malignant tumors (Fig. 19). Tumors 2 cm and smaller in size are considered to be of less risk and are sometimes observed.[63]

EXAMINATION OF SUSPECTED SMALL BOWEL BLEEDING AND OTHER AT-RISK CONDITIONS

Small bowel neoplasms are known to cause small bowel bleeding, and an attempt should be made to exclude them when small bowel bleeding is suspected after negative upper and lower endoscopies. The American College of Gastroenterology has published a clinical guideline on the diagnosis and management of small bowel bleeding and recommends capsule endoscopy as a first-line test if there are no concerns for small bowel obstruction.[23] CT or MR enterography are used as first-line tests in patients with suspected obstruction (eg, known or suspected Crohn disease, prior small bowel surgery, obstructive symptoms, or prior radiation therapy) or as additional tests after negative capsule endoscopy.[23] The rationale for the use of CT enterography is that capsule endoscopy may miss intramural tumors with minimal overlying mucosal abnormalities.[10] Unlike many

other causes of small bowel bleeding that occur predominantly in old or young patients, small bowel tumors can occur in patients of all ages. One meta-analysis examining the yield of capsule endoscopy and double-balloon enteroscopy has estimated that the yield of these examinations for mass lesions of the small bowel is about 10%.[64] The prevalence of small bowel tumors detected by CT or MR enterography in patients with suspected small bowel bleeding is unknown, but one prospective study identified small bowel tumors in 15% (9 of 60).[10] The yield of multiphase CT enterography after negative or nondiagnostic capsule endoscopy has been estimated to be 28% and is higher in patients with a history of prior or current overt small bowel bleeding.[65] In patients with suspected small bowel bleeding, capsule endoscopy and cross-sectional enterography are often used together in a complementary fashion to increase diagnostic yield.[66] In experienced hands, performance of MR enterography seems to be similar or potentially superior to CT enterography in identifying tumors.[10]

Although the most common causes of GI bleeding in adults are vascular lesions, such as angioectasias, which can be treated with balloon-assisted endoscopy, the identification of small bowel neoplasm generally leads directly to surgery. In patients with tumors, surgical extirpation should eliminate or greatly reduce the chance of recurrent small bowel bleeding; patients receiving medical and surgical therapy for specific findings identified at cross-sectional enterography have a lower rate of rebleeding.[67] It is unknown if the routine use of cross-sectional enterography for suspected small bowel bleeding increases

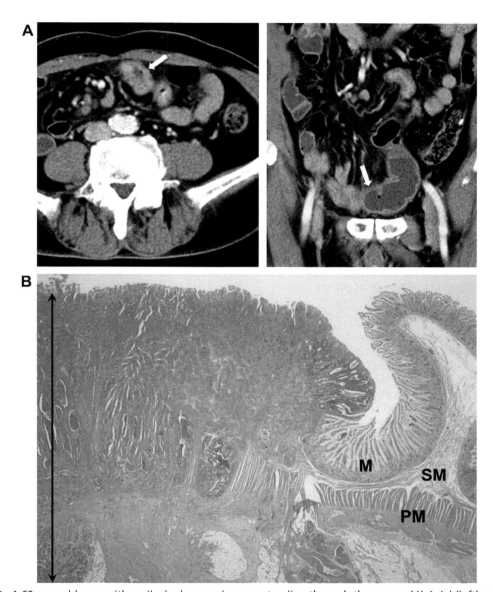

Fig. 12. A 69-year-old man with an ileal adenocarcinoma extending through the serosa. (A) Axial (left) contrast-enhanced CT shows a luminal-encircling mass (arrow). The lesion has extended through the entire thickness of the ileal wall, replacing the normal mural stratification, and shows moderate heterogeneous enhancement. Compare the finding with the thickened ileal wall proximal to the mass caused by obstruction, which maintains the normal stratification (arrow in right). (B) Low-power microscopic view of the surgical specimen shows the replacement of normal mural layers by the transmural extension of the tumor (double arrow) (hematoxylin and eosin stain, original magnification ×12.5). M, mucosa; PM, proper muscle; SM, submucosa.

survival in patients with small bowel tumors; however, one recent retrospective observational study from the Mayo Clinic recently found that after CT enterography was used to routinely examine patients with small bowel bleeding at their institution, the rate of malignant small bowel GISTs remained the same, but the rate of nonmalignant GISTs increased substantially.[62] This finding suggests the possibility that a symptomatic and bleeding small bowel tumor may be more likely to be detected at an earlier stage or lower grade than asymptomatic neoplasms, which may grow undetected.

The appearance of adenocarcinoma, lymphoma, and GIST tumors has already been described. Neuroendocrine neoplasms are one

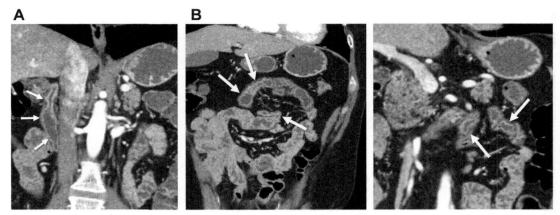

Fig. 13. A 47-year-old man with celiac disease on a gluten-free diet underwent CT enterography. (A) Coronal image through the descending duodenum demonstrates complete loss of duodenal folds (*arrows*), with villous atrophy found at histopathology. (B) Coronal images through the jejunum demonstrate loss of normal jejunal fold pattern, wall thickening, and hyperenhancement, indicating jejunitis (*arrows*). Patient was subsequently diagnosed with type 1 refractory celiac disease.

of the most common small bowel tumors and are frequently detected in patients with small bowel bleeding. They are classified into low-grade tumors (previously called carcinoid tumors) and neuroendocrine carcinomas.[68] Although screening is not performed for small bowel neuroendocrine neoplasms, they are often discovered in patients with suspected small bowel bleeding and are often discovered incidentally at both endoscopy and cross-sectional imaging. Neuroendocrine neoplasms typically occur in distal/terminal ileum, with the small bowel primary presenting as a small enhancing polyp or more characteristically as a plaquelike mass, often with serosal retraction (**Figs. 20 and 21**).[69] Tumor can be singular or multifocal along a bowel segment. Nodal metastases typically cluster around mesenteric vessels (with potential to narrow or occlude them), with advanced mesenteric metastases presenting with a characteristic pattern of rounded soft tissue, punctate calcification, and radiating strands of desmoplasia.

Crohn disease can mimic small bowel tumors; patients with long-standing Crohn disease are at increased risk for these tumors,[70] particularly lymphoma and adenocarcinoma, which can be

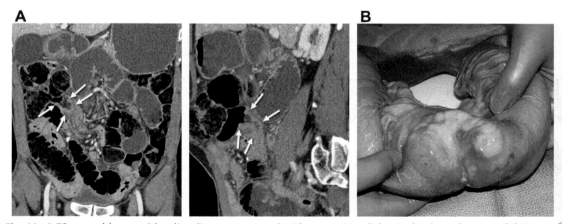

Fig. 14. A 58-year-old man with celiac disease presented with worsening abdominal pain and nausea. (A) Coronal and sagittal CT images taken in the emergency department demonstrate a small bowel obstruction with an annular mass with shouldering and in the mid small bowel (*arrows*). (B) Subsequent segmental resection demonstrated a distal jejunal T-cell lymphoma.

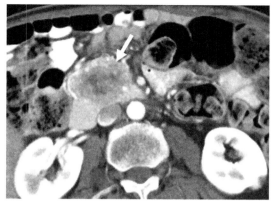

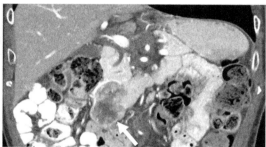

Fig. 15. A 51-year-old man with neurofibromatosis and approximately 6-cm duodenal GIST with intramural and exo-enteric components (*arrows*), confirmed with biopsy and immunohistochemical staining.

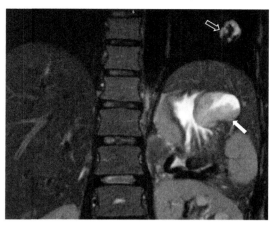

Fig. 17. Coronal MR image in 47-year-old woman with Carney triad showing a recurrent and multifocal and exophytic gastric GIST with necrosis (*solid white arrow*) and a presumed pulmonary chondroma (*open arrow*). Patient has a carotid body tumor resected as a child.

discovered incidentally. Radiological diagnosis of small bowel tumors developing in Crohn disease (**Fig. 22**) is very difficult because the imaging findings are similar to the findings of long-standing Crohn disease, and biopsy should be used when required to distinguish between them. The development of a mass and nodularity at the extraluminal margins of the mass in a location of luminal narrowing/obstruction should be

evaluated carefully regarding the possibility of superimposed malignancy.[29,30]

RADIOLOGIC DIFFERENTIAL DIAGNOSES

Various benign diseases may mimic small bowel cancers on radiological examinations, although most small bowel cancers will likely not be confused with benign diseases. Several chronic inflammatory diseases, such as Crohn disease, tuberculosis, nonsteroidal antiinflammatory drug enteropathy, chronic radiation enteropathy or cryptogenic multifocal ulcerous stenosing enteritis, and chronic ischemic stricture, can present with focal segmental thickening of the small bowel wall that may mimic an adenocarcinoma. As mentioned earlier, shoulderlike or overhanging

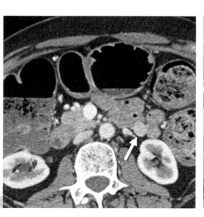

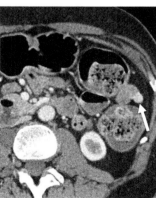

Fig. 16. A 50-year-old woman with suspected small bowel bleeding, negative upper and lower endoscopy, and capsule endoscopy showing small, nonbleeding jejunal arteriovenous malformations. Axial images from CT enterography examination demonstrated multiple enhancing exo-enteric masses measuring between 0.3 and 1.3 cm (*arrows*). At subsequent surgical assessment, 5 small jejunal GISTs at very low risk for recurrence were resected.

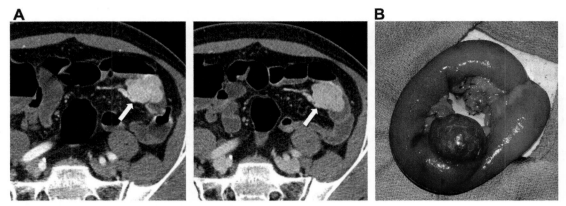

Fig. 18. A 70-year-old man with overt suspected small bowel bleeding with negative upper and lower endoscopy underwent CT enterography. (*A*) Arterial- (left) and enteric-phase (right) CT enterography images demonstrate an avidly enhancing mass (*arrows*) with luminal and exo-enteric components typical of small bowel GIST. (*B*) At surgical extirpation, a 4-cm exophytic mass was found, with histopathology demonstrating a low-risk GIST with 0 mitosis per 50 high power field.

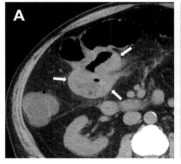
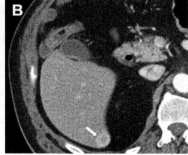

Fig. 19. A 59-year-old man with abdominal pain underwent cross-sectional imaging. (*A*) Unenhanced CT imaging shows large intramural and exo-enteric mass with internal fluid and air (*arrows*). Subsequent resection demonstrated small bowel GIST at high risk for recurrence. (*B*) Approximately 2.5 years later, an enhancing hepatic metastasis (*arrow*) in segment VI was resected.

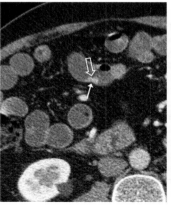
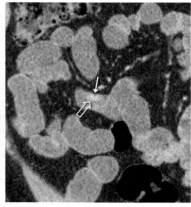

Fig. 20. A 68-year-old man with overt small bowel bleeding and negative upper and lower endoscopies with vascular lesions seen in the ileum on capsule endoscopy. Axial enteric-phase (left) and coronal delayed-phase images (right) demonstrate plaquelike enhancing intramural mass (*open arrows*) with serosal retraction (*small solid arrows*). At surgical resection, a 1.1-cm submucosal neuroendocrine neoplasm invading the muscularis propria was found.

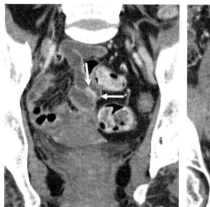
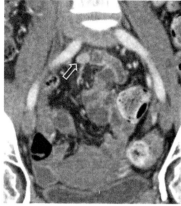

Fig. 21. A 65-year-old woman with iron-deficiency anemia and multiple negative upper and lower endoscopies. A subsequent capsule endoscopy was also negative. Coronal, enteric-phase CT enterography images demonstrate an enhancing plaquelike mass (*solid white arrows*) with nearby enhancing nodes (*open arrow*) adjacent to mesenteric vessels, indicating likely neuroendocrine neoplasm with nearby mesenteric metastases. At surgical resection, a 1.8-cm grade 1 neuroendocrine carcinoma was found, with tumor extending to the perienteric adipose tissue and metastatic carcinoma involving 4 of 8 regional lymph nodes.

appearance of the lesion margin and interruption of the small bowel wall enhancement pattern suggest a malignancy. However, these findings may not be clear-cut in all cases, and diagnostic laparoscopy is occasionally required. Distinguishing features favoring chronic inflammatory conditions include segmental involvement of greater length and involvement of multiple bowel segments with intervening skip areas and other imaging findings of enteric inflammation.[71] Small bowel T-cell lymphoma can often be confused with chronic inflammatory conditions.[55,56] Ectopic pancreas can also present as a mural or exo-enteric mass; this should be considered in mass lesions of the duodenum and jejunum, with MR images often demonstrating an ectopic duct sign (**Fig. 23**).[72,73] Further details on the imaging findings of various cancer-mimicking benign small bowel diseases are beyond the scope of this article and can be found elsewhere.[74–81] In addition to the morphologic differential points, correlation with clinical features is also crucial.

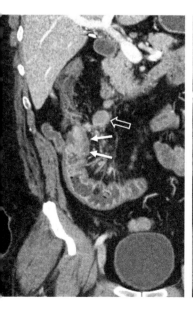
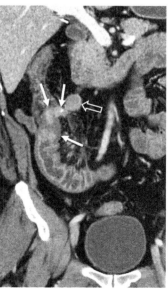

Fig. 22. A 60-year-old man with Crohn disease underwent ileocolonoscopy with biopsy showing chronic active ileitis and colitis and the ileocecal valve and terminal ileum. CT enterography shows masslike luminal enhancement involving the terminal ileum and ileocecal valve and extending into the adjacent mesentery (*solid white arrows*) with adjacent lymphadenopathy (*open arrows*). Subsequent resection demonstrated neuroendocrine neoplasm with regional lymph node metastases.

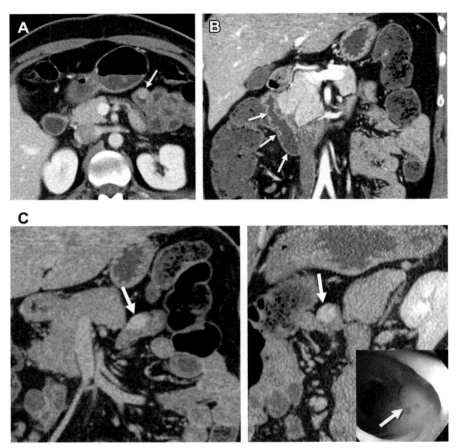

Fig. 23. A 36-year-old woman with pain, nausea, and celiac disease underwent routine abdominopelvic CT. (*A*) An enhancing intramural mass was identified in the proximal jejunum (*arrow*). (*B*) Subsequent multiphase CT enterography shows loss of folds in the descending duodenum (*arrows*), consistent with known celiac disease. (*C*) Coronal delayed images demonstrate an intramural mass (*arrows*), thought to be a small bowel GIST or ectopic pancreas. Subsequent antegrade enteroscopy confirmed a nonbleeding submucosal mass (*arrow in inset*), with biopsy demonstrating pancreatic heterotopia.

SUMMARY

The authors review conditions associated with small bowel cancers and the detection of these tumors at cross-sectional and optical imaging in at-risk patients. CT and MR enterography are being used increasingly in conjunction with capsule endoscopy and balloon-assisted endoscopy in the routine investigation of patients with suspected small bowel bleeding. Although screening and surveillance for small bowel cancers is performed for a small number of patients with conditions predisposing them to small bowel cancer, an increasing number of small bowel tumors are being discovered with the routine use of capsule endoscopy and cross-sectional enterography in patients with suspected small bowel bleeding.

REFERENCES

1. North JH, Pack MS. Malignant tumors of the small intestine: a review of 144 cases. Am Surg 2000;66(1): 46–51.
2. Bilimoria KY, Bentrem DJ, Wayne JD, et al. Small bowel cancer in the United States: changes in epidemiology, treatment, and survival over the last 20 years. Ann Surg 2009;249(1):63–71.
3. Chow JS, Chen CC, Ahsan H, et al. A population-based study of the incidence of malignant small bowel tumours: SEER, 1973-1990. Int J Epidemiol 1996;25(4):722–8.
4. Pan SY, Morrison H. Epidemiology of cancer of the small intestine. World J Gastrointest Oncol 2011;3(3):33–42.
5. Aparicio T, Zaanan A, Mary F, et al. Small bowel adenocarcinoma. Gastroenterol Clin North Am 2016;45(3):447–57.

6. American Cancer Society. Small intestine cancer. Available at: https://www.cancer.org/cancer/small-intestine-cancer.html. Accessed January 25, 2017.

7. American Cancer Society. Cancer statistics center. Available at: http://cancerstatisticscenter.cancer.org. Accessed January 25, 2017.

8. Chang HK, Yu E, Kim J, et al. Adenocarcinoma of the small intestine: a multi-institutional study of 197 surgically resected cases. Hum Pathol 2010;41(8):1087–96.

9. Dabaja BS, Suki D, Pro B, et al. Adenocarcinoma of the small bowel: presentation, prognostic factors, and outcome of 217 patients. Cancer 2004;101(3):518–26.

10. Huprich JE, Fletcher JG, Fidler JL, et al. Prospective blinded comparison of wireless capsule endoscopy and multiphase CT enterography in obscure gastrointestinal bleeding. Radiology 2011;260(3):744–51.

11. Lee SS, Oh TS, Kim HJ, et al. Obscure gastrointestinal bleeding: diagnostic performance of multidetector CT enterography. Radiology 2011;259(3):739–48.

12. Soto JA, Park SH, Fletcher JG, et al. Gastrointestinal hemorrhage: evaluation with MDCT. Abdom Imaging 2015;40(5):993–1009.

13. Baker ME, Hara AK, Platt JF, et al. CT enterography for Crohn's disease: optimal technique and imaging issues. Abdom Imaging 2015;40(5):938–52.

14. Grand DJ, Guglielmo FF, Al-Hawary MM. MR enterography in Crohn's disease: current consensus on optimal imaging technique and future advances from the SAR Crohn's disease-focused panel. Abdom Imaging 2015;40(5):953–64.

15. Amzallag-Bellenger E, Soyer P, Barbe C, et al. Prospective evaluation of magnetic resonance enterography for the detection of mesenteric small bowel tumours. Eur Radiol 2013;23(7):1901–10.

16. Masselli G, Polettini E, Casciani E, et al. Small-bowel neoplasms: prospective evaluation of MR enteroclysis. Radiology 2009;251(3):743–50.

17. Van Weyenberg SJ, Meijerink MR, Jacobs MA, et al. MR enteroclysis in the diagnosis of small-bowel neoplasms. Radiology 2010;254(3):765–73.

18. Soyer P, Aout M, Hoeffel C, et al. Helical CT-enteroclysis in the detection of small-bowel tumours: a meta-analysis. Eur Radiol 2013;23(2):388–99.

19. Masselli G, Di Tola M, Casciani E, et al. Diagnosis of small-bowel diseases: prospective comparison of multi-detector row CT enterography with MR enterography. Radiology 2016;279(2):420–31.

20. Islam RS, Leighton JA, Pasha SF. Evaluation and management of small-bowel tumors in the era of deep enteroscopy. Gastrointest Endosc 2014;79(5):732–40.

21. Appleyard M, Fireman Z, Glukhovsky A, et al. A randomized trial comparing wireless capsule endoscopy with push enteroscopy for the detection of small-bowel lesions. Gastroenterology 2000;119(6):1431–8.

22. Triester SL, Leighton JA, Leontiadis GI, et al. A meta-analysis of the yield of capsule endoscopy compared to other diagnostic modalities in patients with obscure gastrointestinal bleeding. Am J Gastroenterol 2005;100(11):2407–18.

23. Gerson LB, Fidler JL, Cave DR, et al. ACG clinical guideline: diagnosis and management of small bowel bleeding. Am J Gastroenterol 2015;110(9):1265–87 [quiz: 1288].

24. Hakim FA, Alexander JA, Huprich JE, et al. CT-enterography may identify small bowel tumors not detected by capsule endoscopy: eight years experience at Mayo Clinic Rochester. Dig Dis Sci 2011;56(10):2914–9.

25. Cheung DY, Lee IS, Chang DK, et al. Capsule endoscopy in small bowel tumors: a multicenter Korean study. J Gastroenterol Hepatol 2010;25(6):1079–86.

26. Hofman MS, Lau WF, Hicks RJ. Somatostatin receptor imaging with 68Ga DOTATATE PET/CT: clinical utility, normal patterns, pearls, and pitfalls in interpretation. Radiographics 2015;35(2):500–16.

27. Geijer H, Breimer LH. Somatostatin receptor PET/CT in neuroendocrine tumours: update on systematic review and meta-analysis. Eur J Nucl Med Mol Imaging 2013;40(11):1770–80.

28. Lepage C, Bouvier AM, Manfredi S, et al. Incidence and management of primary malignant small bowel cancers: a well-defined French population study. Am J Gastroenterol 2006;101(12):2826–32.

29. Soyer P, Hristova L, Boudghene F, et al. Small bowel adenocarcinoma in Crohn disease: CT-enterography features with pathological correlation. Abdom Imaging 2012;37(3):338–49.

30. Weber NK, Fletcher JG, Fidler JL, et al. Clinical characteristics and imaging features of small bowel adenocarcinomas in Crohn's disease. Abdom Imaging 2015;40(5):1060–7.

31. Wieghard N, Mongoue-Tchokote S, Isaac Young J, et al. Prognosis of small bowel adenocarcinoma in Crohn's disease compares favourably with de novo small bowel adenocarcinoma. Colorectal Dis 2016;19(5):446–55.

32. Vapiwala N. All about small bowel cancer. Available at: https://www.oncolink.org/cancers/gastrointestinal/small-intestine-cancers/all-about-small-bowel-cancer. Accessed January 25, 2017.

33. Syngal S, Brand RE, Church JM, et al. ACG clinical guideline: genetic testing and management of hereditary gastrointestinal cancer syndromes. Am J Gastroenterol 2015;110(2):223–62 [quiz: 263].

34. van Lier MG, Wagner A, Mathus-Vliegen EM, et al. High cancer risk in Peutz-Jeghers syndrome: a systematic review and surveillance recommendations.

Am J Gastroenterol 2010;105(6):1258–64 [author reply 1265].

35. Sokhandon F, Al-Katib S. Multidetector CT enterography of focal small bowel lesions: a radiological-pathological correlation. Abdom Radiol (NY) 2016; 42(5):1319–41.

36. Beggs AD, Latchford AR, Vasen HF, et al. Peutz-Jeghers syndrome: a systematic review and recommendations for management. Gut 2010;59(7): 975–86.

37. Hinds R, Philp C, Hyer W, et al. Complications of childhood Peutz-Jeghers syndrome: implications for pediatric screening. J Pediatr Gastroenterol Nutr 2004;39(2):219–20.

38. Postgate A, Hyer W, Phillips R, et al. Feasibility of video capsule endoscopy in the management of children with Peutz-Jeghers syndrome: a blinded comparison with barium enterography for the detection of small bowel polyps. J Pediatr Gastroenterol Nutr 2009;49(4):417–23.

39. Caspari R, von Falkenhausen M, Krautmacher C, et al. Comparison of capsule endoscopy and magnetic resonance imaging for the detection of polyps of the small intestine in patients with familial adenomatous polyposis or with Peutz-Jeghers' syndrome. Endoscopy 2004;36(12):1054–9.

40. Gupta A, Postgate AJ, Burling D, et al. A prospective study of MR enterography versus capsule endoscopy for the surveillance of adult patients with Peutz-Jeghers syndrome. AJR Am J Roentgenol 2010; 195(1):108–16.

41. Giardiello FM, Trimbath JD. Peutz-Jeghers syndrome and management recommendations. Clin Gastroenterol Hepatol 2006;4(4):408–15.

42. Papadopoulos VD, Nolan DJ. Carcinoma of the small intestine. Clin Radiol 1985;36(4):409–13.

43. Bessette J, Maglinte D, Kelvin F, et al. Primary malignant tumors in the small bowel: a comparison of the small-bowel enema and conventional follow-through examination. AJR Am J Roentgenol 1989;153(4):741–4.

44. Horton KM, Fishman EK. Multidetector-row computed tomography and 3-dimensional computed tomography imaging of small bowel neoplasms: current concept in diagnosis. J Comput Assist Tomogr 2004;28(1):106–16.

45. Shinya T, Inai R, Tanaka T, et al. Small bowel neoplasms: enhancement patterns and differentiation using post-contrast multiphasic multidetector CT. Abdom Radiol (NY) 2017;42(3):794–801.

46. Masselli G, Colaiacomo MC, Marcelli G, et al. MRI of the small-bowel: how to differentiate primary neoplasms and mimickers. Br J Radiol 2012;85(1014): 824–37.

47. Rubio-Tapia A, Ludvigsson JF, Brantner TL, et al. The prevalence of celiac disease in the United States. Am J Gastroenterol 2012;107(10):1538–44 [quiz: 1537, 1545].

48. Al-Bawardy B, Codipilly DC, Rubio-Tapia A, et al. Celiac disease: a clinical review. Abdom Radiol (NY) 2017;42(2):351–60.

49. Lewis NR, Scott BB. Meta-analysis: deamidated gliadin peptide antibody and tissue transglutaminase antibody compared as screening tests for coeliac disease. Aliment Pharmacol Ther 2010; 31(1):73–81.

50. Dickson BC, Streutker CJ, Chetty R. Coeliac disease: an update for pathologists. J Clin Pathol 2006;59(10):1008–16.

51. Oberhuber G. Histopathology of celiac disease. Biomed Pharmacother 2000;54(7):368–72.

52. Rubio-Tapia A, Murray JA. Classification and management of refractory coeliac disease. Gut 2010; 59(4):547–57.

53. Rubio-Tapia A, Hill ID, Kelly CP, et al. ACG clinical guidelines: diagnosis and management of celiac disease. Am J Gastroenterol 2013;108(5):656–76 [quiz: 677].

54. Al-Bawardy B, Barlow JM, Vasconcelos RN, et al. Cross-sectional imaging in refractory celiac disease. Abdom Radiol (NY) 2017;42(2):389–95.

55. Byun JH, Ha HK, Kim AY, et al. CT findings in peripheral T-cell lymphoma involving the gastrointestinal tract. Radiology 2003;227(1):59–67.

56. Kim DH, Lee D, Kim JW, et al. Endoscopic and clinical analysis of primary T-cell lymphoma of the gastrointestinal tract according to pathological subtype. J Gastroenterol Hepatol 2014;29(5): 934–43.

57. American Society of Clinical Oncology. Familial GIST. 2015. Available at: http://www.cancer.net/cancer-types/familial-gist. Accessed January 25, 2017.

58. Rammohan A, Sathyanesan J, Rajendran K, et al. A gist of gastrointestinal stromal tumors: a review. World J Gastrointest Oncol 2013;5(6):102–12.

59. Stratakis CA, Carney JA. The triad of paragangliomas, gastric stromal tumours and pulmonary chondromas (Carney triad), and the dyad of paragangliomas and gastric stromal sarcomas (Carney-Stratakis syndrome): molecular genetics and clinical implications. J Intern Med 2009;266(1): 43–52.

60. Murphy JD, Ma GL, Baumgartner JM, et al. Increased risk of additional cancers among patients with gastrointestinal stromal tumors: a population-based study. Cancer 2015;121(17):2960–7.

61. Levy AD, Remotti HE, Thompson WM, et al. Gastrointestinal stromal tumors: radiologic features with pathologic correlation. Radiographics 2003;23(2): 283–304, 456; [quiz: 532].

62. Vasconcelos R, Dolan SG, Barlow JM, et al. Impact of CT enterography on the diagnosis of small bowel gastrointestinal stromal tumors. Abdom Radiol (NY) 2017;42(5):1365–73.

63. Fletcher CD, Berman JJ, Corless C, et al. Diagnosis of gastrointestinal stromal tumors: a consensus approach. Hum Pathol 2002;33(5):459–65.

64. Pasha SF, Leighton JA, Das A, et al. Double-balloon enteroscopy and capsule endoscopy have comparable diagnostic yield in small-bowel disease: a meta-analysis. Clin Gastroenterol Hepatol 2008; 6(6):671–6.

65. Agrawal JR, Travis AC, Mortele KJ, et al. Diagnostic yield of dual-phase computed tomography enterography in patients with obscure gastrointestinal bleeding and a non-diagnostic capsule endoscopy. J Gastroenterol Hepatol 2012;27(4):751–9.

66. Hara AK, Walker FB, Silva AC, et al. Preliminary estimate of triphasic CT enterography performance in hemodynamically stable patients with suspected gastrointestinal bleeding. AJR Am J Roentgenol 2009;193(5):1252–60.

67. Shin JK, Cheon JH, Lim JS, et al. Long-term outcomes of obscure gastrointestinal bleeding after CT enterography: does negative CT enterography predict lower long-term rebleeding rate? J Gastroenterol Hepatol 2011;26(5):901–7.

68. Klimstra DS, Modlin IR, Coppola D, et al. The pathologic classification of neuroendocrine tumors: a review of nomenclature, grading, and staging systems. Pancreas 2010;39(6):707–12.

69. Levy AD, Sobin LH. From the archives of the AFIP: gastrointestinal carcinoids: imaging features with clinicopathologic comparison. Radiographics 2007; 27(1):237–57.

70. Cahill C, Gordon PH, Petrucci A, et al. Small bowel adenocarcinoma and Crohn's disease: any further ahead than 50 years ago? World J Gastroenterol 2014;20(33):11486–95.

71. Anzidei M, Napoli A, Zini C, et al. Malignant tumours of the small intestine: a review of histopathology, multidetector CT and MRI aspects. Br J Radiol 2011;84:677–90.

72. Kung JW, Brown A, Kruskal JB, et al. Heterotopic pancreas: typical and atypical imaging findings. Clin Radiol 2010;65(5):403–7.

73. Kim DW, Kim JH, Park SH, et al. Heterotopic pancreas of the jejunum: associations between CT and pathology features. Abdom Imaging 2015; 40(1):38–45.

74. Tolan DJ, Greenhalgh R, Zealley IA, et al. MR enterographic manifestations of small bowel Crohn disease. Radiographics 2010;30(2):367–84.

75. Hara AK, Swartz PG. CT enterography of Crohn's disease. Abdom Imaging 2009;34(3):289–95.

76. Kalra N, Agrawal P, Mittal V, et al. Spectrum of imaging findings on MDCT enterography in patients with small bowel tuberculosis. Clin Radiol 2014;69(3): 315–22.

77. Krishna S, Kalra N, Singh P, et al. Small-bowel tuberculosis: a comparative study of MR enterography and small-bowel follow-through. AJR Am J Roentgenol 2016;207(3):571–7.

78. Frye JM, Hansel SL, Dolan SG, et al. NSAID enteropathy: appearance at CT and MR enterography in the age of multi-modality imaging and treatment. Abdom Imaging 2015;40(5):1011–25.

79. Perlemuter G, Guillevin L, Legman P, et al. Cryptogenetic multifocal ulcerous stenosing enteritis: an atypical type of vasculitis or a disease mimicking vasculitis. Gut 2001;48(3):333–8.

80. Chung SH, Park SU, Cheon JH, et al. Clinical characteristics and treatment outcomes of cryptogenic multifocal ulcerous stenosing enteritis in Korea. Dig Dis Sci 2015;60(9):2740–5.

81. Horton KM, Corl FM, Fishman EK. CT of nonneoplastic diseases of the small bowel: spectrum of disease. J Comput Assist Tomogr 1999;23(3): 417–28.

Imaging and Screening of Hereditary Cancer Syndromes

Venkata S. Katabathina, MD[a],*, Christine O. Menias, MD[b],
Srinivasa R. Prasad, MD[c]

KEYWORDS

• Hereditary cancers • Imaging findings • Surveillance

KEY POINTS

• There is a wide spectrum of hereditary cancer syndromes that predispose patients to the early onset of phenotypically distinct tumors in specific organ systems.
• Clinical management of patients with these syndromes is challenging because of a complex interplay of factors, including aggressive tumor histobiology, tumor location, bilateral tumors, advanced disease at presentation, and multiorgan involvement.
• A better understanding of these hereditary syndromes has led to an improved knowledge of underlying tumor genetics and oncological pathways, thus paving the way for molecular diagnostics and targeted therapeutics even in patients with sporadic tumors.
• Laboratory and imaging-based screening strategies allow early diagnosis in asymptomatic patients with a familial predisposition to cancers so as to permit optimal management.

INTRODUCTION

Hereditary cancer syndromes constitute a diverse group of genetic syndromes characterized by the early-onset development of histogenetically distinct neoplasms in specific organ systems in multiple family members.[1,2] These syndromes comprise 3% to 10% of all malignancies in various organ systems.[1] A constellation of clinical syndromes and imaging phenotypes allow characterization of select hereditary cancer syndromes. The finding of specific bilateral tumors and multiorgan involvement may suggest a diagnosis of a hereditary tumor syndrome. A radiologist may be the first physician to alert the clinician to a specific diagnosis of a genetic syndrome based on pathognomonic imaging findings, such as bilateral, multiple renal angiomyolipomas in a patient with

tuberous sclerosis.[1,3] This finding may trigger further genetic tests to establish the diagnosis as well as to screen other family members.

Tumors in patients with hereditary syndromes present significant challenges to patient management because of a complex interplay of various factors, including aggressive tumor biology, tumor location, bilateral tumors, advanced disease, and multiorgan involvement.[2] Increased impetus for a better understanding of tumor genetics and pathways in select hereditary syndromes has led to smarter screening strategies as well as the development of novel molecular diagnostics and therapeutics. Evolving paradigms of prophylactic risk-reducing bilateral salpingo-oophorectomy or, more recently, bilateral salpingectomy in patients with BRCA syndromes provide an excellent example of how

a Department of Radiology, University of Texas Health Science Center at San Antonio, 7703 Floyd Curl Drive, San Antonio, TX 78229, USA; b Department of Radiology, Mayo Clinic, 13400 East Shea Boulevard, Scottsdale, AZ 85259, USA; c Department of Radiology, The University of Texas MD Anderson Cancer Center, 1515 Holcombe Boulevard, Houston, TX 77030, USA
* Corresponding author.
E-mail address: katabathina@uthscsa.edu

Radiol Clin N Am 55 (2017) 1293–1309
http://dx.doi.org/10.1016/j.rcl.2017.06.011
0033-8389/17/© 2017 Elsevier Inc. All rights reserved.

recent advances in pathology and genetics have affected patient management.[4] Detailed studies of these uncommon syndromes have also led to better understanding of histogenesis and the biological diversity of sporadic cancers. The incorporation of poly-ADP-ribose polymerase (PARP) inhibitors in chemotherapy regimens to treat patients with sporadic, ovarian, high-grade serous carcinomas based on the BRCA component of these tumors is a case in point.[5] A plethora of drugs currently available to treat patients with advanced clear cell renal cell carcinomas (RCCs) can be traced to the elucidation of the role of the *VHL* gene in tumorigenesis and the knowledge of impaired VHL–mammalian target of rapamycin (mTOR) pathways in sporadic, metastatic kidney cancers.[6]

A variety of advanced laboratory tests, including genetic tests, are available to establish the diagnosis of hereditary cancer syndromes. Cross-sectional imaging techniques play an integral role in the screening, early diagnosis, surveillance, and management of patients with these syndromes in conjunction with clinical and pathologic findings.[3,7] Unenhanced whole-body magnetic resonance (MR) imaging has recently been shown to be a safe and excellent cancer-screening tool in children with select hereditary cancer predisposition syndromes given its high sensitivity, specific, and negative predictive values as well as the lack of ionizing radiation.[7–10] The screening and surveillance algorithms in select tumor syndromes designed for early diagnosis in asymptomatic patients are also presented in this article (Table 1).

HEREDITARY BREAST AND OVARIAN CANCER SYNDROME

Hereditary breast and ovarian cancer syndrome (HBOC) is an autosomal dominant disorder, associated with increased risk of breast and ovarian cancers.[1,11] The risk of primary peritoneal serous carcinoma; primary fallopian tube carcinoma; and pancreatic, prostate, and colon cancers is also increased.[12] Germline mutations in the tumor suppressor genes, *BRCA1* (chromosome 17q21) and *BRCA2* (chromosome 13q13), which help in maintaining genomic stability through DNA repair, are responsible for the development of HBOC.[1,12] There is a 65% to 75% lifetime risk of breast cancer and 40% to 50% (*BRCA1*) or 10% to 20% (*BRCA2*) risk of ovarian cancer in women with HBOC.[13,14]

Invasive ductal carcinomas are the most common type of breast cancers in HBOC, with significantly higher incidence of triple-negative cancers (estrogen, progesterone, and human epidermal growth factor-2 receptors negative) in *BRCA1* carriers (70% vs 10%–20% of the general population).[15] A well-circumscribed breast mass with sharp margins that mimics a benign lesion is the most common imaging appearance of a BRCA-associated breast cancer on mammogram and ultrasonography (US); malignant calcifications are less frequent on mammography (Fig. 1).[16] Given the benign imaging appearance of cancers, all mammographically detected lesions regardless of imaging features should be biopsied in HBOC. Contrast-enhanced MR can detect early-stage and potentially curable breast cancers in this population.[17]

High-grade serous carcinoma is the most common ovarian malignancy in HBOC and typically manifests at an earlier age compared with sporadic cases; most of these tumors originate from the fimbriated ends of the fallopian tubes (Fig. 2).[4] Although imaging findings of BRCA-associated ovarian serous cancers are similar to sporadic cases, tumors tend to be exquisitely sensitive to PARP inhibitors and platinum agents.[18,19] Primary peritoneal serous carcinoma and primary fallopian tube carcinoma are uncommon malignancies that can develop in HBOC, and show many similarities with serous ovarian cancer; currently, all 3 cancers are grouped as extrauterine pelvic serous carcinomas and are managed in a similar fashion.[18]

HBOC should be suspected in individuals with either a personal or family history of breast cancer diagnosed before the age of 50 years, triple-negative breast cancer, and extrauterine pelvic serous carcinomas.[1] Genetic counseling, followed by appropriate genetic testing, has to be performed in these individuals and their family members. The National Comprehensive Cancer Network (NCCN) recommends breast MR imaging and/or mammogram starting between the ages of 25 and 29 years and discussion of prophylactic mastectomy in HBOC.[20] Screening with a transvaginal sonogram and CA (cancer antigen)-125 levels has not been useful in reducing mortality from ovarian cancer; the NCCN recommends risk-reducing bilateral salpingo-oophorectomy between the ages of 35 and 40 years.[21]

LYNCH SYNDROME

Also known as hereditary nonpolyposis colorectal cancer (CRC), Lynch syndrome (LS) is an autosomal dominant condition that accounts for approximately 3% of CRCs and 2% to 3% of all endometrial cancers.[22] In patients with LS, there is also increased the risk of cancers of the ovary (7%–12%), stomach (5%–13%), small bowel (6%), hepatobiliary system, renal pelvis, ureters, brain, and sebaceous glands (Fig. 3).[22] Germline mutation in one of the several DNA mismatch repair (MMR) genes, MLH1 (chromosome 3p21), MSH2 (chromosome 2p16), MSH6 (chromosome 2p16), and PMS2 (chromosome 7p22), causes LS. These mutations result in defective repair of mismatched nucleotides during DNA replication with the development of microsatellite instability (MSI) and multiple cancers.[23] Among them, deleterious mutations in MLH1 and MSH2 are responsible for 70% to 90% of LS and have the highest risks and the widest array of LS-associated cancers.[23] The Muir-Torre syndrome is a variant of LS, and is characterized by LS-associated cancers, cutaneous keratoacanthomas, and sebaceous tumors.[24]

The lifetime risk of CRC in LS is as high as 75%, and about 50% of cancers develop before the age of 50 years. Increased incidence of synchronous and metachronous cancers, right-sided predominance, a larger size of colonic adenomas, and rapid progression of adenomas to carcinoma, compared with sporadic cases are seen in LS-associated CRCs (Fig. 4).[23] Signet-ring or cribriform histology with abundant mucin production and tumor-infiltrating lymphocytes are seen at histology. Up to 44% of LS with mutations in MSH2 and MSH6 and as many as 25% of CRC survivors may develop endometrial cancer.[22] At pathology, the endometrioid subtype is common with tumor-infiltrating lymphocytes; heterogeneous tumor morphology is commonly seen. On imaging, infiltrating tumors involving the lower uterine segment and endocervical canal in younger women should raise the suspicion of LS (Fig. 5).[11]

The revised Amsterdam criteria are helpful to identify LS mutation carriers: 3 or more relatives with histologically verified LS-associated cancers involving at least 2 generations, and with early-onset cancers diagnosed before the age of 50 years.[23,25,26] This criterion may be remembered by the 3-2-1 rule (3 affected members, 2 generations, and 1 cancer before age 50 years). In addition, revised Bethesda criteria were developed to identify individuals with CRC who should undergo MSI testing.[22,27] However, the concept of universal screening for LS has been proposed and includes the evaluation of MMR deficit (MSI and absence of proteins on immunohistochemistry) in all CRCs and endometrial cancers at the time of initial diagnosis; this strategy has been shown to prevent cancers in unaffected family members.[26,28,29] Annual or bi

colonoscopy is recommended in all mutation carriers of LS, beginning around the age of 25 years or 5 to 10 years before the earliest age of CRC onset in the family.[29,30] Patient education regarding the symptoms of different cancers is helpful for early detection of extracolonic cancers.[30]

FAMILIAL ADENOMATOUS POLYPOSIS

Familial adenomatous polyposis (FAP) is an autosomal dominant disorder characterized by the development of multiple colorectal adenomatous polyps, a high risk of CRC, and multiple extracolonic manifestations.[31] FAP accounts for less than 1% of all CRCs and is caused by the germline mutations in the adenomatous polyposis coli (APC) gene (chromosome 5q21), which functions as a tumor suppressor protein by negatively regulating the β-catenin oncoprotein.[32] FAP can present in 2 phenotypic forms, depending on the site of mutation in the APC gene: classic FAP and attenuated FAP.[32] The development of 100 or more polyps during teenage years is characteristic of classic FAP, and about 50% of them develop adenomas by 15 years and 95% by the age of 35 years (Fig. 6).[33] There is a 100% lifetime risk of CRC, which develops at an average age of 35 years.[33] Attenuated FAP is characterized by fewer polyps (10–99, with an average of 30), later age of onset (mean age of 44 years), right colonic preponderance, and a 70% lifetime risk of CRC.[32,33]

The common extracolonic manifestations in FAP include gastric fundic gland polyps, duodenal polyps, congenital hypertrophy of the retinal pigment epithelium, dental abnormalities, osteomas, and desmoid tumors (10%–15%).[33] Duodenal adenocarcinoma (4%–10%), papillary thyroid carcinoma (2%–3%), hepatoblastoma (1%), and brain tumors (<1%) comprise the extracolonic malignancies in FAP.[31] Computed tomography (CT) and MR imaging play an important role in the initial diagnosis, treatment follow-up, and long-term surveillance of both colonic and extracolonic cancers. Desmoid fibromatoses commonly develop in the abdominal wall or mesentery, show infiltrative growth, and frequently recur after surgical resection (Fig. 7).[31]

Annual sigmoidoscopy or colonoscopy should be initiated in patients with classic FAP and their first-degree relatives at the age of 12 to 14 years and continued until colectomy is performed.[26] Colonoscopy is indicated at 18 to 20 years in attenuated FAP cases and repeated every 2 years.[32] Upper gastrointestinal

Table 1
Select hereditary cancer syndromes with genetic abnormality, associated cancers, and screening guidelines

Syndrome	Genes (Chromosomal Locus)	Common Cancers	Other Common Manifestations	Cancer Screening Guidelines
Hereditary breast and ovarian cancer syndrome	BRCA1 (17q21) BRCA2 (13q13)	Breast cancer and high-grade serous cancer of the ovary	Peritoneal serous carcinoma; primary fallopian tube carcinoma; pancreatic, prostate, and colon cancers	Annual breast MR imaging and/or mammogram starting between the ages of 25–29 y
Lynch syndrome	MLH1 (3p21) MSH2 (2p16) MSH6 (2p16) PMS2 (7p22)	Colorectal and endometrial cancers	Cancers of the ovary, stomach, and small bowel	Annual colonoscopy in all mutation carriers, beginning at the age of 25 y or 5–10 y before the earliest age of colon cancer onset in the family
FAP	APC (5q21)	Multiple colorectal adenomatous polyps and colorectal carcinoma	Gastric and duodenal polyps, osteomas, and desmoid tumors	Annual colonoscopy in patients with classic FAP and their first-degree relatives at the age of 12–14 y Annual upper GI endoscopy and neck US starting at 25–30 y
Li-Fraumeni syndrome	TP53 (17p13)	Sarcomas, breast cancers, brain tumors, hematologic cancers, and adrenal cortical carcinomas	—	Annual mammography with or without breast MR imaging, starting at age 20–25 y Annual whole-body MR imaging examination is increasingly being considered
Cowden syndrome	PTEN gene (10q21)	Breast, thyroid, renal, and endometrial cancers	Trichilemmomas, macrocephaly, Lhermitte-Duclos disease, benign thyroid nodules, fibrocystic breast disease, multiple GI polyps, and uterine fibroids	Annual renal US at 40 y and repeating every 1–2 y Annual endometrial biopsy and/or the transvaginal US starting at age 30 y and colonoscopy starting at 35–40 y
Hereditary diffuse gastric cancer	E-cadherin (16q22)	Aggressive diffuse, infiltrating gastric cancer (signet-ring type)	—	Prophylactic gastrectomy in asymptomatic carriers of CDH1 gene and intensive annual endoscopic surveillance in those who decline gastrectomy Annual breast MR imaging with or without mammogram starting at 30 y

Syndrome	Gene			
von Hippel-Lindau disease	VHL (3p25)	Cerebellar/spinal cord hemangioblastomas, retinal angiomas, clear cell RCCs, pheochromocytomas and pancreatic neuroendocrine tumors	Complex renal cysts, pancreatic cysts, endolymphatic sac tumors, and epididymal cystadenomas	Annual abdominal US starting at the age of 8 y and abdominal MR imaging in suspected pheochromocytomas. Annual brain and spine MR imaging with contrast starting at the age of 16 y and MR imaging of the auditory canal if there are abnormal findings
Birt-Hogg-Dube syndrome	Folliculin (17p11)	Cutaneous fibrofolliculomas, bilateral pulmonary cysts, and multiple renal oncocytic tumors	Pneumothorax	Abdominal CT/MR imaging and chest CT starting at 21 y and repeated at least every 3 y
MEN syndrome type 1	MEN1 (11q13)	Parathyroid adenomas, pancreatic neuroendocrine tumors, and pituitary adenomas	Facial angiofibromas, collagenomas, adrenal cortical adenomas, and lipomas	Head MR imaging starting at age 5 y and repeating every 3 years and annual pancreatic CT/MR imaging starting at the age of 20 y
MEN syndrome type 2	RET (10q11)	Medullary thyroid carcinoma and pheochromocytoma	Primary hyperparathyroidism, lichen amyloidosis, and Hirschsprung disease	Genetic counseling, RET gene testing is mandatory for at-risk family members and prophylactic thyroidectomy before age 5 y if possible
Hereditary PGL 1	SDHD gene (11q23)	Head and neck paragangliomas, mostly benign	—	All patients with multiple head and neck paragangliomas should be tested for mutations in the SDHD gene
Hereditary PGL 4	SDHB gene (11p35)	Abdominal and pelvic paragangliomas, mostly malignant	RCC and GI stromal tumors	All patients with metastatic paragangliomas should be tested for mutations in the SDHB gene
TSC	TSC1 gene (9q34) and TSC2 gene (16p13)	Subependymal giant cell astrocytomas	Renal angiomyolipomas and cysts, and intracranial findings (subependymal nodules and cortical tubers)	Brain and abdominal MR imaging in all TSC patients at the time of diagnosis and high-resolution chest CT is suggested in women 18 y of age or older

In addition to screening guidelines discussed in this table, there are many clinical and laboratory findings that can help in early identification of malignancies in hereditary cancers syndromes, which are discussed in detail elsewhere in this article.

Abbreviations: FAP, familial adenomatous polyposis; GI, gastrointestinal; MEN, multiple endocrine neoplasia; PGL, paraganglioma syndrome; TSC, tuberous sclerosis complex; US, ultrasonography.

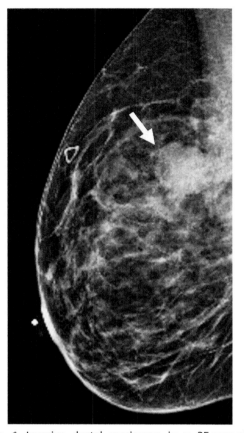

Fig. 1. Invasive ductal carcinoma in a 35-year-old woman with *BRCA1* mutations. Digital mammogram image in mediolateral oblique view shows a high-density mass with irregular margins (*arrow*) consistent with invasive ductal carcinoma.

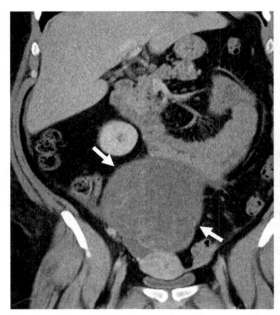

Fig. 3. Endometrioid subtype of ovarian cancer in a 37-year-old woman with LS. Coronal, contrast-enhanced CT image depicts a multiseptated cystic mass in the right ovary (*arrows*).

endoscopy is to be started when colorectal polyposis is diagnosed or at 25 to 30 years and should be performed ly.[26,33] Neck palpation with or without the US is indicated starting at 25 to 30 years for identifying thyroid cancers.[26] Individuals with a positive family history of desmoids and prior abdominal surgery should undergo periodic abdominal imaging with either CT or MR imaging.[33]

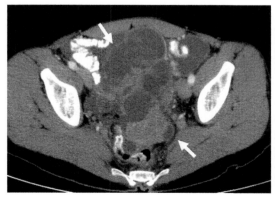

Fig. 2. High-grade serous carcinoma of the ovary in a 46-year-woman with *BRCA1* mutations. Axial contrast-enhanced CT image of the pelvis shows heterogeneously enhancing mixed solid-cystic masses in the pelvis (*arrows*).

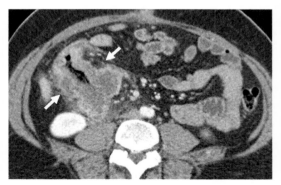

Fig. 4. Adenocarcinoma of the ascending colon in a 42-year-old man with LS. Axial, contrast-enhanced CT image of the abdomen shows irregular, lobulated wall thickening of the ascending colon (*arrows*) consistent with cancer.

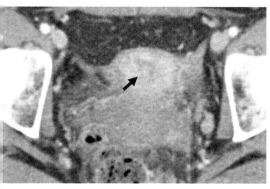

Fig. 5. Endometrioid subtype of endometrial cancer in a 33-year-old woman with LS. Axial, contrast-enhanced CT image of the pelvis shows a heterogeneously enhancing, infiltrating endometrial mass (*arrow*).

LI-FRAUMENI SYNDROME

Li-Fraumeni syndrome (LFS) is an autosomal dominant condition manifested by multiple cancers at an unusually early age, including sarcomas, breast cancers, brain tumors, hematologic cancers, and adrenal cortical carcinomas among the most common tumors (**Figs. 8** and **9**).[9,34] Germline mutations in the tumor suppressor gene *TP53* (chromosome 17p13), which helps in the elimination of abnormal DNA-containing cells during cell cycle, are responsible for the development of LFS.[35] Given the high penetrance of the mutated TP53 gene, the lifetime risk of cancer is estimated to be about 90% by the age 60 years in women and 75% in men.[36] Patients with LFS show an increased risk of radiation-induced cancers; radiation therapy is commonly avoided in these patients.[37] Sarcomas account for 25% of all tumors in LFS. All types of bone and soft tissue sarcomas can develop except Ewing sarcoma; osteosarcomas are the most common sarcomas.[35] Breast cancer is common in premenopausal women and shows amplification of *HER-2* at the molecular level. High-grade gliomas and choroid plexus carcinomas can present either in childhood or in young adults.[34] Approximately 10% of LFS carriers may develop adrenal cortical carcinomas.[38]

A comprehensive clinical, biochemical, and imaging surveillance protocol has been proposed for early tumor detection, which can improve long-term surveillance.[9] Imaging studies such as whole-body MR imaging, brain MR imaging, breast MR imaging, mammography, and abdominal/pelvic US play a pivotal role in this protocol.[9,36] Annual physical examination, breast self-examination beginning at 18 years, annual mammography with or without breast MR imaging, starting at age 20 to 25 years, and other targeted tumor surveillance based on family history of cancer has been recommended in LFS carriers.[36] Annual whole-body MR imaging examination is increasingly being considered as a screening test in LFS and other hereditary cancer syndromes.[8,9]

COWDEN SYNDROME

Cowden syndrome (CS) is an autosomal dominant condition caused by germline mutations in the *PTEN* gene (chromosome 10q21) and is associated with an increased risk of breast, thyroid, renal, colon, and endometrial cancers as well as hamartomatous lesions in multiple organ systems.[39] The protein from the *PTEN* gene acts as a negative controller of mTOR and PI3K (phosphoinositide 3-kinase)-AKT (protein kinase B) pathways in the process of cellular

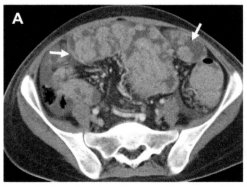
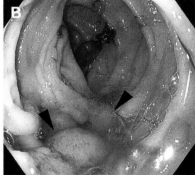

Fig. 6. Multiple colonic polyps in a 20-year-old woman with FAP syndrome. (*A*) Axial contrast-enhanced CT image of the abdomen shows innumerable polyps (*arrows*) in the colon. (*B*) Optical colonoscopy image confirms the findings of multiple colonic polyps (*arrowheads*).

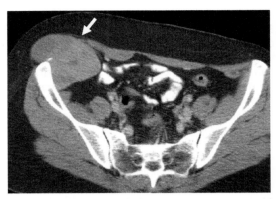

Fig. 7. Abdominal wall desmoid in a 25-year-old woman with FAP syndrome. Axial contrast-enhanced CT image of the abdomen shows a heterogeneously enhancing soft tissue mass in the right anterior abdominal wall (arrow), which biopsy proved to be a desmoid fibromatosis.

proliferation.[40] Trichilemmomas, palmoplantar keratosis, facial papules, and oral papillomas are common dermatologic and mucosal lesions in CS.[39] The benign lesions of CS for which imaging studies play an important role include macrocephaly, Lhermitte-Duclos disease (dysplastic cerebellar gangliocytoma), benign thyroid nodules, Hashimoto thyroiditis, vascular malformations/hemangiomas, fibrocystic breast disease, multiple gastrointestinal polyps, uterine fibroids, and endometriosis (Figs. 10 and 11).[41] Breast cancer is the most common malignancy in patients with CS; there is an estimated 25% to 50% lifetime risk in women diagnosed with CS.[39,41] Up to 34% of patients with CS may develop thyroid cancer; age at diagnosis less

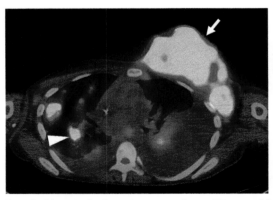

Fig. 8. Metastatic breast cancer in a 28-year-old woman with LFS. Axial ^{18}F-fluorodeoxyglucose (FDG) PET-CT image shows a large left breast mass (arrow) and multiple lung metastases (arrowhead) with increased FDG activity.

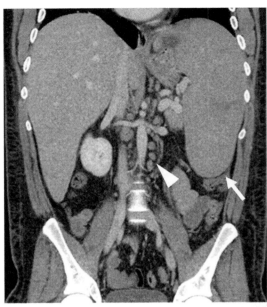

Fig. 9. T-cell lymphoma in a 24-year-old man with LFS. Coronal contrast-enhanced CT image of the abdomen shows marked hepatosplenomegaly (arrow) and retroperitoneal lymphadenopathy (arrowhead).

than 18 years, follicular histology, and male gender suggest the possibility of PTEN mutations.[39] The lifetime risks of endometrial and renal cancers in patients with CS are 28% and 34% respectively; papillary RCC is the most common histologic subtype (see Figs. 10 and 11).[40] Up to 20% of patients may develop colon cancer during their lifetimes.

Annual comprehensive physical examination starting at 18 years of age with particular attention to breast and thyroid is commonly used. Annual renal US at 40 years and repeating every 1 to 2 years is recommended. Annual endometrial biopsy and/or transvaginal US starting at age 30 years and colonoscopy starting at 35 to 40 years, as well as follow-up depending on number and type of polyps, have also been recommended in patients with CS.[39,40]

HEREDITARY DIFFUSE GASTRIC CANCER

Hereditary diffuse gastric cancer (HDGC) is an autosomal dominant disorder with high penetrance, caused by germline mutations in the E-cadherin (CDH1) tumor suppressor gene (chromosome 16q22).[42] The lifetime risk of an aggressive diffuse type of gastric cancer is found in 70% of men and 55% of women, with an average age of 38 years.[43] Gastric cancers are often multifocal and located beneath an intact mucosal

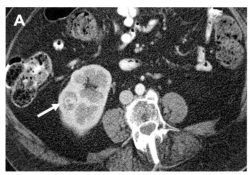
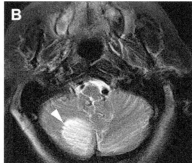

Fig. 10. CS in a 32-year-old man. (A) Axial contrast-enhanced CT image of the abdomen shows an enhancing right renal mass (arrow), which was proved to be a papillary RCC on biopsy. (B) Axial T2-weighted MR image of the brain shows a well-defined, hyperintense area in the right cerebellar hemisphere with widened cerebellar folia giving rise to a striated appearance (arrowhead) consistent with Lhermitte-Duclos disease (dysplastic cerebellar gangliocytoma).

surface and often signet-ring type with tumor cells containing abundant mucin.[43] About 40% of women with *CDH1* mutations may develop lobular breast cancer during their lifetimes.[42] At imaging, diffuse irregular gastric wall thickening (linitis plastica appearance) with lymphadenopathy, invasion into adjacent organs, and distant metastatic disease is the characteristic feature of HDGC, especially if the patient is less than 40 years of age (Fig. 12).

The presence of diffuse gastric cancer in a family member less than 50 years of age with associated lobular breast cancer in the same or another family member is a reliable indicator of *CDH1* mutation in the family; all other family members should undergo genetic counseling.[44] Given the high penetrance, prophylactic gastrectomy is recommended in asymptomatic carriers of the CDH1 gene and intensive annual endoscopic

surveillance in those who decline gastrectomy.[42,44] Annual breast MR imaging with or without mammogram is recommended, starting at the age of 30 years.[42]

VON HIPPEL-LINDAU DISEASE

von Hippel-Lindau disease (VHL) is an autosomal dominant disorder that results from germline mutations in the *VHL* tumor suppressor gene (chromosome 3p25) and is characterized by benign and malignant tumors in multiple organs.[45] The *VHL* gene plays a pivotal role in the regulation of the intracellular oxygen-sensing pathway. Inactivation of this gene causes unbridled upregulation of multiple somatic and vascular growth factors, including vascular endothelial growth factor, leading to the development of vascular tumors.[46] Cerebellar and spinal cord

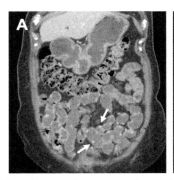
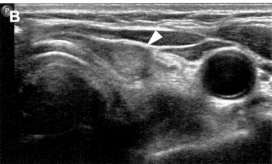

Fig. 11. CS in a 43-year-old woman after right hemithyroidectomy for follicular adenoma. (A) Coronal contrast-enhanced CT image of the abdomen shows multiple enhancing small bowel polyps (arrows). (B) Axial US image of the neck shows a homogeneously isoechoic nodule in the left lobe (arrowhead), which was proved to be a second follicular adenoma on percutaneous fine-needle aspiration.

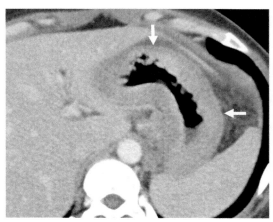

Fig. 12. Hereditary diffuse gastric carcinoma in a 46-year-old woman. Axial contrast-enhanced CT of the abdomen shows diffuse gastric wall thickening giving rise to linitis plastica appearance (*arrows*). The diagnosis of the signet-ring cell type of gastric cancer was proved by histopathologic examination.

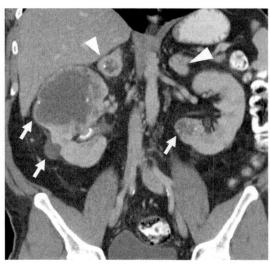

Fig. 14. A 28-year-old man with VHL. Coronal contrast-enhanced CT image of the abdomen shows multiple complex renal cysts and RCCs (*arrows*), and bilateral adrenal pheochromocytomas (*arrowheads*).

hemangioblastomas, retinal angiomas, endolymphatic sac tumors, clear cell RCCs, complex renal cysts, pheochromocytomas, pancreatic cysts and pancreatic neuroendocrine tumors (PNETs), and epididymal cystadenomas are common neoplasms in VHL syndrome (**Figs. 13** and **14**).[46] The pancreas (35%–77%), central nervous system (CNS) (44%–72%), and kidneys (25%–60%) are the most commonly involved organs in VHL syndrome.[45]

Because most VHL-associated tumors show characteristic findings on imaging studies, radiologists play a major role in the initial diagnosis, surveillance of asymptomatic carriers, and posttreatment follow-up.[46] VHL should be suspected in individuals with more than 1 CNS hemangioblastoma, or 1 hemangioblastoma with 1 visceral disorder, or any manifestation with a known family history.[47] Annual abdominal US starting at the age of 8 years and abdominal MR imaging in patients with biochemical abnormalities has been recommended in *VHL* gene carriers.[45] Annual MR imaging of the brain and spine with contrast is to be considered starting at the age of 16 years and MR imaging of the auditory canal if there are abnormal findings on audiological assessment.[47] Clinical neurologic examination with a special focus on the retina, general physical examination, and laboratory testing for urine and serum metanephrine levels form an integral part of the VHL surveillance program.[45]

BIRT-HOGG-DUBE SYNDROME

Birt-Hogg-Dube syndrome (BHD) is an autosomal dominant disorder characterized by the development of cutaneous fibrofolliculomas, bilateral pulmonary cysts, and multiple renal tumors.[48] Germline mutations in the tumor suppressor *Folliculin* (*FLCN*) gene located on chromosome 17p11 are responsible for BHD development. The folliculin protein is shown to modulate the AKT-mTOR pathway, which is essential for cell growth.[48,49] Fibrofolliculomas are the most common clinical findings in patients BHD; they can occur in up to 90% of patients more than 25 years of age and appear as whitish papules on the face, neck, and upper torso (**Fig. 15**).[50]

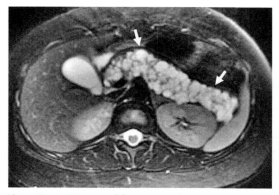

Fig. 13. A 37-year-old man with VHL. Axial T2-weighted MR image of the abdomen shows multiple pancreatic cysts replacing the parenchyma (*arrows*).

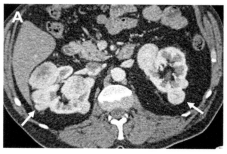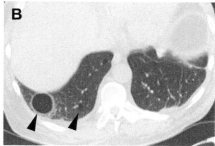

Fig. 15. A 33-year-old man with BHD. (*A*) Contrast-enhanced CT of the abdomen shows multiple enhancing masses in both kidneys (*arrows*), proved to be hybridomas at pathology. (*B*) Axial contrast-enhanced chest CT shows multiple cysts in the right lung base (*arrowheads*).

About 70% to 85% of individuals with BHD develop multiple pulmonary cysts of varying sizes and shape, which tend to be located in the lower lobes in basilar and mediastinal regions with numerous nonenhancing septations in the larger cysts on CT (see **Fig. 15**).[48,51] About 30% of patients with BHD present with spontaneous pneumothorax from a ruptured lung cyst by the average age of 36 years.[49,51] Renal neoplasms may develop in 12% to 34% of patients, with a mean age of presentation at 50 years. Renal tumors are often bilateral and multifocal with hybrid oncocytic/chromophobe RCCs and chromophobe RCCs comprising up to 85% of them.[52] Renal masses show homogeneous enhancement, a central scar, and scattered areas of necrosis, based on variable cellularity and hemorrhagic/cystic areas.[52–54] At-risk family members of patients with BHD are recommended to undergo contrast-enhanced abdominal CT or MR imaging starting at 20 or 21 years of age, which should be repeated at least every 3 years.[48] Chest CT is also recommended at the same time to evaluate for pulmonary cysts.[45,50] Although imaging surveillance is recommended for renal tumors less than 3 cm, larger tumors need to be treated with nephron-sparing procedures.[48]

MULTIPLE ENDOCRINE NEOPLASIA SYNDROMES

Multiple endocrine neoplasia (MEN) syndromes are autosomal dominant cancer syndromes, characterized by the simultaneous occurrence of neoplasms in 2 or more endocrine organs.[55] MEN syndromes are categorized into 2 main types: MEN1 and MEN2.[56]

Also known as Wermer syndrome, MEN1 results from inactivating mutations of the *MEN1* tumor suppressor gene (chromosome 11q13) and is characterized by the development of tumors of

the parathyroid gland (>95%), pancreas (30%–70%), and pituitary gland (30%–40%).[55] Other common neoplasms in MEN1 include facial angiofibromas, collagenomas, adrenal cortical adenomas, and lipomas.[57] Parathyroid adenomas are the most common tumors in MEN1 and are the initial manifestation in most patients who present with hypercalcemia and increased serum parathyroid hormone levels. They appear as homogeneously hypoechoic focal lesions on US with increased vascularity in the periphery.[58] Asymmetric focal radiotracer uptake with retention on delayed imaging on technetium-sestamibi nuclear medicine scan is the characteristic feature of the parathyroid adenoma.[59]

PNETs, the most common pancreatic neoplasms, are responsible for significant mortality and morbidity in MEN1 syndrome. PNETs include gastrinomas (more than half of the cases), insulinomas, and nonfunctioning tumors.[59] Gastrinomas may be seen in the duodenal wall. At CT/MR imaging, intense contrast enhancement during the arterial phase of multiphase CT/MR imaging is one of the characteristic features of PNETs (**Fig. 16**).[59,60] Whole-body imaging techniques such as somatostatin receptor (octreotide scan) imaging and fluorodeoxyglucose-PET scan help in detecting distant metastases and assessing treatment response (**Fig. 17**).[59,61] Gastrin hypersecretion from duodenal/pancreatic gastrinomas can result in Zollinger-Ellison syndrome, which is characterized on imaging by diffuse, enhancing gastric fold thickening, multiple gastric/duodenal/jejunal ulcers, and esophageal strictures from reflux disease (**Fig. 18**).[60] There is a high incidence of anterior pituitary tumors in women with MEN1, with prolactinomas being the most common pituitary tumors in MEN1 (65%), followed by somatotrophinomas (25%).[55,58] Contrast-enhanced brain MR is the imaging modality of choice for identifying both

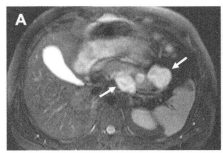
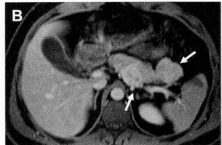

Fig. 16. A 45-year-old woman with MEN type 1 syndrome. (*A, B*) Axial T2-weighted and contrast-enhanced T1-weighted MR images of the abdomen show multiple T2 hyperintense masses that show homogeneous enhancement after gadolinium administration (*arrows*). These lesions were proved to be low-grade neuroendocrine tumors at pathology.

microadenomas and macroadenomas in the pituitary.[61] Annual serum prolactin levels, fasting glucose levels starting at age 5 years, serum calcium and parathyroid hormone levels starting at age 8 years, and gastrin levels starting at age 20 years are recommended in *MEN1* mutation carriers.[57,62] Head MR imaging starting at age 5 years and repeating every 3 years and annual pancreatic CT/MR imaging starting at the age of 20 years or earlier if abnormal serum indicators of PNETs are suggested.[57,62]

MEN2 syndrome is caused by gain-of-function mutations of *RET* proto-oncogene, located on chromosome 10q11, which encodes the receptor tyrosine kinase and includes 3 subtypes: MEN2A, MEN2B, and familial medullary thyroid cancer (FMTC).[63] Also known as Sipple syndrome, MEN2A is the most common type, characterized by the development of medullary thyroid

carcinoma (MTC) (100%), pheochromocytoma (>50%), and primary hyperparathyroidism (15%–30%).[63,64] MTC is usually the first manifestation of MEN2A and can appear between 5 and 25 years of age. Cutaneous lichen amyloidosis and Hirschsprung disease are rare clinical findings in MEN2A.[63] MEN2B is the least common and most aggressive subtype, characterized by the earlier occurrence of most aggressive MTC, multiple neuromas, and the diffuse ganglioneuromatosis of the gastroenteric mucosa (40%).[63,64] MTC is the only manifestation in FMTC subtype of MEN2, and there should be at least 4 affected persons in the same family; MTC has a more benign clinical course and better prognosis.[58] On US, MTC appears as a solid, hypoechoic

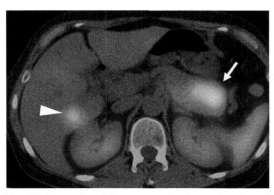

Fig. 17. The role of Octreoscan in the evaluation of pancreatic neuroendocrine tumors in MEN1 syndrome. Axial image of the indium-111 Octreoscan shows increased radiotracer uptake in the pancreatic tail (*arrow*) and the liver parenchyma (*arrowhead*) consistent with hepatic metastasis.

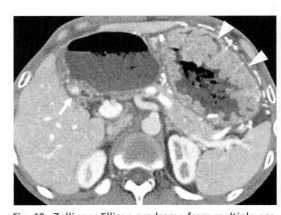

Fig. 18. Zollinger-Ellison syndrome from multiple gastrinomas in 37-year-old woman with MEN type 1 syndrome. Axial contrast-enhanced CT image of the abdomen shows an enhancing nodule in the first part of the duodenum (*arrow*) and diffuse, enhancing gastric mucosal thickening (*arrowheads*), consistent with Zollinger-Ellison syndrome. There are multiple gastrinomas in the other parts of the duodenum (not shown here).

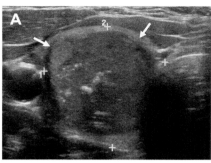
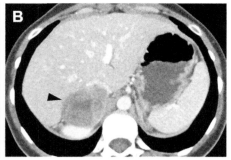

Fig. 19. A 39-year-old woman with MEN type 2A syndrome. (*A*) Axial US of the neck shows a heterogeneous, hypoechoic nodule in the right thyroid lobe with scattered calcifications (*arrows*), which was proved to be MTC on biopsy. (*B*) Axial contrast-enhanced CT image of the abdomen depicts a hypodense mass in the right adrenal gland (*arrowhead*), which was pathologically verified to be a pheochromocytoma.

mass with increased vascularity, and scattered microcalcifications and macrocalcifications (**Fig. 19**).[65] CT and MR imaging are helpful in assessing local invasion, nodal disease, and distant metastases. Whole-body radionuclide imaging with different tracers permits accurate staging, treatment response, and long-term surveillance.[65] Appropriate genetic counseling, followed by *RET* gene testing, is mandatory for at-risk family members and prophylactic thyroidectomy before age 5 years, if possible, may prevent the development of MTC.[64]

HEREDITARY PHEOCHROMOCYTOMA AND PARAGANGLIOMA SYNDROMES

Hereditary pheochromocytoma and paraganglioma syndromes (PGLs) are a group of autosomal dominant disorders characterized by the development of multiple paragangliomas and pheochromocytomas.[66] PGLs are caused by germline mutations in the genes encoding for 4 subunits of the succinate dehydrogenase (SDH) mitochondrial complex (*SDHA*, *SDHB*, *SDHC*, and *SDHD*), which is a major component of the Krebs cycle and electron transport chain.[66] There are 4 types of PGL syndromes: types 1, 2, 3, and 4, which result from mutations of *SDHD*, *SDHAF2* (helps in flavination of subunit A), *SDHC*, and *SDHB* genes respectively.[67] Among them, PGL type 1 and 4 are common and are discussed later.

PGL1 syndrome is caused by inactivating mutations in the *SDHD* gene (chromosome 11q23) and is associated with the development of multifocal, bilateral head and neck paragangliomas (parasympathetic chain) in up to 80% of patients, with a mean age of presentation of 30 years.[67,68] Most of these tumors are benign and nonsecretory so individuals with PGL1 are asymptomatic and

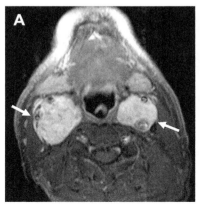
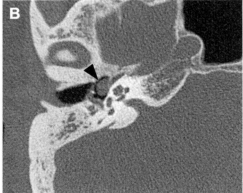

Fig. 20. A 53-year-old man with hereditary PGL 1 (*SDHD* gene mutations). (*A*) Axial contrast-enhanced T1-weighted image of the neck shows homogeneously enhancing, bilateral carotid body paragangliomas (*arrows*). (*B*) Axial high-resolution CT image of the right temporal bone shows a glomus tympanicum in the right middle ear cavity (*arrowhead*).

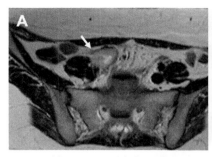
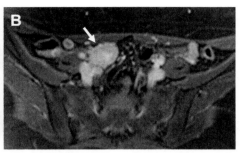

Fig. 21. A 33-year-old woman with hereditary PGL 4 (*SDHB* gene mutations). (*A*) Axial T2-weighted and (*B*) contrast-enhanced T1-weighted MR images of the pelvis show a T2-hyperintense mass in the right common iliac region that shows homogeneous enhancement after contrast administration, which was proved to be a pelvic paraganglioma (*arrows*) on surgical excision.

commonly diagnosed on imaging studies.[69] At CT/ MR imaging, intensely enhancing masses in the carotid body, along with the vagal nerve branches, and jugular foramina are the characteristic features of PGL1 (**Fig. 20**).[70]

PGL4 syndrome develops because of inactivating mutations in the *SDHB* gene, located on chromosome 11p35, and is characterized by abdominal and pelvic sympathetic paragangliomas, followed by pheochromocytomas that can cause symptoms from catecholamine secretion and mass effect on the adjacent organs.[67,68] Primary tumors are typically large and show malignancy risk up to 70%, and distant metastatic disease is common.[68] Heterogeneously enhancing masses with areas of necrosis and hemorrhage are common imaging findings in PGL4 (**Fig. 21**).[70] There is also increased risk of RCC, gastrointestinal stromal tumors, and papillary thyroid cancer in patients with PGL4 (**Fig. 22**).[67] All patients with metastatic paragangliomas should be tested for mutations in the *SDHB* gene.[67]

TUBEROUS SCLEROSIS COMPLEX

Tuberous sclerosis complex (TSC) is an autosomal dominant condition caused by inactivating mutations of the *TSC1* gene (chromosome 9q34, encodes hamartin) and/or *TSC 2* genes (chromosome 16p13, encodes tuberin); tuberin-hamartin complex functions as a tumor suppressor by suppression of the mTOR pathway.[71] CNS lesions in TSC are the primary cause of mortality and morbidity and include cortical and cerebellar tubers, radial migration lines, subependymal nodules, and subependymal giant cell astrocytomas.[72] Gadolinium-enhanced MR imaging of the brain is the imaging modality of choice for diagnosis, screening, and monitoring of

intracranial lesions (**Fig. 23**).[73] Renal lesions are seen in up to 60% of patients with TSC and include angiomyolipomas (AMLs) and renal cysts (see **Fig. 23**).[73] Renal AMLs larger than 4 cm or with intralesional aneurysms larger than 5 mm carry increased risk of spontaneous rupture and require prophylactic embolization.[73] Other lesions in TSC include cardiac rhabdomyomas, lung/retroperitoneal lymphangioleiomyomatosis, hepatic AMLs, and sclerotic lesions in the bones.[71] Recent studies suggest that a spectrum of distinctive renal tumors occurs in patients with TSC; tumors occur at a younger age compared with the general population.[73] Contrast-enhanced brain and abdominal MR imaging are recommended in all patients with TSC at the time of diagnosis and high-resolution chest CT is suggested in women 18 years of age or older.[74]

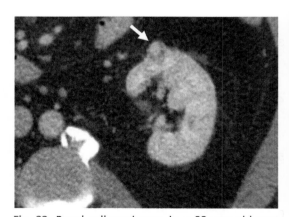

Fig. 22. Renal cell carcinoma in a 33-year-old man with hereditary PGL 4 (*SDHB* gene mutations). Axial contrast-enhanced CT image of the abdomen shows a homogeneously enhancing mass in the left kidney (*arrow*), which was proved to be a clear cell RCC.

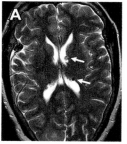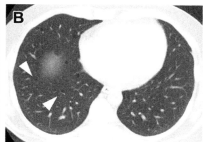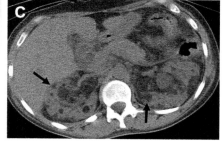

Fig. 23. A 24-year-old woman with tuberous sclerosis. (*A*) Axial T2-weighted MR image of the brain shows multiple subependymal nodules (*white arrows*). (*B*) Axial unenhanced chest CT image shows multiple right lung cysts (*arrowheads*). (*C*) Axial, unenhanced CT image of the abdomen shows bilateral, multiple renal angiomyolipomas (*black arrows*).

SUMMARY

There is a wide spectrum of hereditary cancer syndromes that are characterized by distinctive genophenotypic manifestations. Based on the characteristic imaging findings, the radiologist may be the first physician to suspect a syndromic basis of distinctive multisystem tumors in a given patient leading to accurate diagnosis. Radiologists play a pivotal role in the screening, initial diagnosis, management, and long-term surveillance of patients with hereditary cancer syndromes and their at-risk family members. Improved knowledge of screening and surveillance guidelines of common hereditary cancer syndromes permits optimal patient care.

REFERENCES

1. Garber JE, Offit K. Hereditary cancer predisposition syndromes. J Clin Oncol 2005;23(2):276–92.
2. Nagy R, Sweet K, Eng C. Highly penetrant hereditary cancer syndromes. Oncogene 2004;23(38): 6445–70.
3. Shinagare AB, Giardino AA, Jagannathan JP, et al. Hereditary cancer syndromes: a radiologist's perspective. AJR Am J Roentgenol 2011;197(6): W1001–7.
4. Nik NN, Vang R, Shih Ie M, et al. Origin and pathogenesis of pelvic (ovarian, tubal, and primary peritoneal) serous carcinoma. Annu Rev Pathol 2014;9: 27–45.
5. Gadducci A, Guerrieri ME. PARP inhibitors in epithelial ovarian cancer: state of art and perspectives of clinical research. Anticancer Res 2016;36(5): 2055–64.
6. Massari F, Ciccarese C, Santoni M, et al. Metabolic alterations in renal cell carcinoma. Cancer Treat Rev 2015;41(9):767–76.
7. Monsalve J, Kapur J, Malkin D, et al. Imaging of cancer predisposition syndromes in children. Radiographics 2011;31(1):263–80.
8. Anupindi SA, Bedoya MA, Lindell RB, et al. Diagnostic performance of whole-body MRI as a tool for cancer screening in children with genetic cancer-predisposing conditions. AJR Am J Roentgenol 2015;205(2):400–8.
9. Villani A, Shore A, Wasserman JD, et al. Biochemical and imaging surveillance in germline TP53 mutation carriers with Li-Fraumeni syndrome: 11 year follow-up of a prospective observational study. Lancet Oncol 2016;17(9):1295–305.
10. Jasperson KW, Kohlmann W, Gammon A, et al. Role of rapid sequence whole-body MRI screening in SDH-associated hereditary paraganglioma families. Fam Cancer 2014;13(2):257–65.
11. Ballinger LL. Hereditary gynecologic cancers: risk assessment, counseling, testing and management. Obstet Gynecol Clin North Am 2012;39(2):165–81.
12. Welcsh PL, King MC. BRCA1 and BRCA2 and the genetics of breast and ovarian cancer. Hum Mol Genet 2001;10(7):705–13.
13. Antoniou A, Pharoah PD, Narod S, et al. Average risks of breast and ovarian cancer associated with BRCA1 or BRCA2 mutations detected in case series unselected for family history: a combined analysis of 22 studies. Am J Hum Genet 2003;72(5):1117–30.
14. King MC, Marks JH, Mandell JB, New York Breast Cancer Study Group. Breast and ovarian cancer risks due to inherited mutations in BRCA1 and BRCA2. Science 2003;302(5645):643–6.
15. Mavaddat N, Barrowdale D, Andrulis IL, et al. Pathology of breast and ovarian cancers among BRCA1 and BRCA2 mutation carriers: results from the consortium of investigators of modifiers of BRCA1/2 (CIMBA). Cancer Epidemiol Biomarkers Prev 2012;21(1):134–47.
16. Schrading S, Kuhl CK. Mammographic, US, and MR imaging phenotypes of familial breast cancer. Radiology 2008;246(1):58–70.
17. Passaperuma K, Warner E, Causer PA, et al. Long-term results of screening with magnetic resonance

imaging in women with BRCA mutations. Br J Cancer 2012;107(1):24–30.

18. Katabathina VS, Amanullah FS, Menias CO, et al. Extrauterine pelvic serous carcinomas: current update on pathology and cross-sectional imaging findings. Radiographics 2016;36(3):918–32.

19. Swisher EM, Sakai W, Karlan BY, et al. Secondary BRCA1 mutations in BRCA1-mutated ovarian carcinomas with platinum resistance. Cancer Res 2008; 68(8):2581–6.

20. Hartmann LC, Lindor NM. The role of risk-reducing surgery in hereditary breast and ovarian cancer. N Engl J Med 2016;374(5):454–68.

21. Daly MB, Pilarski R, Axilbund JE, et al. Genetic/familial high-risk assessment: breast and ovarian, version 2.2015. J Natl Compr Canc Netw 2016;14(2): 153–62.

22. Cohen SA, Leininger A. The genetic basis of Lynch syndrome and its implications for clinical practice and risk management. Appl Clin Genet 2014;7: 147–58.

23. Lynch HT, Lynch J. Lynch syndrome: genetics, natural history, genetic counseling, and prevention. J Clin Oncol 2000;18(21 Suppl):19S–31S.

24. Ponti G, Ponz de Leon M. Muir-Torre syndrome. Lancet Oncol 2005;6(12):980–7.

25. Kalady MF, Heald B. Diagnostic approach to hereditary colorectal cancer syndromes. Clin Colon Rectal Surg 2015;28(4):205–14.

26. Syngal S, Brand RE, Church JM, et al. ACG clinical guideline: genetic testing and management of hereditary gastrointestinal cancer syndromes. Am J Gastroenterol 2015;110(2):223–62 [quiz: 263].

27. Jenkins MA, Hayashi S, O'Shea AM, et al. Pathology features in Bethesda guidelines predict colorectal cancer microsatellite instability: a population-based study. Gastroenterology 2007;133(1):48–56.

28. Palomaki GE, McClain MR, Melillo S, et al. EGAPP supplementary evidence review: DNA testing strategies aimed at reducing morbidity and mortality from Lynch syndrome. Genet Med 2009;11(1):42–65.

29. Giardiello FM, Allen JI, Axilbund JE, et al. Guidelines on genetic evaluation and management of Lynch syndrome: a consensus statement by the US Multi-Society Task Force on Colorectal Cancer. Am J Gastroenterol 2014;109(8):1159–79.

30. Lindor NM, Petersen GM, Hadley DW, et al. Recommendations for the care of individuals with an inherited predisposition to Lynch syndrome: a systematic review. JAMA 2006;296(12):1507–17.

31. Al-Sukhni W, Aronson M, Gallinger S. Hereditary colorectal cancer syndromes: familial adenomatous polyposis and lynch syndrome. Surg Clin North Am 2008;88(4):819–44, vii.

32. Brosens LA, Offerhaus GJ, Giardiello FM. Hereditary colorectal cancer: genetics and screening. Surg Clin North Am 2015;95(5):1067–80.

33. Leoz ML, Carballal S, Moreira L, et al. The genetic basis of familial adenomatous polyposis and its implications for clinical practice and risk management. Appl Clin Genet 2015;8:95–107.

34. Ossa CA, Molina G, Cock-Rada AM. Li-Fraumeni syndrome. Biomedica 2016;36(2):182–7.

35. Correa H. Li-Fraumeni syndrome. J Pediatr Genet 2016;5(2):84–8.

36. McBride KA, Ballinger ML, Killick E, et al. Li-Fraumeni syndrome: cancer risk assessment and clinical management. Nat Rev Clin Oncol 2014;11(5): 260–71.

37. Heymann S, Delaloge S, Rahal A, et al. Radio-induced malignancies after breast cancer postoperative radiotherapy in patients with Li-Fraumeni syndrome. Radiat Oncol 2010;5:104.

38. Malkin D. Li-Fraumeni syndrome and p53 in 2015: celebrating their silver anniversary. Clin Invest Med 2016;39(1):E37–47.

39. Mester J, Eng C. Cowden syndrome: recognizing and managing a not-so-rare hereditary cancer syndrome. J Surg Oncol 2015;111(1):125–30.

40. Uppal S, Mistry D, Coatesworth AP. Cowden disease: a review. Int J Clin Pract 2007;61(4):645–52.

41. Gustafson S, Zbuk KM, Scacheri C, et al. Cowden syndrome. Semin Oncol 2007;34(5):428–34.

42. Tan RY, Ngeow J. Hereditary diffuse gastric cancer: what the clinician should know. World J Gastrointest Oncol 2015;7(9):153–60.

43. Hansford S, Kaurah P, Li-Chang H, et al. Hereditary diffuse gastric cancer syndrome: CDH1 mutations and beyond. JAMA Oncol 2015;1(1):23–32.

44. Pinheiro H, Oliveira C, Seruca R, et al. Hereditary diffuse gastric cancer - pathophysiology and clinical management. Best Pract Res Clin Gastroenterol 2014;28(6):1055–68.

45. Nielsen SM, Rhodes L, Blanco I, et al. Von Hippel-Lindau disease: genetics and role of genetic counseling in a multiple neoplasia syndrome. J Clin Oncol 2016;34(18):2172–81.

46. Shanbhogue KP, Hoch M, Fatterpaker G, et al. von Hippel-Lindau disease: review of genetics and imaging. Radiol Clin North Am 2016;54(3): 409–22.

47. Schmid S, Gillessen S, Binet I, et al. Management of von Hippel-Lindau disease: an interdisciplinary review. Oncol Res Treat 2014;37(12):761–71.

48. Schmidt LS, Linehan WM. Molecular genetics and clinical features of Birt-Hogg-Dube syndrome. Nat Rev Urol 2015;12(10):558–69.

49. Hasumi H, Baba M, Hasumi Y, et al. Birt-Hogg-Dube syndrome: clinical and molecular aspects of recently identified kidney cancer syndrome. Int J Urol 2016;23(3):204–10.

50. Menko FH, van Steensel MA, Giraud S, et al. Birt-Hogg-Dube syndrome: diagnosis and management. Lancet Oncol 2009;10(12):1199–206.

51. Agarwal PP, Gross BH, Holloway BJ, et al. Thoracic CT findings in Birt-Hogg-Dube syndrome. AJR Am J Roentgenol 2011;196(2):349–52.

52. Zamora CA, Rowe SP, Horton KM. Case 218: Birt-Hogg-Dube syndrome. Radiology 2015;275(3): 923–7.

53. Raman SP, Johnson PT, Allaf ME, et al. Chromo-phobe renal cell carcinoma: multiphase MDCT enhancement patterns and morphologic features. AJR Am J Roentgenol 2013;201(6):1268–76.

54. Ishigami K, Jones AR, Dahmoush L, et al. Imaging spectrum of renal oncocytomas: a pictorial review with pathologic correlation. Insights Imaging 2015; 6(1):53–64.

55. Carling T. Multiple endocrine neoplasia syndrome: genetic basis for clinical management. Curr Opin Oncol 2005;17(1):7–12.

56. Thakker RV. Multiple endocrine neoplasia type 1 (MEN1) and type 4 (MEN4). Mol Cell Endocrinol 2014;386(1–2):2–15.

57. Carroll RW. Multiple endocrine neoplasia type 1 (MEN1). Asia Pac J Clin Oncol 2013;9(4):297–309.

58. Grajo JR, Paspulati RM, Sahani DV, et al. Multiple endocrine neoplasia syndromes: a comprehensive imaging review. Radiol Clin North Am 2016;54(3): 441–51.

59. Scarsbrook AF, Thakker RV, Wass JA, et al. Multiple endocrine neoplasia: spectrum of radiologic ap-pearances and discussion of a multitechnique imag-ing approach. Radiographics 2006;26(2):433–51.

60. Lewis RB, Lattin GE Jr, Paal E. Pancreatic endocrine tumors: radiologic-clinicopathologic correlation. Ra-diographics 2010;30(6):1445–64.

61. Knaus CM, Patronas NJ, Papadakis GZ, et al. Multi-ple endocrine neoplasia, type 1: imaging solutions to clinical questions. Curr Probl Diagn Radiol 2016; 45(4):278–83.

62. Brandi ML, Gagel RF, Angeli A, et al. Guidelines for diagnosis and therapy of MEN type 1 and type 2. J Clin Endocrinol Metab 2001;86(12):5658–71.

63. Marini F, Falchetti A, Del Monte F, et al. Multiple endocrine neoplasia type 2. Orphanet J Rare Dis 2006;1:45.

64. Taieb D, Kebebew E, Castinetti F, et al. Diagnosis and preoperative imaging of multiple endocrine neoplasia type 2: current status and future direc-tions. Clin Endocrinol (Oxf) 2014;81(3):317–28.

65. Ganeshan D, Paulson E, Duran C, et al. Current up-date on medullary thyroid carcinoma. AJR Am J Roentgenol 2013;201(6):W867–76.

66. Kantorovich V, King KS, Pacak K. SDH-related pheo-chromocytoma and paraganglioma. Best Pract Res Clin Endocrinol Metab 2010;24(3):415–24.

67. Martins R, Bugalho MJ. Paragangliomas/pheochro-mocytomas: clinically oriented genetic testing. Int J Endocrinol 2014;2014:794187.

68. King KS, Pacak K. Familial pheochromocytomas and paragangliomas. Mol Cell Endocrinol 2014; 386(1–2):92–100.

69. Ingram M, Barber B, Bano G, et al. Radiologic appearance of hereditary adrenal and extraadrenal paraganglioma. AJR Am J Roentgenol 2011; 197(4):W687–95.

70. Barber B, Ingram M, Khan S, et al. Clinicoradiologi-cal manifestations of paraganglioma syndromes associated with succinyl dehydrogenase enzyme mutation. Insights Imaging 2011;2(4):431–8.

71. Lam HC, Nijmeh J, Henske EP. New developments in the genetics and pathogenesis of tumours in tu-berous sclerosis complex. J Pathol 2017;241(2): 219–25.

72. Rovira A, Ruiz-Falco ML, Garcia-Esparza E, et al. Recommendations for the radiological diagnosis and follow-up of neuropathological abnormalities associated with tuberous sclerosis complex. J Neurooncol 2014;118(2):205–23.

73. Krishnan A, Kaza RK, Vummidi DR. Cross-sectional imaging review of tuberous sclerosis. Radiol Clin North Am 2016;54(3):423–40.

74. Krueger DA, Northrup H, International Tuberous Sclerosis Complex Consensus Group. Tuberous sclerosis complex surveillance and management: recommendations of the 2012 International Tuber-ous Sclerosis Complex Consensus Conference. Pe-diatr Neurol 2013;49(4):255–65.

1 Publication Title	2 Publication Number	3 Filing Date
RADIOLOGIC CLINICS OF NORTH AMERICA	596 – 510	9/18/2017

4 Issue Frequency	5 Number of Issues Published Annually	6 Annual Subscription Price
JAN, MAR, MAY, JUL, SEP, NOV	6	$474.00

7 Complete Mailing Address of Known Office of Publication (Not printer) (Street, city, county, state, and ZIP+4®)

ELSEVIER INC.
230 Park Avenue, Suite 800
New York, NY 10169

Contact Person: STEPHEN R. BUSHING
Telephone (Include area code): 215-239-3688

8 Complete Mailing Address of Headquarters or General Business Office of Publisher (Not printer)

ELSEVIER INC.
230 Park Avenue, Suite 800
New York, NY 10169

9 Full Names and Complete Mailing Addresses of Publisher, Editor, and Managing Editor (Do not leave blank)

Publisher (Name and complete mailing address)

ADRIANNE BRIGIDO, ELSEVIER INC.
1600 JOHN F KENNEDY BLVD. SUITE 1800
PHILADELPHIA, PA 19103-2899

Editor (Name and complete mailing address)

JOHN VASSALLO, ELSEVIER INC.
1600 JOHN F KENNEDY BLVD. SUITE 1800
PHILADELPHIA, PA 19103-2899

Managing Editor (Name and complete mailing address)

PATRICK MANLEY, ELSEVIER INC.
1600 JOHN F KENNEDY BLVD. SUITE 1800
PHILADELPHIA, PA 19103-2899

10 Owner (Do not leave blank. If the publication is owned by a corporation, give the name and address of the corporation immediately followed by the names and addresses of all stockholders owning or holding 1 percent or more of the total amount of stock. If not owned by a corporation, give the names and addresses of the individual owners. If owned by a partnership or other unincorporated firm, give its name and address as well as those of each individual owner. If the publication is published by a nonprofit organization, give its name and address.)

Full Name	Complete Mailing Address
WHOLLY OWNED SUBSIDIARY OF REED/ELSEVIER, US HOLDINGS	1600 JOHN F KENNEDY BLVD. SUITE 1800 PHILADELPHIA, PA 19103-2899

11. Known Bondholders, Mortgagees, and Other Security Holders Owning or Holding 1 Percent or More of Total Amount of Bonds, Mortgages, or Other Securities. If none, check box ▶ ☐ None

Full Name	Complete Mailing Address
N/A	

12. Tax Status (For completion by nonprofit organizations authorized to mail at nonprofit rates) (Check one)
The purpose, function, and nonprofit status of this organization and the exempt status for federal income tax purposes:
☒ Has Not Changed During Preceding 12 Months
☐ Has Changed During Preceding 12 Months (Publisher must submit explanation of change with this statement)

13 Publication Title	14. Issue Date for Circulation Data Below
RADIOLOGIC CLINICS OF NORTH AMERICA	JULY 2017

15. Extent and Nature of Circulation			Average No. Copies Each Issue During Preceding 12 Months	No. Copies of Single Issue Published Nearest to Filing Date
a. Total Number of Copies (Net press run)			1489	1178
b. Paid Circulation (By Mail and Outside the Mail)	(1)	Mailed Outside-County Paid Subscriptions Stated on PS Form 3541 (include paid distribution above nominal rate, advertiser's proof copies, and exchange copies)	860	791
	(2)	Mailed In-County Paid Subscriptions Stated on PS Form 3541 (include paid distribution above nominal rate, advertiser's proof copies, and exchange copies)	0	0
	(3)	Paid Distribution Outside the Mails Including Sales Through Dealers and Carriers, Street Vendors, Counter Sales, and Other Paid Distribution Outside USPS®	336	323
	(4)	Paid Distribution by Other Classes of Mail Through the USPS (e.g. First-Class Mail®)	0	0
c. Total Paid Distribution (Sum of 15b (1), (2), (3), and (4))			1196	1114
d. Free or Nominal Rate Distribution (By Mail and Outside the Mail)	(1)	Free or Nominal Rate Outside-County Copies included on PS Form 3541	70	64
	(2)	Free or Nominal Rate In-County Copies included on PS Form 3541	0	0
	(3)	Free or Nominal Rate Copies Mailed at Other Classes Through the USPS (e.g. First-Class Mail)	0	0
	(4)	Free or Nominal Rate Distribution Outside the Mail (Carriers or other means)	0	0
e. Total Free or Nominal Rate Distribution (Sum of 15d (1), (2), (3) and (4))			70	64
f. Total Distribution (Sum of 15c and 15e)			1266	1178
g. Copies not Distributed (See Instructions to Publishers #4 (page #3))			223	0
h. Total (Sum of 15f and g)			1489	1178
i. Percent Paid (15c divided by 15f times 100)			94.47%	94.57%

* If you are claiming electronic copies, go to line 16 on page 3. If you are not claiming electronic copies, skip to line 17 on page 3.

16. Electronic Copy Circulation	Average No. Copies Each Issue During Preceding 12 Months	No. Copies of Single Issue Published Nearest to Filing Date
a. Paid Electronic Copies ▶	0	0
b. Total Paid Print Copies (Line 15c) + Paid Electronic Copies (Line 16a) ▶	1196	1114
c. Total Print Distribution (Line 15f) + Paid Electronic Copies (Line 16a) ▶	1266	1178
d. Percent Paid (Both Print & Electronic Copies) (16b divided by 16c × 100) ▶	94.47%	94.57%

☒ I certify that 50% of all my distributed copies (electronic and print) are paid above a nominal price.

17. Publication of Statement of Ownership

☒ If the publication is a general publication, publication of this statement is required. Will be printed ☐ Publication not required
in the NOVEMBER 2017 issue of this publication.

18. Signature and Title of Editor, Publisher, Business Manager, or Owner		Date
STEPHEN R. BUSHING – INVENTORY DISTRIBUTION CONTROL MANAGER	*[signature]*	9/18/2017

I certify that all information furnished on this form is true and complete. I understand that anyone who furnishes false or misleading information on this form or who omits material or information requested on the form may be subject to criminal sanctions (including fines and imprisonment) and/or civil sanctions (including civil penalties).

PS Form **3526**, July 2014 (Page 1 of 4 (see instructions page 4)) PSN 7530-01-000-9931   PRIVACY NOTICE: See our privacy policy on www.usps.com.

PS Form **3526**, July 2014 (Page 3 of 4)   PRIVACY NOTICE: See our privacy policy on www.usps.com.

Moving?

Make sure your subscription moves with you!

To notify us of your new address, find your **Clinics Account Number** (located on your mailing label above your name), and contact customer service at:

Email: journalscustomerservice-usa@elsevier.com

800-654-2452 (subscribers in the U.S. & Canada)
314-447-8871 (subscribers outside of the U.S. & Canada)

Fax number: 314-447-8029

**Elsevier Health Sciences Division
Subscription Customer Service
3251 Riverport Lane
Maryland Heights, MO 63043**

*To ensure uninterrupted delivery of your subscription, please notify us at least 4 weeks in advance of move.

ELSEVIER

Printed and bound by CPI Group (UK) Ltd, Croydon, CR0 4YY

08/05/2025

01864703-0020